Liver Metastases

Biology, Diagnosis and Treatment

Springer
London
Berlin
Heidelberg
New York
Barcelona
Budapest
Hong Kong
Milan
Paris
Santa Clara
Singapore
Tokyo

O.J. Garden, J.G. Geraghty and D.M. Nagorney (Eds)
R.A. Audisio and H.S. Stoldt (Associate Eds)

Liver Metastases

Biology, Diagnosis and Treatment

With 43 figures, 18 in colour

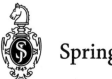 Springer

Dr. O.J. Garden
Professor of Hepatobiliary Surgery, Department of Surgery, University of Edinburgh, Royal Infirmary, Lauriston Place, Edinburgh EH3 9YW, UK

Dr. J.G. Geraghty
Consultant Surgeon, Professorial Department of Surgery, Nottingham City Hospital, Hucknall Road, Nottingham NG5 1PB, UK

Dr. D.M. Nagorney
Professor of Surgery, Mayo Clinic, 200 First Street SW, Rochester, Minnesota, MN 55905, USA

Associate Editors

Dr. R.A. Audisio
Deputy Director of General Surgery, European Institute of Oncology, Via Ripamonti 435, 20133 Milan, Italy

Dr. H.S. Stoldt
Consultant Surgeon, Department of Surgical Oncology, European Institute of Oncology, Via Ripamonti 435, 20141 Milan, Italy

British Library Cataloguing in Publication Data
Liver metastases: biology, diagnosis and treatment
    1. Liver metastases   2. Liver metastases – Diagnosis   3. Liver metastases – Treatment
    I. Garden, O James   II. Geraghty, J.G.   III. Nagorney, D.M.
    616.9'94'36
    ISBN-13:978-1-4471-1508-3   e-ISBN-13:978-1-4471-1506-9
    DOI: 10.1007/978-1-4471-1506-9

Library of Congress Cataloging-in-Publication Data
Liver metastases: biology, diagnosis, and treatment / O.J. Garden, J.G. Geraghty, and
    D.M. Nagorney (eds.).
        p.   cm.
    Includes bibliographical references and index.
    ISBN-13:978-1-4471-1508-3 (alk. paper)
    1. Liver metastasis. I. Garden, O. James. II. Geraghty, J.G. (James G.), 1955–. III. Nagorney, D.M. (David M.),
    1950–.
    [DNLM: 1. Liver Neoplasms – secondary.   2. Liver Neoplasms – diagnosis.   3. Liver Neoplasms – therapy.
    4. Neoplasm Metastases.
    WI 735 L7848   1998]
    RC280.L5L5855   1998
    616.99'436–dc21
    DNLM/DLC
    for Library of Congress   97-52056

© Springer-Verlag London Limited 1998
Softcover reprint of the hardcover 1st edition 1998

The use of registered names, trademarks, etc. in this publication does not imply, even in the absence of a specific statement, that such names are exempt from the relevant laws and regulations and therefore free for general use.

Product liability: The publisher can give no guarantee for information about drug dosage and application thereof contained in this book. In every individual case the respective user must check its accuracy by consulting other pharmaceutical literature.

Typeset by EXPO Holdings, Malaysia

28/3830-543210 Printed on acid-free paper

Contents

Contributors

Adson, Martin A.
Professor of Surgery Emeritus
Mayo Medical School
200 First Street Southwest
Rochester
Minnesota MN 55905
USA

Bignami, Paola
Istituto Nazionale Tumori
Via G. Veneziana 1
20133 Milano
Italy

Blumgart, Leslie H.
Department of Surgery, Hepatobiliary Service
Memorial Sloan-Kettering Cancer Center
1275 York Avenue
New York NY 10021
USA

Burnhill, Ruth
Palliative Care Program
European Institute of Oncology
Via Ripamonti 435
20141 Milano
Italy

Chinol, Marco
Division of Nuclear Medicine
European Institute of Oncology
Via Ripamonti 435
20141 Milano
Italy

Dallavalle, Giuseppe
Medical Oncology
Ospedale S Carlo Borromeo
Via Pio II, 3
20153 Milano
Italy

Doci, Roberto
Istituto Clinico Humanitas
Via Manzoni 56
20089 Rozzano (Mi)
Italy

Fidler, Isiah J.
Professor and Chairman,
Department of Cell Biology
University of Texas
MD Anderson Cancer Center
1515 Holcombe Boulevard, Box 173
Houston
Texas 77030
USA

Flye, M. Wyne
Professor of Surgery,
Molecular Microbiology and Immunology
Washington University School of Medicine
Suite 5103, One Barnes Hospital Plaza
St Louis
Missouri MO 63110
USA

Fong, Yuman
Department of Surgery, Hepatobiliary Service
Memorial Sloan-Kettering Cancer Center
1275 York Avenue
New York NY 10021
USA

Garden, O. James
Professor of Hepatobiliary Surgery
University Department of Surgery
Royal Infirmary
Edinburgh EH3 9YW
UK

Gennari, Leandro
Istituto Clinico Humanitas
Via Manzoni 56
20089 Rozzano (Mi)
Italy

Geraghty, James G.
Consultant Surgeon
Professorial Department of Surgery
Nottingham City Hospital
Hucknall Road
Nottingham NG5 1PB
UK

Greco, Carlo
Department of Radiation Oncology
European Institute of Oncology
Via Ripamonti 435
20141 Milano
Italy

John, Timothy G.
Consultant Surgeon
Department of Surgery
North Hampshire Hospital
Basingstoke
Hants RG24 9NA
UK

Karpoff, Howard M.
Department of Surgery, Hepatobiliary Service
Memorial Sloan-Kettering Cancer Center
1275 York Avenue
New York NY 10021
USA

Labianca, Roberto
Medical Oncology
Ospedale S Carlo Borromeo
Via Pio II, 3
20153 Milano
Italy

Lang, Hauke
Klinik für Abdominal und
Transplantationschirurgie
Medizinische Hochschule Hannover
Carl Neuberg Str. 1
30625 Hannover
Germany

Leen, Edward
Consultant Radiologist
Department of Radiology
Glasgow Royal Infirmary
Queen Elizabeth Building
Alexandra Parade
Glasgow G31 2ER
UK

Leiser, Mark J.
Assistant Professor of Surgery
Department of Surgery
University of Texas
Southwestern Medical Center
5323 Harry Hines Boulevard
Dallas TX 75235-9156
USA

Madhavan, Krishnakumar
Consultant Surgeon
Department of Surgery
Royal Infirmary
Edinburgh EH3 9YW
UK

Minsky, Bruce D.
Department of Radiation Oncology
Memorial Sloan-Kettering Cancer Center
1275 York Avenue
New York
NY 10021
USA

Nagorney, David M.
Professor of Surgery
Division of General Surgery
Mayo Clinic
200 First Street Southwest
Rochester
Minnesota MN 55905
USA

Nordlinger, Bernard
Hôpital Ambroise Parê
Chirurgie générale digestive et oncologique
9 avenue Charles De Gaulle
92104 Boulogne Cedex
France

Oldhafer, Karl Jürgen
Klinik für Abdominal und
Transplantationschirurgie
Medizinische Hochschule Hannover
Carl Neuberg Str. 1
30625 Hannover
Germany

Pagnelli, Giovanni
Division of Nuclear Medicine
European Institute of Oncology
Via Ripamonti 435
20141 Milano
Italy

Pessi, M. Adelaide
Medical Oncology
Ospedale S Carlo Borromeo
Via Pio II, 3
20153 Milano
Italy

Pichlmayr, Rudolf
(Died August 29, 1997)
Professor of Surgery
Klinik für Abdominal und
Transplantationschirurgie
Medizinische Hochschule Hannover
Carl Neuberg Str. 1
30625 Hannover
Germany

Radinsky, Robert
Department of Cell Biology
University of Texas
MD Anderson Cancer Center
1515 Holcombe Boulevard, Box 173
Houston
Texas 77030
USA

Redhead, Doris N.
Consultant Radiologist
Department of Radiology
Royal Infirmary
Lauriston Place
Edinburgh EH3 9YW
UK

Sbanotto, Alberto
Palliative Care Program
European Institute of Oncology
Via Ripamonti 435
20141 Milano
Italy

Schlitt, Hans-Jürgen
Klinik für Abdominal und
Transplantationschirurgie
Medizinische Hochschule Hannover
Carl Neuberg Str. 1
30625 Hannover
Germany

Stoldt, H. Stephan
Consultant Surgeon
Department of Surgical Oncology
European Institute of Oncology
Via Ripamonti 435
20141 Milano
Italy

Ventafridda, Vittorio
WHO Collaborating Center
for Cancer Control and Palliative Care
European Institute of Oncology
Via Ripamonti 435
20141 Milano
Italy

Giuseppina, Zamparelli
Medical Oncology
Ospedale S Carlo Borromeo
Via Pio II, 3
20153 Milano
Italy

Introduction

Martin A. Adson

1

I have framed the introduction to this text by looking backward to two personal events: my surgical introduction to the liver and my more recent retirement from it. These benchmarks gave focus to my reading, placed progress in frames of time, and offer some historical perspective. The value of reflection about the treatment of liver metastases forty years ago may be questioned by readers who now study liver metastases at the molecular level; but it is not good to be isolated from the past, and others who intervene grossly with new instruments may find understanding in surgical memory. These reflections are personal, but less personal than metastatic cancer which must be treated in the *context* of personal relationships – with patients and colleagues.

My surgical training was completed in 1955 but was incomplete 'liver-wise' because most of my teachers had little need and less inclination to trespass on the liver. However, my mentor, Dr. John McMaster Waugh, often took out things that others left behind. In 1963, a year after his untimely death, his personal experience with resection of hepatic metastases from a variety of visceral cancers was published. Operative mortality was 4% and 20% of his 25 patients lived for five or more years.

Despite that favourable report, such efforts did not become the conventional wisdom of that day, because such operations were not convenient and in ordinary hands their risk was unacceptable. Nevertheless, John Waugh had established an institutional precedent and obligation to patients referred for management of metastatic tumours of the liver. I found myself in a lonely gap between institutional and personal obligation. John Waugh was no longer here; I had been surgically and metaphysically close to him; and none of my colleagues seemed to be much interested in the liver. I had

shared only a small part of my mentor's surgical experience with the liver (which on no day involved resection of the huge tumours that I was then asked to see). Also, at that time, like most young surgeons, I did not feel ordinary and was extraordinarily reluctant to leave in place a tumour that might reasonably be taken out when nothing else useful might be done. That attitude was reinforced by close association with surgical pathologists whose expert interpretation of frozen sections was clinically enhanced by frequent visits with surgeons in the operating room. I recall asking Drs. David Dahlin and Malcolm Dockerty for help with a surgical judgement when they said simply: 'If you leave that in, don't you think it will grow?' That whimsical remark was offered within a very special relationship. I had studied surgical pathology with both of them and we all knew that their knowledge and experience was just one aspect of surgical judgment.

That was particularly true when surgeons and surgical pathologists were dealing with a 'new' clinico-pathological entity for which the benefits of surgical treatment were unknown. Surgically inviting hepatic metastases, once clinically obscure, were made newly visible by evolving diagnostic technology, newly vulnerable to changing surgical attitudes, and more often referred after discovery during another surgeon's operation.

Most surgeons removed small superficial lesions safely. However, the reported risk of removing larger lesions was formidable; and the unreported risk of this endeavour was unacceptable. In this circumstance, a so-called general surgeon had to decide whether to become a liver surgeon or not. In the early 1960s, that transition involved two major concerns: one strategic (what should be done), and the other tactical (what could be done). It was difficult to make a case for the removal of any hepatic metastasis when in every case we were ignorant of the tumour's stage. However, there were no therapeutic alternatives, some evidence for surgical success, and nothing to suggest that patients might be helped by watching such tumours grow. Moreover, surgeons were not by their *nature* sufficiently scientific or dispassionate enough to participate in prospective controlled therapeutic trials. Surgeons, then as now, were driven by intuition, curiosity, or professed wisdom (a complex I came to recognize as one form of *surgical momentum*) to remove whatever growth might contribute to their patient's death. This empirical approach was determined by the invisibility of micrometastases and undetectability of subcentimetre (or somewhat larger) lesions hidden deep within the liver. Then, as now, each patient's prognosis was determined more by micrometastases unseen and left in place than by tumours taken out.

In 1967, in consideration of 'diagnostic measures', I wrote: 'The ideal diagnostic procedure is one that would afford precise localization of lesions in relationship to hepatic vasculature *and* recognition of the smallest significant lesions', – and went on to comment on the limitations of diagnostic measures available in those days. The short list included: the inaccessibility of many lesions to percutaneous biopsy with the Vim–Silverman needle – the vague images rendered on hepatic scintiscans utilizing rose bengal ^{131}I; the greater sensitivity of (but carcinogenic potential of) radiographic techniques utilizing thorium dioxide (thorotrast); and the encouraging early experience with and comparative value of selective celiac arteriography and hepatic portography utilizing the splenic pulp or the umbilical vein. There was no longer list!

At that time, when surgical strategy was founded on a bewilderment that left *benefit* unknown, so was the *risk* of major resectional liver surgery either unknown, unadmitted, or widely unpublicized. Therefore, my second major concern – a tactical uneasiness involving problems with haemostasis – related to the size and location of metastatic tumours of patients whom I was more often being asked to see. Having forgotten some of what I felt then person by person and case by case, my fading memory has been restored by reading word by word papers that I had written and published back then. I am now struck by the uncommon openness of those early personal accounts.

My earliest reported experience with *Hepatic Lobectomy* published in 1965 reflected my concern about technical shortcomings: 'The absence of death from operative hemorrhage in this group of patients is gratifying but misleading. The quantity of blood lost was moderate in four cases, significant from the standpoint of risk (but still compatible with a surgeon's dignity) in three, but shamefully excessive in four.' I added Dr. Robert R. Jones' name to that paper because as I admitted in the rest of that paragraph: 'That these last four patients survived is more a reflection of the size of our blood bank than evidence of any really satisfactory surgical method for hemostasis.' In those early days, Bob's intuition as a clinical anaesthesiologist transcended all ordinary knowledge of physiology. He contributed to the lack of operative deaths in that first reported series of patients each time he said: 'I think I better get another six-pack of blood.'

Such surgical embarrassment was determined almost exclusively by the proximity of large tumours to major veins. Vascular inflow occlusion (the Pringle manoeuvre) had no effect upon bleeding from the distorted, displaced, or adherent vena cava or the major hepatic vein which drained the hepatic remnant to be saved. Unfortunately, one had to discover such things alone when most surgeons were reluctant to write about their own misadventures.

There was a sparse but growing literature about major hepatic resections in the late 1950s and early 1960s. Unfortunately, there was in it an element of misleading journalistic enthusiasm. Noteworthy are the few prideful case reports of selected surgical successes culled from unreported disastrous happenings within the authors' total experience. Also, the haemostatic techniques offered then for safe resection ignored many anatomical realities and lacked the sophistication and honesty essential for success today. All too often trouble (bleeding!) could not be avoided by 'finger fracture' or 'mattress sutures' through non-existent tumour-free margins, or other bywords of that day.

The critical problems with major veins were just a part of a more fundamental ignorance of the unique nature of hepatic anatomy. I had been attracted to gastroenterological surgery because, having a father who was a neurosurgeon, I thought that the viscera might be more closely linked to meaningful human activity than were the mind or brain – and then came to feel that the liver was located most closely to the soul. I was disappointed to find out that the liver was an opaque, bloody sponge interposed between both splanchnic and systemic circulations.

It is now possible to contend with these complex relationships in ways considered in this book. But *then* an anatomy that was only beginning to be understood could be learned not from hearsay – but only by operating on it.

Today many fellowships away from home are attractive opportunities for apprenticeship and exposure to knowledge and experience unavailable nearby. I thought about and hoped for such opportunities then but simply did not know where to go.

The next thirty years involved a seasoning of liver surgery. With experience the uneasiness of those first encounters with severe operative haemorrhage turned slowly to an attentive confidence. Anatomical abstractions became familiar realities, the map became the territory and external support complemented that internal security: As more patients were seen to live longer after hepatic metastasectomy and when no therapeutic alternatives were found, surgical referral of such patients and approval of such uncommon operations became commonplace. This acceptance along with acknowledgement of the complexity and risk of major operations on the liver fostered recognition of hepatobiliary surgery as a speciality worldwide. In time many more surgeons in more countries became involved and, as authors, more became forthcoming about judgemental and technical uncertainties. This more open acknowledgement of problems gave rise to solutions. Improved haemostatic techniques, new instruments, and more general application of anatomical sophistication became part of a growing productive *internationalization* of liver surgery.

In the mid-1980s the resultant momentum was heartening and exhilarating. Soon so many leaders appeared that it became most important to be a good attentive follower! That multinational momentum has found expression in this book, and is evidence of progress developing more rapidly within a global community. Also evident is an equally important diversity derived in part from realistic concerns about the limitations of resectional surgery. Perceptions and perspective are distorted by the fragmentation of medical practice, the consuming intensity of each specialist's obligations, and the motivational need for a sense of self-worth. Few physicians and fewer surgeons know much about the total population from which their individual practices are derived and even a general oncologist sees only a partial sample of a selected few. In this circumstance even increased understanding of one's day to day responsibilities is perceived as progress.

My own view of the flow of progress as a participant in change for over thirty years was determined by total involvement in the problems of and solutions for patients referred (selectively) one by one – punctuated by disappointment or transient satisfaction that came either with each separate failure or with a goal achieved. That recurring exercise, modified by more understanding, better performance, and personal growth, along with improving supporting services was *in fact* progress of a sort. However, these were changes of order not of kind and, in retrospect, were slow, unidimensional and very unscientific at beset. At the time of my retirement ten years ago, most of the risk had gone out of the risk/benefit proposition offered patients, but the chance of benefit was only slightly improved and still unpredictable for individuals. Most of the progress involved imaging technologies which could predict failure better than success. More patients were spared unnecessary operations by disclosure of smaller, previously undetectable metastases that in earlier years would have been seen as late postoperative recurrence. Thus better, more appropriate operations were being done for a somewhat smaller proportion of the total population of patients with liver metastases. Nevertheless my own capacity for rationalization was taxed by the inability to offer better odds. A patient's willingness to go through an inconvenient, discomforting, costly ordeal for one chance in four (or less) for real help or cure was better than having no chance at all (and very far from today's ethical considerations of futility). Nevertheless the disproportionate relationship between that surgical ordeal (with its need for the stamina of both patient and surgeon) and the incidence of long-term failure of resectional surgery for the great majority of patients so treated became unsatisfying and less sustaining. The treatment of liver metastases had become a dominant and domineering obligation. I retired from an unchanging risk/benefit equation that had not become the kind of purpose, meaning and fulfillment that I had set out to find forty years before.

It was my clinical curiosity about *surgical* progress since that time that determined acceptance of the invitation to write this foreword. Fortunately, my reluctance (and inability) to appraise scientific contributions was reinforced by editorial license and grace to consider primarily changes related to my own experience in consideration of the many chapters of this book.

The considerable surgical progress during the last ten years has involved refinements of surgical technique, better haemostasis, application of segmental anatomy, adaptation of a variety of ablative procedures, and improvement of the techniques and pharmacology of liver transplantation. Although laparoscopic techniques have reduced the cost and discomforts of some diagnostic procedures, in their application to major (resectional) procedures there is need to distinguish between cleverness and wisdom. Unfortunately, like progress in the preceding thirty years, these too are changes of order not of kind. They fail to overcome the inherent limitations of the surgical therapeutic model: the search for anatomical solutions to biological problems – which is further compromised by ignorance of each tumour's stage. This brings to mind Womak's Law: 'Doing a bad operation well does not make it a good operation.' Application of this judgement to each 'curative' hepatic resection that fails to cure may be too severe; but in that light the most substantive change has been the surgical acquisition of a radiographical technique. The availability of intra-operative ultrasound puts in the surgeon's hands the ability – and the responsibility – to find any ultrasonographic image that might either spare the patient the intended operation or modify the one proposed. Data showing consequent improvement of survival rates is not yet available.

Given a level of safety of major hepatic resections that has changed little in experienced hands during the past twenty-five years, and the disappointment to be found in the focal piecemeal extirpation of systemic disease, the recent progress most relevant to the potential surgical *patient* is the improvement of pre-operative diagnostic technology along with the radiologist's expertise. The fact that many subcentimetre lesions are now in range of several imaging techniques must contribute daily to some reduction in the performance of previously unavoidable ineffective operations.

Doris Redhead's consideration of 'diagnosis' in Chapter 5 is concise, comprehensive and clinically acute. Although 'None of the pre-operative techniques allows the detection of microscopic metastasis', experience with the Doppler perfusion index (DPI), which reveals changes in the ratio of hepatic arterial to total blood flow that appear to occur even in the presence of occult metastases, is encouraging. As one who long ago found excitement in the need for a surgeon and radiologists, given new vision, to learn relevant surgical anatomy together – and, who

also enjoyed the fact that each new imaging machine attracted a few new colleagues to that relationship, the author's assurance that 'Hepatic surgeons and radiologists are *interactive* in the drive to achieve 100% diagnostic accuracy' lets me hope that valued relationships will not be left out by change.

Although resectional surgery and some focal ablative techniques are now the only curative modalities, their success depends too much upon a specific stage of the metastatic process that is too seldom seen. The most precise extirpative and ablative techniques fail as tactical exercises because blind strategic planning is so poor. Success correlates better with an indeterminable stage of the metastatic process than with the extent or technical excellence of the focal procedure done. Unfortunately, poor strategy trumps good tactics.

There is simply no way for surgical perfection to challenge the sophistication, determination, and apparent caprice of the metastatic cancer cell. That threat will be met only when the pathobiology of metastasis at the molecular level is better understood. Once considered to be 'the ultimate expression of cellular anarchy', the metastatic process is now seen as a highly selective stepwise interaction between cells with a metastatic potential and host-organ defences. The ways in which metastasizing cells might be discouraged by inhibition of their invasive or proliferative potential, their capacity for angiogenesis, resistance to chemotherapeutic agents or regulation of carcinoembryonic antigen are considered well in the six non-surgical chapters of this book.

Looking back past the benchmarks that for me have put progress in frames of time, I wish that somewhere during that passing time I could have looked backward at the kind of understanding of the pathobiology of metastatic cancer that would have enabled me to do more good operations that made better sense.

Finally, with regard for the contents of this book, the inclusion of a chapter on palliation is an important addition which I hope will be extended some day to consider the suffering beyond physical pain that must be acknowledged and in some way softened for the patient who has metastatic cancer. It is a matter of dealing with the disease in *context* – in relation to patients and their illnesses. My retreat from the practice of surgery has been incomplete because some visits to hospitals and operating rooms were required for confinement as a patient and for more painful involvement as a parent. These experiences confirmed many long-standing subjective non-scientific concerns about the obligations of physicians and surgeons – and have broadened my perspective. Therefore, I do not apologize for the personal nature of this account when it is the nature of the person who chooses to become a clinical oncologist that determines the blend of science and humanity that the patient with cancer is looking for and requires.

I think that some scientists (who will contribute largely to more effective clinical practice) deal very directly with cancer cells – singly, in clumps or clusters, or sometimes in a mouse; but the rest of us as clinical oncologists relate to cancer through *relationships* with patients and with colleagues who share our concern, frustration, and bewilderment. The *science* of oncology has done little to affect the length of life or comfort of patients who have liver metastases. Therefore, until something really helpful can be done, the way in which our *humanity* is brought to the relationship with patients who hope for more than we can give is as important – and most often *more* important – than is the offering of a pretended science. The common denominators of all metastatic cancers are pain, fear and loss and the common denominator of involved physicians is concern. Neither these terrifying components of cancer nor the efforts of defenders can be measured or controlled scientifically, but disregard of this reciprocal relationship by physicians or surgeons is a denial of moral obligation. Abandonment in the context of medical practice is a form of spiritual malpractice.

There is no specific formula for the relationship required when science is found wanting, but palliation of suffering of this kind must begin with *acknowledgement*. This involves what Reynolds Price has called 'Mere human connection', a capacity for affection and a willingness to share one's importance and strength with the person whose importance is threatened by the cancer that you have been trained to treat.

The Natural History of Metastases to the Liver

Mark J. Lieser and David M. Nagorney

2

The liver is the repository of metastatic deposits from virtually any primary tumour site and type. Although most discussions of hepatic metastases focus on those of colorectal origin because of their higher incidence of liver metastases, primaries including sarcomas, breast, kidney and neuroendocrine tumours also metastasize to the liver. According to Tumour, Node, Metastisis classification, tumour deposits in the liver by definition denote distant disease. Thus, the presence of hepatic metastases always indicates a worsening of prognosis, and a significant decrease in the likelihood of cure.

Worldwide, colorectal carcinoma is the fourth most common malignancy following cancers of the lung, breast and prostate. Approximately 150 000 Americans are diagnosed with colorectal cancer per year, and over 50 000 deaths per year are attributed to this entity.[1] Many of these patients die with metastatic disease to the liver – in fact, 60–80% of patients with progression of disease have hepatic metastases. Of these, the liver is the initial site of recurrence in approximately 15%, and approximately 35% of patients will develop hepatic metastases during the course of their disease.[2]

Obviously, then, spread of colorectal cancer to the liver is an ominous finding signifying advanced disease. Since the 1960s, there have been numerous studies attempting to document the natural course of these liver metastases. Although the earliest of these studies demonstrated a dismal prognosis, subsequent series have shown a more varied natural history.[2]

Because of the apparent uncertainty over the true course of this disease, there has been controversy regarding optimum treatment. As no chemotherapeutic regimen has demonstrated curative benefit in treatment of colorectal carcinoma metastatic to the liver, knowledge of this disease's natural history is critical for determining whether surgical extirpation of these lesions is efficacious.

Incidence of Disease

Studies of the natural history of colorectal metastases are dependent on the sensitivity of the diagnostic tools employed by the clinician. Synchronous metastases, those recognized at the time of the diagnosis of the primary tumour, have occurred with a frequency of approximately 19%.[3] Metachronous metastases, those appearing after diagnosis of the primary tumour, were, in fact, most probably present microscopically at the initial presentation of the primary or were seeded at operation.[4] Thus, depending on the sensitivity of the diagnostic modality used, metastases may be classified as synchronous or metachronous. In one study of 71 patients who underwent computed tomography (CT) or ultrasonography (US) postoperatively, 17 (24%) were found to have hepatic metastases despite an ostensibly tumour-free liver intraoperatively.[5] Thus, data differentiating synchronous from metachronous metastases should be viewed with some scepticism. In fact, older series tend to report higher incidences of metachronous lesions, probably due to the use of less sensitive tests and a less vigorous attempt to detect them.

The accuracy of conventional CT or ultrasonography in detecting hepatic metastases has been reported to be between 40 and 60%.[6] Machi, Olsen and Stadler all demonstrated that newer diagnostic techniques, such as intraoperative ultrasonography (IOUS), increase the number of metastatic lesions classified as synchronous.[6–8] Machi *et al.*, followed

187 patients with colorectal cancer. In this group there were a total of 104 hepatic metastases in 45 patients. Pre-operative CT scans detected 49 of these metastatic lesions, and pre-operative US detected 43. Using a combination of CT and US in each patient, 53 (or 51%) of all tumours were diagnosed. Surgical exploration and palpation found an additional 29 tumours, but failed to detect 13.[6]

Intraoperative ultrasonography, however, detected an additional 22 tumours that were not found by either pre-operative study or by palpation. In addition, all tumours that were found by pre-operative CT or US, were seen by IOUS.[6] However, IOUS and even palpation of the liver which are often difficult to perform through the lower abdominal incisions used in many colonic operations, may preclude the wide application of these accurate modalities.

Goligher, based on post-mortem examinations of patients who died in the early postoperative period, concluded that approximately 16% of patients who were considered disease free by inspection and palpation had occult metastases.[9] In contrast, Hogg estimated the frequency at 5% and Gray at 7.7%.[10,11] Two of these series, however, are over 40 years old, and the intra-operative description of the liver was based on palpation and visual inspection alone.[9,10] Two more recent series have shown an incidence of synchronous metastases at 18.1% and 19.4%, respectively.[3,12] Lower postoperative mortality rates make it unlikely that similar autopsy studies will further substantiate these findings.

Rate of Growth

The growth rate of tumours is based on a formula described by Gompertz in 1825 for actuarial uses.[13] Gompertzean growth when applied to neoplasms proposes that the exponential growth rate of tumours slows as the tumour mass reaches a size of approximately one gram.[14]

Few studies have been conducted to calculate the growth rate of colorectal cancer, much less hepatic metastases from colorectal primaries.[80] In fact, only one study has attempted to calculate the age and growth of colorectal metastases to the liver. Finlay et al. estimated growth of liver metastases based on serial CT scans of untreated lesions. They calculated the mean age of overt metastases (detected at

laparotomy) to be 3.7 ± 0.9 years and of occult metastases to be 2.3 ± 0.4 years.[15]

Finlay's study, although unique, is not without flaws. First, liver masses were often assessed using only two CT scans per patient which were obtained at variable intervals. More problematic is the fact that tumour doubling times had wide variations: for overt metastases it was 48–321 days (mean = 155) and for occult metastases it was 30–192 days (mean = 86). Even using Gompertzian growth characteristics, the calculations of tumour age using this data is suspect due to its lack of uniformity.[15] Furthermore, relying on strict Gompertzean characteristics is fraught with potential pitfalls. Growth rate in biological systems is a complex process, dependent on numerous factors including the proportion of cells dividing at any given time, available nutrients, the time of a complete cell cycle, the degree of cell death, and the presence of promoting or inhibitory factors.[16] In addition, tumour growth can be disturbed by host defences, other therapies and hormonal levels.[14] Relying on a set formula also ignores other unanswered questions such as whether the metastatic process is a continuous one or an 'on–off' phenomenon from the primary, and whether metastases begin from a single cell or a clump of tumour cells deposited in the liver.[15] Finally, studies of the growth characteristics of breast cancer have recently challenged the concept that tumour growth can be assumed to proceed in such a predictable fashion.[17]

One ostensible reason for the high incidence of metastases to the liver is that it is the first filter of blood flow from the bowel. However, not every malignant cell that passes through the liver implants there. The metastatic process is highly selective and not random; obviously tumours require unique characteristics to become metastases. Tumours need to invade the surrounding stroma, gain access to lymphatics or the vascular tree, survive the body's immune system, stop in the bed of the 'target organ', extravasate into its parenchyma, develop their own blood supply, and begin to grow.[18]

Studies have demonstrated that tumour cells implanted in the portal system of rats are more likely to implant in the liver in the face of liver trauma or resection.[19] This finding is consistent with the concept that liver injury results in the release of tissue factors to promote growth, regeneration, and repair of the liver. These factors promote the colonization and growth of metastatic tumour cells that express receptors for these growth factors.[20]

Tumour cells with a high metastatic potential have been shown to express increased levels of metalloproteinases that enable them to degrade the basement membrane and extracellular matrix.[21] Once they have escaped the primary tumour site and entered the bloodstream, tumour cells need to adhere to the microvasculature of the target organ. Tumour cells that survive to develop into metastases express specific adhesion molecules that promote liver metastases. These include ganglioside $GM_2 B_1$ integrins and CD44.[22-24]

Finally, tumours with high metastatic potential appear to express higher levels of factors that promote angiogenesis such as vascular endothelial growth factor.[25,26] Thus, the metastatic process does not appear to be random, but a complex one in which a select population of tumour cells express an array of factors that enable them to escape the primary tumour, adhere to the target organ and thrive in this new milieu.

The clinical relevance of these adhesion molecules and growth factors has yet to be established. Although they clearly exist and influence the natural history of tumours, their predictive value for determining prognosis or refining indications for and types of adjuvant therapy have not been explored.

Risk Factors for Development of Hepatic Metastases

From the numerous published series of patients with recurrent colorectal cancer, some risk factors for development of hepatic metastases have been determined. Probably the strongest risk factor for development of hepatic metastases from colorectal cancer is the stage of the primary tumour. The incidence of hepatic metastases increases with greater depth of invasion of the tumour and with increased lymph node involvement.[26] Although venous invasion of the tumour correlates with increased risk of metastases, whether it is an independent prognostic factor because venous invasion correlates with tumour stage is unclear.[27,28]

Because of differing patterns of venous drainage, i.e. portal versus systemic, it has been proposed that a colonic primary presents a greater risk factor for hepatic metastases than does a rectal primary. Two series totaling over 3000 patients each showed a trend toward higher incidence from colon primaries, although statistical significance was lacking.[3,12] In contrast, Pickren's study of autopsies of patients succumbing to colorectal cancer showed a 56.8% incidence of liver metastases from colonic primaries versus 45.9% from rectal primaries ($P < 0.005$).[29] The significance of origin of the primary as a risk factor is controversial. Similarly, it is noteworthy that colorectal cancers rarely metastasize to cirrhotic livers. This observation has been attributed to decreased hepatic blood flow from the portal circulation via collaterals which arise to compensate portal hypertension.[30] Consequently, portal venous collaterals provide alternative routes for tumour dissemination. Furthermore, the cirrhotic liver itself may not provide an environment which fosters tumour growth even if accessed.

Survival of Unresected Metastases

Numerous reports over the past four decades have attempted to chronicle the natural history of untreated liver metastases. In published series from 1954 to 1995 the median survival of patients with untreated hepatic metastases ranges from 4.5 months to 19 months. However, most series report survival of less than one year, and five-year survival is rare.[27,31-53] Indeed, less than 1% of the total reported patients among these 24 series survived five years (Table 2.1). As of 1988, there were only 14 reports in the medical literature of five-year survivors without resection.[54] In one recent series, Stangl et al. prospectively followed over 1000 patients with liver metastases from colorectal cancer. Four hundred and eighty-four of them opted to forego any form of therapy. Of this group the median survival was 7.5 months and 1% survived five years.[52] These poor survival statistics are understandable because in addition to representing loss of local control, the presence of liver metastases also indicates a biologically aggressive tumour.

No controlled, prospective study has compared the natural history of untreated colorectal metastases to the liver with those that are resected. However several concurrent series have provided such comparison, though selection factors for management of untreated patients will forever remain obscure. Although the indications and merits of

Table 2.1   Survival of patients with unresected, untreated hepatic metastases from colorectal carcinoma

Study (year)	Patients (number)	Median survival	Five-year survival (%)
		(months)	
Stearns and Brinkley[31] (1954)	50	18	1
Bacon and Markin[32] (1964)	110	10.6	0
Pestana et al.[33] (1964)	353	9	3
Jaffe et al.[34] (1968)	177	5	0
Bengmark and Hafstrom[35] (1969)	38	5.7	0
Oxley and Ellis[36] (1969)	112	12	1
Cady et al.[37] (1970)	269	13*	1
Abrams and Lerner[38] (1971)	58	5.9	2
Nielson et al.[39] (1971)	103	6.8	3
Baden and Anderson[40] (1975)	105	10	3
Wood et al.[42] (1976)	104	6.6*	2
Wanebo et al.[43] (1978)	125	19	0
Bengtsson et al.[44] (1981)	155	4.5	0
Goslin et al.[45] (1982)	125	12.5	0
Lahr et al.[46] (1983)	175	6.1	1
Wagner et al.[47] (1984)	252	19	2
Finan et al.[48] (1985)	90	10.3	0
DeBrauw et al.[49] (1989)	83	8.4	1
Palmer et al.[50] (1989)	30	12	N.S.
Scheele et al.[51] (1990)	921 (unresectable)	6.9	0
	62 (resectable)	14.2	
Stangl et al.[52] (1994)	484	7.5	1
Rougier et al.[53] (1995)	318	5.7	N.S.

* Mean survival.

hepatic resection are discussed elsewhere (Chapter 6), these series do provide data regarding the natural history of untreated patients. Wilson and Adson's study from the Mayo Clinic compared two groups of 60 patients.[41] Each group had hepatic metastases of comparable number and extent. One group underwent presumptive curative resection, while the other underwent biopsy only. The resected group had a five-year survival of 25%, but the biopsied group had no five-year survivors.

A second report by Adson compared 141 patients who underwent resection with 70 who had technically resectable disease but whose tumours were not removed.[47] Only 2.5% of the non-resected patients survived five years, while 25% of the resected group did. Unfortunately, due to the retrospective nature of this study, resectability can only be inferred from recorded descriptions of the number and anatomical location of the metastases. Scheele compared 921 patients judged unresectable with 62 patients judged resectable but who did not undergo surgery and 183 patients who underwent potentially curative liver resection.[51] No patient in either of the non-operative groups survived five years. The median survival of

the unresectable group was shorter (6.9 months versus 14 months), which may have been related to the extent of liver involvement. However, the resected group had a five-year survival of 38%.

Furthermore, over the past decade, hepatic resection techniques have become more refined with a concomitant decrease in intra-operative and post-operative mortality to <5%. With resection so safe and with the replete accumulated, albeit retrospective, evidence pointing to a benefit from resection, it would be difficult to conduct a true randomized prospective study comparing resection to no treatment, and it is unlikely that such a study could be performed ethically.

One might assume that more recent series would show improved survival due to earlier detection of metastases with improved imaging and diagnostic techniques. In particular, use of newer diagnostic tools mentioned earlier such as IOUS and CT portography probably allows for demonstration of an artificial increase in survival for both resected and unresected patients, because metastatic lesions are diagnosed earlier in their course.[6–8] The findings of many retrospective studies been challenged because diagnostic modalities changed over the duration of study. The impact of such a trend, however, has yet to be uniformly demonstrated. In fact, Rougier *et al.*, in a recent large series of unresected patients showed a median survival for patients with one to two liver lesions of 9.9 months – a survival worse than earlier studies of similar patient populations.[53] This poorer outcome probably reflects the fact that patients with the best functional status have been preselected for surgical resection. Despite the absence of such a trend, the variability in median survival in part reflects the wide array of diagnostic tools available to clinicians.

The premise that the accuracy of imaging may bias observed survival of unresected metastases has a modicum of support. As noted earlier, Machi's series with good follow-up has demonstrated that intra-operative ultrasonography detects unknown lesions in approximately 10% of cases.[6] Kemeny *et al.* report that CT accurately predicts tumour location and number only 43% of the time.[55] Surgical exploration is better at detecting metastases than CT or US, but IOUS is better than all three.[6] The precise role and accuracy of other, newer diagnostic modalities is debatable.

CT portography (CTAP) can detect lesions less than 15 mm in diameter that are not seen by CT or US.[56] However, CTAP has a false-positive rate as high as 17%.[57] MRI is more sensitive and accurate for detecting lesions <20 mm than CT, but not as sensitive as CTAP. For lesions >20 mm MRI and CT are equivalent.[58]

Finally, even newer modalities for detecting liver metastases are allowing the imaging of these lesions in even earlier stages. Radioimmunoguided surgery (RIGS), in which a gamma detector is employed intra-operatively to detect metastases which have been marked with a radiolabelled monoclonal antibody has been touted as a means of detecting hepatic metastases even earlier.[59,60] Burak *et al.* report RIGS using CC83, the antibody with the highest affinity coefficient, demonstrated a sensitivity of 100%. In 17 patients with 27 tumour sites, pre-operative CT identified only 13 (44%).[59] B72.2, another antibody with a lower tumour affinity, demonstrated a sensitivity of 78%.[60] Although there were 12 false-positives in Burak's series, 10 were in lymph nodes that, the authors postulate, probably contained microscopic foci of cancer that would have been detected with more sensitive staining

Table 2.2 Prognostic determinants in patients with unresected, untreated hepatic metastases from colorectal carcinoma

Author	Stearns[31] (1954)	Jaffe[34] (1968)	Bengmark[35] (1969)	Oxley[36] (1969)	Cady[37] (1970)	Abrams[38] (1971)	Wilson[41] (1976)	Wood[42] (1976)	Wanebo[43] (1978)	Bengston[44] (1981)	Goslin[45] (1982)	Wagner[47] (1984)	Finan[48] (1985)	Palmer[50] (1989)	Stangl[52] (1994)	Rougier[53] (1995)
Patient characteristics																
age	–	–	–	–	–	–	–	–	–	negative	negative	–	–	–	negative	positive
weight loss	–	–	–	–	positive	–	–	–	–	–	positive	–	positive	–	–	–
sex	–	–	–	–	positive	negative	–	–	–	–	negative	–	–	–	negative	negative
other symptoms	–	–	–	–	positive	–	–	–	–	–	–	–	positive	–	–	–
performance status	–	–	–	–	–	–	–	–	–	–	positive	–	–	positive	–	positive
Lab values elevated																
alkaline phosphatase	–	positive	positive	positive	–	–	–	–	–	positive	positive	–	positive	positive	positive	positive
SGOT/LDH	–	–	–	positive	–	–	–	–	–	–	positive	–	–	positive	–	positive
WBC	–	–	–	–	–	–	–	–	–	–	–	–	positive	–	positive	–
CEA	–	–	–	–	–	–	–	–	–	–	positive	–	–	–	positive	positive
Primary tumour																
stage	–	–	–	–	positive	–	–	–	–	–	–	positive	positive	–	positive	–
grade	–	positive	–	–	–	–	–	–	–	–	positive	positive	positive	–	positive	–
? resected	positive	negative	negative	–	positive	positive	–	–	positive	positive	–	–	positive	–	positive	positive
site: colon vs. rectum	–	positive	positive	–	positive	–	–	–	–	–	negative	–	–	–	negative	–
Metastases																
grade	–	–	–	–	–	–	–	–	–	–	–	–	positive	–	–	–
number	–	–	–	–	–	–	positive	–	positive	–	positive	–	–	–	positive	positive
% liver involved	–	positive	–	–	–	–	–	positive	positive	positive	positive	–	–	positive	positive	positive
distant metastases	positive	negative	–	–	positive	–	–	–	–	–	–	–	–	–	positive	positive

Key: positive = significant prognostic variable; negative = not a significant prognostic variable; – = not studied.

Table 2.3 Prognostic determinants in patients with unresected hepatic metastases from colorectal carcinoma treated with chemotherapy

Author (1980)	Lahr[46] (1983)	Kemeny[61] (1983)	Bedikian[62] (1986)	Ekberg[63] (1989)	Chang[64] (1989)	Kemeny[65] (1991)	Fortner[66] (1984)	Graf[67] (1991)	Lavin[68] (1980)
Patient characteristics									
age	negative	positive	–	negative	negative	negative	negative	–	–
weight loss	–	–	–	–	–	positive	–	–	positive
sex	negative	negative	positive	negative	positive	negative	negative	–	–
other symptoms	positive	–	–	–	–	–	–	–	–
performance status	positive	–	positive	–	–	–	–	–	–
Lab values elevated									
alkaline phosphatase	positive	positive	positive	positive	positive	positive	negative	–	–
SGOT/LDH	positive	positive	–	negative	positive	positive	negative	–	–
WBC	–	positive	–	–	–	positive	–	–	–
CEA	negative	positive	–	–	positive	negative	negative	–	–
Primary tumour									
stage	–	–	positive	negative	negative	–	negative	–	–
grade	negative	–	–	negative	negative	–	–	–	–
? resected	positive	–	positive	–	–	–	–	positive	–
site: colon vs. rectum	negative	negative	–	negative	negative	negative	negative	positive	–
Metastases									
grade	–	–	–	–	–	–	–	–	–
number	positive	–	–	negative	–	–	–	–	–
% liver involved	–	–	–	positive	positive	positive	positive	–	–
distant metastases	–	–	–	positive	positive	–	–	negative	positive

Key: positive = significant prognostic variable;
negative = not a significant prognostic variable;
- = not studied.

techniques. Thus, newer and more sensitive imaging modalities may provide greater resolution of liver lesions and depict metastases in earlier and more varied stages of development.

Determinants of Prognosis

The variability in reported survival with unresected liver metastases has implied heterogeneity in the patient population. Several factors, consequently, have been identified as correlates to survival (Tables 2.2 and 2.3).

Laboratory Values/Patient Characteristics

Alkaline Phosphatase

Of all laboratory values, serum alkaline phosphatase has been shown as an independent predictor of survival in untreated patients in the most studies.[34–36,44,45,48,50,52,53] Finan's series demonstrated a threefold increase in length of survival if alkaline phosphatase was <13 KAU.[48] Similarly, Stangl *et al.* reported a median survival of 9.9 months with alka-

line phosphatase values <105 U/litre, 7.2 months for alkaline phosphatase of 106–315 U/litre, and 3.9 months for alkaline phosphatase >315 U/litre.[52] Serum alkaline phosphatase has also correlated with survival in all but one series of patients treated with chemotherapy (Table 2).[46,61–65]

Carcinoembryonic Antigen (CEA)

Serum CEA level measured at the time of detection of liver metastases has correlated with survival, though this finding has not been consistent.[45,52,53,61,64] In an early study of patients treated with chemotherapy by Kemeny *et al.*, patients with normal CEA (<5 ng/ml) had a median survival of 23 months versus 9.2 months for those with an elevated CEA. Interestingly, a subsequent 1989 study by Kemeny *et al.* did not confirm the significance of CEA elevations.[61] Stangl's series did demonstrate a significant difference in median survival (10.1 months versus 7.3 months), but only if CEA values were stratified less than or greater than 50 ng/ml, respectively.[52]

Other Laboratory Values

While various other laboratory data, including liver function tests, have been measured by various investigators, no survival correlation as strong as

CEA and alkaline phosphatase has been demonstrated. Lactase dehydrogenase and white blood cell count have correlated with survival in some series, but this is generally thought to be a reflection of the extent of liver involvement and less of an independent variable.[36,45,46,50,52,53,61,65,66]

Age/Gender

Most series – either of untreated patients or patients treated with chemotherapy – do not show age or gender as a significant prognostic variable. In two of the chemotherapy series gender was significant.[62,64] However, in Bedikian's series[62] the survival difference was minimal (females, 7 months; males, 5 months), and in Chang's series[64] the gender difference was not significant with multivariate analysis.

Other Patient Characteristics

Performance status correlates with survival. It should be noted, however, that performance status is both a function of the tumour load in the liver and of the patient's general well-being. Other parameters such as weight loss and the presence of symptoms have been found to be of prognostic value as they are reflective of performance status.[37,45,46,50,53,61,62,65]

Resection of the Primary Tumour

Most studies have shown that prognosis is improved if the primary is resected even in the presence of synchronous metastases.[31,34,35,38,39,43,44,46,52,53,62,67] Whether this data is confounded by the fact that the primary is more likely to be resected if there is less liver involvement is uncertain. Two recent studies that controlled for this factor, however, have demonstrated a survival benefit from resection regardless of the degree of hepatic involvement.[52,53]

Characteristics of the Metastases

The most significant prognostic factor of untreated hepatic metastases from colorectal cancer is the extent of liver replaced by tumour. The series of Finan, Palmer, Wagner, Goslin, Stangl and Wood, all confirm metastatic extent as a significant predictor of survival.[42,45,47,48,50,52] Finan et al. demonstrated a median survival of 16.4 months of <20% of the liver was involved versus 5.6 months with >20% involvement.[48] Wagner had a mean survival of 24, 16 and 11 months with solitary, multiple but unilateral, and bilateral involvement, respectively.[47] The disparity between these two studies probably lies in the imprecise nature of Wagner's classification system. Hence, a patient with bilateral involvement could theoretically have a smaller fraction of liver overtaken with tumour. Nevertheless, both series confirm the premise that length of survival correlates with the absolute amount of tumour in the liver. Finally, Stangl's data report a 10.8 month median survival with <25% liver involvement versus 5.9 months with >25% involvement.[52] All series of chemotherapeutically treated lesions similarly found significance in this variable.[63–66]

Number of Metastases

The number of metastases has also significantly correlated with survival in studies by Stangl, Nielson, Rougier, Goslin and Finan of untreated metastases.[39,45,48,52,53] This factor has probably been most extensively studies in the surgically treated population in which it was also found significant with survival inversely correlating to the number of metastases. These findings have led some surgeons to propose over four lesions as a contraindication to resection, a subject of some controversy.

Histological Grade of Metastases

Although the relationship of the grade of the primary tumour to survival has been studied often, the correlation of the grade of the metastases to survival has not been adequately evaluated in of untreated patients.

Presence of Symptoms

The presence of symptoms relating to the metastases such as pain or weight loss has correlated with survival in both Cady and Finan's studies of untreated patients.[37,48] Finan et al. have reported a median survival of 6.2 months if the patient had weight loss >3 kg versus 13.0 months without weight loss.[48] Similarly, all four series of patients who underwent chemotherapy that evaluated weight loss found an adverse correlation with survival.[46,62,65,68]

Lymph Node Status

Because the presence of metastases in perihepatic lymph nodes has been a strong negative predictor of survival and usually contraindicates resection, this factor has not been assessed in untreated patients. However, in Fortner and Ekberg's series of patients treated chemotherapeutically the presence of disease in perihepatic lymph nodes is a poor prognostic finding.[63,66]

Extrahepatic Disease

The presence of extrahepatic disease is a uniformly poor prognostic factor in untreated patients.[31,34,37,52,53] This factor was demonstrated as early as Stearns' series in 1954 and was reaffirmed recently in Rougier's series.

Genotypic Characteristics

Although molecular biological techniques have been extensively applied in the study of the natural history and prognosis of colonic primaries, this technology has less frequently been applied to metastases. Cady et al. performed flow cytometric analysis on 51 resected liver specimens containing hepatic metastases of colorectal origin.[69] They demonstrated a significant difference in five-year survival between patients with diploid metastases and those with nondiploid metastases (20% vs. 0%, respectively). Similarly, Tsushima et al. analysed the DNA content of 88 resected colorectal metastases. Although there was no statistical difference in five-year survival between patients with diploid and polyploid metastases, survival of patients with aneuploid metastases was 20% compared to 32% for the diploid group ($P < 0.05$).[70] Finally, though not presenting any data regarding prognosis, Kastrinakis et al. characterized the p53 gene status of 18 matched colorectal primaries and their corresponding liver metastases.[71] Mutations of p53, a tumour suppressor gene, are the most common findings in human cancers. In four patients, no p53 alterations were detected in either the primary or the metastasis. In eight patients, both the primary and the liver lesion contained alterations in p53. However, in six patients, only the liver metastasis contained a p53 mutation. The authors hypothesize that p53 altered cells have an advantage in establishing a metastatic focus.

Characteristics of the Primary Tumor

Primary Tumour Stage

The studies by Stangl, Finan, Wagner and Cady all found the stage of the primary tumour was prognostically significant in patients with untreated metastases, though Cady's more recent series did not.[37,47,48,52,69] In Finan's study median survival was 16.7 months compared with 10.8 months for Duke's B and C tumours respectively.[48] Of five studies of patients treated with chemotherapy alone, only Bedikian's has found the stage of the primary as significant.[62]

Primary Tumour Grade

Goslin, Wagner, Jaffe and Finan have found that grade of the primary tumour correlates with survival in patients with untreated hepatic metastases.[34,45,47,48] According to Finan's data, median survival decreased from 13 to 7 months with a grade of well/moderate and poor respectively.[48]

Primary Tumour Location

Only two early studies have shown a survival difference between colonic and rectal primaries.[34,37] More recent series by Goslin and Stangl, however, did not find the site of primary cancer as significant.[45,52] As noted earlier, these proposed differences are based on the theoretical premise that rectal primaries will metastasize more diffusely due to both portal and systemic venous drainage.

It is acknowledged that survival beyond five years with hepatic metastases is rare, and that the only patients disease-free at five years are those status postresection. Thus to standardize and optimize patient care, numerous staging systems for these lesions have been proposed, although none have been uniformly adopted. Reflecting the fact that one of the strongest predictors of survival is the percent of liver involved with tumour, all of the staging

Table 2.4 Proposed staging systems for hepatic metastases from colorectal cancer*

1. Fortner *et al.* (1984)
   I   PHR: ≤50%
   II   PHR: 55 to 80%
   II   PHR: >80%
   A   No extrahepatic involvement or prior chemotherapy
   B   Either nodal metastases and/or prior chemotherapy

2. Gennari *et al.* (1984)
   H_1 PHR: ≤25%
   H_2 PHR: 25 to 50%
   H_3 PHR: >50%
   s   single metastasis
   m   multiple metastasis to one anatomic lobe
   b   bilateral metastases
   I   infiltration of adjacent organs or structures
   F   impairment of liver function

Staging:
   I H_{Is}
   II $H_{1m, b}$ H_{2s}
   III $H_{2m, b}$ $H_{3s, m, b}$
   IV   A   Minimal intraabdominal extrahepatic disease (detected only at laparotomy)
        B   Extrahepatic disease

3. van de Velde *et al.* (1986)
   P_1 PHR: 25%
   P_2 PHR: 25 to 75%
   P_3 PHR: >75%
   E   concurrent extrahepatic disease
   S   symptoms attributable to liver metastases

Staging:
   O   Curatively resected metastases
   I P_1, no E or S
   II P_2, no E or S
   III P_3, no E or S
   any P, +E, any S
   any P, any E, +S

* PHR = percent hepatic replacement.

systems incorporate this characteristic (Table 2.4).[66,72,73] Gennari *et al.* noted that in prior series there was a clear prognostic difference when patients were divided into groups based on <25%, 25–50% and >50% hepatic replacement by tumour. This became the basis for their staging system.[72] Fortner *et al.* developed a similar staging system with different groupings also based on the percent hepatic replacement by metastases.[66] In their series of patients treated with intra-arterial chemotherapy, 24 month survival was 37% and 10% for stages Ia and Ib, respectively; 6% and 4% for IIa and IIb, respectively; and 0% for all else.

Non-Colorectal Primaries

Among the non-colorectal tumours that metastasize to the liver are those originating in the gallbladder, breast, stomach, sarcomas, melanoma, renal cell carcinoma, adrenocortical carcinoma, carcinoid and neuroendocrine tumours.[74] It is more difficult to describe the natural history of these liver metastases because of their lower incidence, infrequent reports and patterns of tumour spread.

Patients with non-colorectal, non-neuroendocrine liver metastases have a poorer prognosis than those with colorectal primaries. It is difficult to determine with any accuracy the risk factors for development of these metastases because of their low frequency. For example, the incidence of liver metastases from retroperitoneal sarcomas is 14%, and that of soft tissue sarcomas less than 10%. Median survival in untreated patients is approximately 12 months.[75] For the other aforementioned malignancies, the presence of liver metastases portends a median survival between 2 and 8 months.[74] Because these tumours present more infrequently there is only anecdotal data regarding the efficacy of surgical resection.

The data regarding neuroendocrine tumours that metastasize to the liver are both more extensive and more promising. Carcinoids are the most common neuroendocrine malignancy that metastasize to the liver;[76] 95% of all carcinoids arise from the appendix, rectum or the small bowel, and 40% arise within 2 feet of the ileocecal valve.[77] Up to 40% of patients with gastrinoma or glucagonoma develop liver metastases, whereas less than 5% of patients with carcinoid or insulinoma do.[76] Carcinoid tumours rarely metastasize if the primary is less than 2 cm.[77]

Neuroendocrine tumours are characterized by production of specific hormones or amines that produce clinical signs/symptoms that can act as tumour markers. Carcinoid syndrome occurs only in the presence of hepatic metastases. (Other neuroendocrine malignancies such as islet cell tumours, may cause hormone-related symptoms from small primaries.)[77] These liver metastases are usually bilobar, and thus are less frequently amenable to complete resection. Neuroendocrine tumours, however, are generally slow growing; hence five-year survival even in the presence of liver metastases is common.[76] In Moertel's series of 183 patients at the

Mayo Clinic followed from the onset of symptoms from their carcinoid primary until death, the average duration of disease was nine years.[77] The five-year survival with untreated liver metastases in this report was 30%. A 35% five-year survival with untreated metastases from islet cell tumours has been reported which is far longer than the rare five-year survivor with colorectal metastases.[78] Because of the indolent natural history of these metastases, hepatic resection to debulk these tumours is often appropriate because the patient has potential for prolonged survival even in the presence of residual disease.[79]

Summary

The liver is the most common site of metastases from colorectal carcinoma. In view of the incidence of colon cancer worldwide, and the number of patients who either present with or subsequently develop hepatic metastases, knowledge of their risk factors, natural history and prognosis are of increasing importance to the clinician.

The strongest risk factor for developing liver metastases is the stage of the primary tumour. The most important prognostic factor in patient outcome is the fraction of liver overtaken by tumour.

There remains disagreement regarding the rate of growth of liver metastases and the median survival once they are detected. Some of this confusion arises from an evolving array of diagnostic tools employed in evaluating the liver. Further investigation into prognostic variables such as molecular biological characteristics of metastases is needed to enable improved prediction of patient outcome, and to facilitate targeted therapy of these lesions. Because of the increased safety of hepatic resection, further studies of large populations with untreated liver metastases are unlikely.

Neuroendocrine tumours are the second most common malignancies that spread to the liver. They are usually bilobar, but slow growing, with five-year survival being more common than with colorectal metastases. Finally, an array of other carcinomas and sarcomas metastasize to the liver. Their infrequency makes evaluation of natural history and prognosis difficult.

References

1. Parker SL, Tong T, Bolden S, Wingo PA. Cancer statistics, 1996. *CA Cancer J Clin* 1996; **46:**5–27.
2. Levitan N, Hughes KS. Management of non-resectable liver metastases from colorectal cancer. *Oncology* 1990; **4:**77–84.
3. Kune GA, Kune S, Field B *et al.* Survival in patients with large bowel cancer. A population-based investigation from the Melbourne Colorectal Cancer Study. *Dis Colon Rectum* 1990; **33:**938–946.
4. Turnbull RB, Jr., Kyle K, Watson FR, Spratt J. Cancer of the colon: The influence of the no touch isolation technique on survival rates. *Ann Surg* 1967; **166:**420–427.
5. Finlay IG, McArdle CS. Occult hepatic metastases in colorectal carcinoma. *Br J Surg* 1986; **73:**732–735.
6. Machi J, Isomoto H, Kurohiji T *et al.* Accuracy of intraoperative ultrasonography in diagnosing liver metastases from colorectal cancer: Evaluation with postoperative follow-up results. *World J Surg* 1991; **15:**551–557.
7. Olsen AK. Intraoperative ultrasonography and the detection of liver metastases at laparotomy. *Aust NZ J Surg* 1980; **50:**524–526.
8. Stadler J, Holscher AH, Adolf J. Intraoperative ultrasonographic detection of occult liver metastases in colorectal cancer. *Surg Endosc* 1991; **5:**36–40.
9. Goligher JC. The operability of carcinoma of the rectum. *BMJ* 1941; 393–397.
10. Hogg L, Pack GK. Diagnostic accuracy of hepatic metastases at laparotomy. *Arch Surg* 1956; **72:**251–252.
11. Gray BN. Surgeon accuracy in the diagnosis of liver metastases at laparotomy. *Aust NZ J Surg* 1980; **50:**524–526.
12. Faivre J, Rat P, Arveux P. Epidemiology of liver metastases from colorectal cancer. In: Nordlinger B, Jaeck D (eds) *Treatment of Hepatic Metastases of Colorectal Cancer* 1992:33–8. Paris: Springer Verlag.
13. Gompertz B. On the nature of the function expressive of the law of human mortality and on the new mode of determining the value of life contingencies. *Phil Trans R Soc London* 1825; **115:**513–585,
14. Norton L, Simon R. Growth curve of an experimental solid tumor following radiotherapy. *J Natl Cancer Inst* 1977; **58:**1735–1741.
15. Finlay IG, Meek D, Brunton F, McArdle CS. Growth rates of hepatic metastases in colorectal carcinoma. *Br J Surg* 1988; **75:**641–644.
16. Baserga R. The cell cycle. *NEJM* 1981; **304:**453–459.
17. Retsky MW, Swartzendruber DE, Bame PD, Wardwell RH. Computer model challenges breast cancer treatment strategy. *Cancer Invest* 1994; **12:**559–567.
18. Radinsky R, Ellis LM. Molecular determinants in the biology of liver metastases. *Surg Oncol Clin NA* 1996; **5:**215–230.
19. Loizidou MC, Lawrence RJ, Holt S *et al.* Facilitation by partial hepatectomy of tumor growth within the rat liver following the intraportal injection of syngeneic tumor cells. *Clin Exp Metastasis* 1991; **9:**335–349.
20. Michalopoulos GK. Liver regeneration: Molecular mechanisms of growth control. *FASEB J* 1990; **4:**176–187.
21. Levy A, Cioce V, Sobel ME *et al.* Increased expression of the 72 kDa type IV collagenase in human colonic adenocarcinoma. *Cancer Res* 1991; **51:**439–444.
22. Coulombe J, Pelletier G. Gangliosides and organ-specific metastatic colonization. *Int J Cancer* 1993; **53:**104–109.
23. Fujita S, Suzuki J, Kinoshita M *et al.* Inhibition of cell attachment, invasion and metastasis of human carcinoma cells by anti-integrin beta-1 subunit antibody. *Jpn J Cancer Res* 1992; **83:**1317–1326.

24. Tanabe KK, Ellis LM, Saya H. Expression of the CD44R1 adhesion molecule is increased in human colon adenocarcinomas and metastases. *Lancet* 1993; **341**:725–726.

25. Ellis LM, Liu W. Vascular endothelial growth factor (VEGF) expression and alternate splicing in non-metastatic and metastatic human colon cancer cell lines. *Proc AACR* 1995; **36**:A525.

26. Taylor I, Mullee MA, Campbell MJ. Prognostic index for the development of liver metastases in patients with colorectal cancer. *Br J Surg* 1990; **77**:499–501.

27. Morris MJ, Newland RC, Pheils MT, Macpherson JG. Hepatic metastases from colorectal carcinoma: an analysis of survival rates and histopathology. *Aust NZ J Surg* 1977; **47**:365–368.

28. Tsuchiya A, Ando Y, Kikuchi Y, Kanazawa M et al. Venous invasion as a prognostic factor in colorectal cancer. *Surg Today* 1995; **25**:950–953.

29. Pickren JW, Tsukada Y, Lane WW. Liver metastasis: Analysis of autopsy data. In: Weiss L, Gilbert HA, (eds) *Liver Metastasis* 1982; 222–28. Boston: Hall Medical,

30. Uetsuji S, Yamamura M, Yamamichi K et al. Absence of colorectal cancer metastases to the cirrhotic liver. *Am J Surg* 1992; **164**:176–177.

31. Stearns MW, Brinkley GJ. Palliative surgery for cancer of the rectum and colon. *Cancer* 1954; **7**:1016–1019.

32. Bacon HE, Martin PV. The rationale of palliative resection for primary cancer of the colon complicated by liver and lung metastases. *Dis Colon Rectum* 1964; **7**:211–217.

33. Pestana C, Reitemeyer RJ, Moertel CG et al. The natural history of carcinoma of the colon and rectum. *Am J Surg* 1964; **108**:826–829.

34. Jaffe BM, Donegan WL, Watson F et al. Factors influencing survival in patients with untreated hepatic metastases. *Surg Gynecol Obstet* 1968; **127**:1–11.

35. Bengmark S, Hafstrom L. The natural history of primary and secondary malignant tumors of the liver: I. The prognosis for patients with hepatic metastases from colonic and rectal carcinoma at laparotomy. *Cancer* 1969; **23**:198–202.

36. Oxley EM, Ellis H. Prognosis of carcinoma of the large bowel in the presence of liver metastases. *Br J Surg* 1969; **56**:149–152.

37. Cady B, Monson DO, Swinton NW. Survival of patients after colonic resection for carcinoma with simultaneous liver metastases. *Surg Gynecol Obstet* 1970; **131**:697–700.

38. Abrams MS, Lerner HJ. Survival of patients at Pennsylvania Hospital with hepatic metastases from carcinoma of the colon and rectum. *Dis Colon Rectum* 1971; **14**:431–434.

39. Nielson J, Barlslev I, Jensen HE. Carcinoma of the colon with liver metastases. *Acta Chir Scand* 1971; **137**:463–465.

40. Baden H, Anderson B. Survival of patients with untreated liver metastases from colorectal cancer. *Scand J Gastroenterol* 1975; **10**:221–223.

41. Wilson SM, Adson MA. Surgical treatment of hepatic metastases from colorectal cancers. *Arch Surg* 1976; **111**:330–334.

42. Wood CB, Gillis CR, Blumgart LH. A retrospective study of the natural history of patients with liver metastases from colorectal cancer. *Clin Oncol* 1976; **2**:285–288.

43. Wanebo HJ, Semoglon C, Attiyeh F et al. Surgical management of patients with primary operable colorectal cancer and synchronous liver metastases. *Am J Surg* 1978; **135**:81–84.

44. Bengston G, Carlsson G, Hafstrom L et al. Natural history of patients with untreated liver metastases from colorectal cancer. *Am J Surg* 1981; **141**:586–589.

45. Goslin R, Steele G, Zamcheck N et al. Factors influencing survival in patients with hepatic metastases from adenocarcinoma of the colon and rectum. *Dis Colon Rectum* 1982; **25**:749–754.

46. Lahr CJ, Soong S-J, Cloud G et al. A multifactorial analysis of prognostic factors in patients with liver metastases from colorectal carcinoma. *J Clin Oncol* 1983; **1**:720–726.

47. Wagner JS, Adson MA, van Heerden JA et al. The natural history of hepatic metastases from colorectal cancer: A comparison with resective treatment. *Ann Surg* 1984; **199**:502–508.

48. Finan PJ, Marshall RJ, Cooper EH et al. Factors affecting survival in patients presenting with synchronous hepatic metastases from colorectal cancer: A clinical and computer analysis. *Br J Surg* 1985; **72**:373–377.

49. DeBrauw LM, DeVelde CJH, Bouwhuis-Hoogerwerf ML. Diagnostic evaluation and survival analysis of colorectal cancer patients with liver metastases. *J Surg Oncol* 1989; **7**:1407–1418.

50. Palmer M, Petrelli NJ, Herrera L. No treatment option for liver metastases from colorectal adenocarcinoma. *Dis Colon Rectum* 1989; **32**:698–701.

51. Scheele J, Stangl R, Altendorf-Hofmann A. Hepatic metastases from colorectal carcinoma: Impact of surgical resection on the natural history. *Br J Surg* 1990; **77**:1241–1246.

52. Stangl R, Altendorf-Hofmann A, Charnley RM, Scheele J. Factors influencing the natural history of colorectal liver metastases. *Lancet* 1994; **343**:1405–1410.

53. Rougier P, Milan C, Lazorthes F, et al. Prospective study of prognostic factors in patients with unresected hepatic metastases from colorectal cancer. *Br J Surg* 1995; **82**:1397–1400.

54. Hughes KS, Rosenstein RB, Songhorabodi S et al. Resection of the liver for colorectal carcinoma metastases. *Dis Colon Rectum* 1988; **31**:1–4.

55. Kemeny MM, Hogan JN, Ganteaune L, Goldberg DA, Terz JJ. Preoperative staging with computerized axial tomography and biochemical tests in patients with hepatic metastases. *Ann Surg* 1986; **203**:169–172.

56. Ferrucci JT. Liver tumor imaging – current concepts. *Radiol Clin N A* 1994; **32**:39–54.

57. Soyer P, Bluenke DA, Hruban RH et al. Hepatic metastases from colorectal cancer: Detection and false positive findings with helical CT during arterial portography. *Radiology* 1994; **193**:71–74.

58. Thoeni RF. Clinical applications of magnetic resonance imaging of the liver. *Invest Radiol* 1990; **26**:266–273.

59. Burak WE Jr., Schneebaum S, Kim JA et al. Pilot study evaluating the intraoperative localization of radiolabeled monoclonal antibody CC83 in patients with metastatic colorectal carcinoma. *Surgery* 1995; **118**:103–108.

60. Bertsch DJ, Burak WE Jr., Young DC et al. Radioimmunoguided surgery system improves survival for patients with recurrent colorectal cancer. *Surgery* 1995; **118**:634–639.

61. Kemeny N, Brown DW. Prognostic factors in advanced colorectal carcinoma: the importance of lactic dehydrogenase, performance status and white blood cell count. *Am J Med* 1983; **74**:786–794.

62. Bedikian AY, Chen TT, Malaky MA et al. Prognostic factors influencing survival of patients with advanced colorectal cancer: Hepatic artery infusion versus systemic intravenous chemotherapy for liver metastases. *J Clin Oncol* 1984; **2**:174–180.

63. Ekberg J, Tranberg KG, Lunstedt C et al. Determinant of survival after intra-arterial infusion of 5-fluorouracil for liver metastases from colorectal cancer. A multivariate analysis. *J Surg Oncol* 1986; **31**:246–254.

64. Chang AE, Steinberg SM, Culnane M et al. Determinants of survival in patients with unresectable colorectal liver metastases. *J Surg Oncol* 1989; **40**:245–251.

65. Kemeny N, Niedwiecki D, Shurgot B et al. Prognostic variables in patients with hepatic metastases from colorectal cancer: Importance of medical assessment of liver involvement. *Cancer* 1989; **63**:742–747.

66. Fortner JG, Silva JS, Cox EB et al. Multivariate analysis of a personal series of 247 patients with liver metastases from col-

orectal cancer. II. Treatment by intrahepatic chemotherapy. *Ann Surg* 1984; **199**:317–323.

67. Graf W, Glimelius B, Pahlman L *et al.* Determinants of prognosis in advanced colorectal cancer. *Eur J Cancer* 1991; **27**:1119–1123.

68. Lavin P, Mittleman A, Douglass H *et al.* Survival and response to chemotherapy for advanced colorectal adenocarcinoma: An Eastern Cooperative Oncology Group Report. *Cancer* 1980; **46**:1536–1543.

69. Cady B, Stone MD, McDermott WV Jr. *et al.* Technical and biologic factors in disease-free survival after hepatic resection for colon cancer metastases. *Arch Surg* 1992; **127**:561–569.

70. Tsushima K, Nagorney DM, Rainwater LM *et al.* Prognostic significance of nuclear deoxyribonucleic acid ploidy patterns in resected hepatic metastases from colorectal carcinoma. *Surgery* 1987; **102**:635–643.

71. Kastrinakis WV, Ramchurren N, Rieger KM *et al.* Increased incidence of *p53* mutations is associated with hepatic metastasis in colorectal neoplastic progression. *Oncogene* 1995; **100**:647–652.

72. Gennari L, Doci R, Bozzetti F *et al.* Proposal for staging liver metastases. *Recent Results Cancer Res* 1986; **100**:80–84.

73. van de Velde CJH. The staging of hepatic metastases arising from colorectal cancer. *Recent Results Cancer Res* 1986; **100**:85–90.

74. Kavolius J, Fong Y, Blumgart LH. Surgical resection of metastatic liver tumors. *Surg Oncol Clinics* 1996; **5**:337–352.

75. Jaques DP, Coit D, Casper E *et al.* Hepatic metastases from soft tissue sarcoma. *Ann Surg* 1995; **221**:392–397.

76. Ihse I, Person B, Tibblin S. Neuroendocrine metastases of the liver. *World J Surg* 1995; **19**:76–82.

77. Moertel CG. An odyssey in the land of small tumors. *J Clin Oncol* 1987; **5**:1503–1522.

78. Thompson GB, van Heerden JA, Grant CS. Islet cell carcinomas of the pancreas: a twenty year experience. *Surgery* 1988; **104**:1011–1017.

79. Que FG, Nagorney DM, Batts KP *et al.* Hepatic resection for metastatic neuroendocrine carcinoma. *Am J Surg* 1995; **169**:36–43.

80. Norstein J, Silen W. Natural history of liver metastases from colorectal carcinoma. *Gastrointest Surg* 1997; **1**:398–407.

The Biology of Liver Metastasis

Robert Radinsky and Isaiah J. Fidler

3

Introduction

Metastasis – the spread of malignant tumour cells from a primary neoplasm to distant parts of the body where they multiply to form new growths – is a major cause of death from cancer. The treatment of metastatic cancer poses a major problem to clinical oncologists, because the presence of multiple metastases makes complete eradication by surgery, radiation or drugs nearly impossible. For most tumours, the presence of liver metastasis renders the patient essentially incurable. Modification of current treatment regimens is unlikely to significantly impact on the natural history of this disease. A better understanding of the biology of liver metastases and the molecular events leading to the metastatic phenotype is essential if new and innovative therapeutic approaches are to be developed to treat this disease.

For many reasons, the liver is the site of metastases from cancers of diverse and distant organs, in particular those of the gastrointestinal tract. This phenomenon may be due to the liver's place as the first visceral organ that malignant cells of gastrointestinal origin encounter following release into capillaries, postcapillary venules and subsequently the portal circulation. However, the interaction or lodgement of circulating tumour cells within an organ is not by itself sufficient for the formation of metastasis. Rather, metastasis is a highly selective process whereby only cells of the necessary genotype and phenotype are capable of completing all steps in the metastatic process. In addition, host organ interactions with the metastatic tumour cell play a crucial role in the survival of cells with metastatic potential and their ability to form metastases. The phenomenon of site-specific metastasis to

the liver extends to other primary tumours as well. The incidence of liver metastases from primary melanoma, breast and ocular melanoma is greater than metastases to any other single organ, even though these tumours do not directly drain into the portal circulation.[1] Although numerous primary cancers metastasize to the liver, metastasis of primary colorectal carcinomas to the liver will be used as a paradigm in this chapter since recent data from our laboratories and others have characterized this model extensively.

Insight into the molecular mechanisms regulating the pathobiology of cancer metastasis as well as a better understanding of the interaction between the metastatic cell and the organ-specific microenvironment should provide a foundation for the design of new therapeutic approaches. Furthermore, the development of *in vivo* and *in vitro* models that will allow for the isolation and characterization of cells possessing metastatic potential within both primary tumours and metastases will be invaluable in the design of more effective and safe therapeutic modalities. In this chapter, we summarize data dealing with the biology of cancer metastasis with special emphasis on recent reports from our laboratories demonstrating that the organ microenvironment can profoundly influence the biological behaviour of metastatic tumour cells, including resistance to chemotherapy,[2–5] the production of degradative enzymes,[6–8] angiogenesis,[9–11] induction of carcinoembryonic antigen[12] and tumour cell proliferation in liver.[13–16] These data support the concept that the microenvironment of different organs (in this case, liver) can influence the biological behaviour of tumour cells at different steps of the metastatic process. These findings have obvious implications for the therapy of neoplasms in general and metastases in particular.

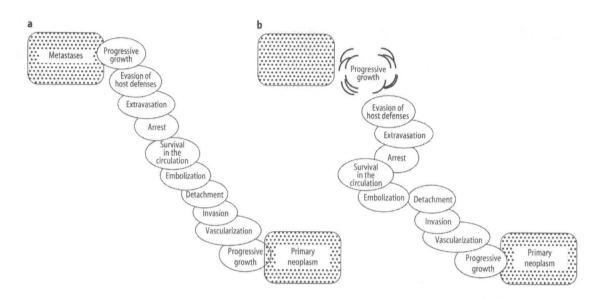

Figure 3.1. Sequential linked steps in the pathogenesis of tumour cell metastasis. Tumour cells must complete every step in the process to produce clinically relevant metastases. These steps include the progressive growth and vascularization of the primary neoplasm, tumour cell invasion of the surrounding tissue and detachment from the primary tumour, embolization and survival in the circulation, arrest and extravasation in the target tissue, evasion of host defences, and finally proliferation at the secondary site of implantation. Failure to complete one or more steps disrupts the linkage and eliminates the cell. A. Metastatic cell. B. Non-metastatic tumor cell deficient in the final step of metastasis, i.e. progressive growth ability at the secondary metastatic site.

The Metastatic Cascade

Metastasis is a highly selective, non-random process favoring the survival of a minor subpopulation of metastatic cells that preexists within the primary tumour mass.[16,17] To produce clinically relevant metastases, tumour cells from this subpopulation must complete a sequence of interrelated steps (Figure 3.1). This process begins with the invasion of the surrounding normal stroma either by single tumour cells with increased motility or by groups of cells from the primary tumour. Once the invading cells penetrate the vascular or lymphatic channels, they may grow there, or a single cell or clumps of cells may detach and be transported within the circulatory system. Tumour emboli must survive the host's immune and non-immune defences and the turbulence of the circulation, arrest in the capillary bed of compatible organs, extravasate into the organ parenchyma, survive, proliferate and establish a micrometastasis. Growth of these small tumour lesions requires the development of a vascular supply and continuous evasion of host defense cells. Failure to complete one or more steps of the process (e.g. inability to invade/extravasate, inability to grow progressively in a distant organ's parenchyma,

etc.) eliminates the cells (Figure 3.1). To produce clinically relevant distant metastases, the successful metastatic cell must therefore exhibit a complex phenotype that is regulated by transient or permanent changes at the DNA and/or mRNA level(s).[13-17]

There is now wide acceptance that many malignant tumours, including colon carcinomas, contain heterogeneous subpopulations of cells. This heterogeneity is exhibited in a wide range of genetic, biochemical, immunological and biological characteristics such as growth rate, antigenic and immunogenic status, cell surface receptors and products, enzymes, karyotypes, cell morphologies, invasiveness, drug resistance and metastatic potential. It is likely that specific tumour cells or colonies within the larger heterogeneous tumour specimen are the forerunners of distant metastases.[18]

Host and Tumour Interactions in the Process of Liver Metastasis

Numerous examples exist in which malignant tumours metastasize to specific organs.[19,20] As early as 1889, Paget proposed that the growth of metastases is due to the specific interaction of particular tumour cells with particular organ environments.[21] This hypothesis, supported both experimentally[19] and clinically,[22] may explain metastatic colonization patterns that cannot be due solely to mechanical lodgement and/or anatomical considerations.[23] There is considerable evidence that the microenvironment of each organ influences the implantation, invasion, survival and growth of particular tumour cells, meaning that the outcome of metastasis is influenced by both the intrinsic properties of the tumour cell and host-specific factors. Therefore, the successful metastatic cell must today be viewed as a cell receptive to its environment.[16]

Metastasis of Human Colon Carcinoma

Cancer of the colon and rectum is the second most prevalent cause of cancer deaths in men and the third most common in women.[24] The majority of patients with colon cancer present with either Dukes' stage B or C disease. Overall survival for patients undergoing surgical excision of Dukes' stage B and C diseases is 60–85% and 40–60%, respectively. Approximately 55% of colorectal cancers will recur within five years. In spite of surgery to remove the primary tumour, half will recur regionally, and up to 80% will produce distant metastases. The liver is the most common site of distant metastases.[25] Surgical treatment of these metastases is effective as a curative therapy only in a small number of cases,[26] and chemotherapy and radiation therapy are largely palliative.[27] Survival once metastases are diagnosed tends to be short, averaging 9.8 months.[28] Therefore, diagnosis of patients with colon cancer at an early or premalignant stage and the identification of patients likely to relapse following surgery alone are crucial goals. Given how little is known about the genetic alterations associated with metastasis,[29] an increased understanding of the molecular mechanisms mediating this process is a primary goal of cancer research aimed at improving treatment for liver metastasis.

Models for Human Colon Carcinoma Liver Metastasis

Two criteria must be met in the design of an appropriate model for human cancer metastasis. It must use metastatic cells, and these cells must grow in a relevant organ environment. Many investigators have reported on the implantation of human tumour cells into the subcutis of nude mice, but in the majority of cases the growing tumours failed to produce metastases.[16] Since the most common site of colon carcinoma metastasis is the liver, our laboratory sought to develop a reproducible model of hepatic metastases. Tumor cells from colon carcinoma surgical specimens were implanted into the spleens of nude mice.[16,30–33] The growth of colon cancer in the liver directly correlated with the metastatic potential of the cells, i.e. cells from surgical specimens of primary human colon carcinoma (HCC) classified as Dukes' stage D or from liver metastases produced significantly higher numbers of colonies in the liver of nude mice than cells from a Dukes' stage B tumour.[31,32] All tumour cells recovered from the nude mouse livers were of human origin by karyotype and isoenzyme analyses. Radioactive distribution analyses of colon cancer cells demonstrated that shortly after intrasplenic injection the tumour cells reached the liver.[33] Hence, the production of HCC tumours in the livers of nude mice was determined by the ability of HCC cells to proliferate in the liver parenchyma rather than by the ability of the cells to reach the liver.[33] The mere presence of viable tumour cells in a particular organ does not always predict that the cells will be able to proliferate and produce metastases.[16]

The classification of primary colon carcinoma as a Dukes' stage B tumour denotes that the lesions are confined to the wall of the colon; in contrast, patients with tumours classified as Dukes' stage D present with metastases in the lymph nodes and visceral organs.[34] If Dukes' stage B tumours are an earlier manifestation of primary colon cancer than Dukes' stage D tumours, then we could postulate that the composition of Dukes' stage B tumours contain few metastatic cells, whereas Dukes' stage D tumours contain many. The experiments described above assessing liver metastatic potential in the intrasplenic assay of nude mice supported this hypothesis.[16,30–33] Additional experiments were carried out to select and isolate cells directly with increasing liver-metastasizing potential from heterogeneous primary colon cancers.[31] Briefly, cells derived from a surgical specimen of a Dukes' stage B_2 primary colon carcinoma were established in culture or injected into the subcutis, caecum and spleen of nude mice. Progressively growing tumours were isolated and established in culture.

Implantation of these four culture-adapted cell lines into the cecum or spleen of nude mice produced very few liver tumour foci. HCC cells from these few liver metastases were expanded into culture and reinjected into the spleen of nude mice to provide a source for further cycles of selection. Importantly, with each successive *in vivo* selection cycle, the metastatic ability of the isolated and propagated cells increased. Four cycles of selection yielded cell lines with a very high metastatic efficiency in nude mice.[31] In parallel studies using a surgical specimen of a Dukes' stage D primary colon cancer, cells from highly metastatic cell lines were isolated, but successive selection cycles for growth in the liver only slightly increased metastatic properties.[31,32] These results demonstrate that highly metastatic cells can be selected from primary colon cancers and that orthotopic implantation of these cells in nude mice is a valid model for determining metastatic potential.[15,30–33,35,36]

If a human tumour is biologically heterogeneous, some of its cells may possess a growth advantage, depending on whether it is transplanted to the skin, the caecum, the liver or the kidney of nude mice. Recent data utilizing a genetically tagged HCC cell population validates this statement.[37] Distinct colon carcinoma clones differentially expressing specific mRNA transcripts for metastasis-related genes were the forerunners of the liver metastases.[37] The importance of orthotopic implantation of human neoplasms is also supported by results in other human tumour model systems, including melanoma (into the skin),[38] mammary carcinomas (into the mammary fatpad),[39] pancreatic carcinoma (into the pancreas),[40] and lung cancer (into the bronchi).[41] The correct *in vivo* model system for human spontaneous metastasis therefore allows the interaction of the tumour cells with their relevant organ environment.[16]

Organ-derived Growth Factors

A mechanism for site-specific tumour growth involves interactions between receptive metastatic cells and the organ environment, possibly mediated by local growth factors (Figure 3.2). Although the involvement of particular peptide growth factors in organ-specific metastasis is open to question, these factors are known to mediate the growth of normal and neoplastic cells.[42] Evidence supporting the influence of organ-specific growth factors on metastasis has been obtained, in part, from experiments

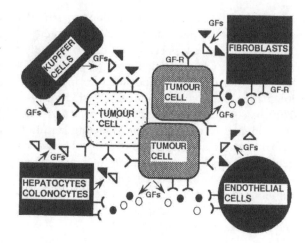

Figure 3.2. A model for the paracrine regulation of metastatic colon carcinoma cells in the liver. Paracrine regulation of tumour cells can involve stimulation or inhibition by growth factors in the extracellular environment. Candidate stimulatory ligands include TGF-α, which is produced by hepatocytes in response to trauma. Experimental evidence indicates that this physiological regulator of liver regeneration works through an autocrine loop in hepatocytes and through a paracrine mechanism in adjacent non-parenchymal cells through the EGF-R. Another candidate mitogen, HGF, is synthesized and secreted from liver endothelial, Kupffer and Ito cells, which is consistent with its paracrine action in the growth regulation of liver as well as colonic epithelium.[50–52] Furthermore, after liver damage, a rapid increase in HGF production is observed in the Ito and Kupffer cells in parallel to the down-regulation of its receptor, c-Met, in hepatocytes.[52] Hence, homeostatic processes such as inflammation and repair that follow damage to an organ facilitate the proliferation of normal, and, in some cases, tumour cells possessing the appropriate receptors. Tumour cells can also release factors that can affect the host cells resulting in a reciprocal relationship between the tumour cells and host cells, in the tumour microenvironment.[13] Key: growth factors (GFs); growth factor receptor (GF-R). (Modified from Radinsky.[13]

on the effects of organ-conditioned medium on the growth of particular neoplastic cells. The presence of stimulatory or inhibitory factors in a particular tissue correlated with the site-specific pattern of metastasis and has been reviewed.[13,15,16,19,20] To date, only a few of these organ-derived growth factors have been isolated and purified to homogeneity, as opposed to quite a few tissue-specific inhibitors.[15,19] All together, this evidence suggests a role for organ-derived paracrine growth factors in the regulation of tumour cell proliferation (Figure 3.2). Once the new factors are sufficiently purified, more definitive analyses of organ-specific paracrine factors involved in site-specific metastasis will be possible.[13,16,19]

Different concentrations of hormones in individual organs, differentially expressed local factors, or paracrine growth factors may all influence the growth of malignant cells at particular sites[19,20] (Figure 3.2). For example, specific peptide growth factor are concentrated in distinct tissue environments. One example is insulin-like growth factor-I (IGF-I). IGF-I is synthesized in most mammalian tissue, its highest concentration being in the liver.[43] This growth factor controls cell cycle progression through G_1.[44] A recent study demonstrated that carcinoma cells metastatic to the liver were growth stimulated by hepatocyte-derived IGF-I in direct proportion to IGF-I-receptor density on the metastatic versus non-metastatic tumour cells; the correlation suggests a potential mechanism of selection in the process of liver colonization.[45] Another example is transforming growth factor (TGF)-β. The principal sources of this peptide are the platelets and bone, suggesting it has roles in healing and bone-remodelling processes.[13] Many transformed cells produce increased levels of TGF-β and simultaneously lose their sensitivity to its growth inhibitory effects.[46] Interestingly, moderately or highly metastatic murine fibrosarcoma cells were growth-stimulated by TGF-β_1, while non-metastatic and transformed cells of the identical lineage were growth inhibited, similar to the non-transformed parental cell lines.[47] Clonal stimulation or inhibition of human colon and renal carcinoma cells by TGF-β_1 has also been observed and correlated with differential expression of its receptors.[48] The mechanisms responsible for altered growth factor responses are currently under investigation. At the least, these results indicate that the receptive metastatic cell (as compared to its nonmetastatic counterparts) may acquire altered responses to growth factor signals. This has been reviewed.[13,16,19,20]

Tissue-specific Repair Factors

Host factors (autocrine or paracrine) that control organ repair and/or regeneration may also affect the proliferation of malignant tumour cells. It is interesting to speculate that metastatic cells may therefore proliferate in secondary organs that produce compatible growth factors; that is, growth factors similar to those involved in the cellular regulation of the normal tissue from which the primary tumour originated (Figure 3.2). For example, colon carcinoma cells utilize and respond to specific growth factors that regulate normal colonic epithelium.[49,50]

Some of these identical factors also regulate homeostasis and tissue renewal and repair in the liver (e.g. TGF-α and hepatocyte growth factor [HGF] (Figure 3.2).[51,52] Do these same factors and receptors participate in the regulation of HCC growth in the liver? There is evidence they do. For instance, after partial hepatectomy (60%), the liver undergoes rapid cell division termed 'regeneration.' Recently, we transplanted HCC cells into nude mice that had been subjected to either partial hepatectomy (60%), nephrectomy or control abdominal surgery.[53] Those implanted subcutaneously demonstrated accelerated growth in partially hepatectomized mice but not in nephrectomized or control mice. Conversely, human renal carcinoma cells (HRCC) established as micrometastases in the lungs of nude mice underwent significant growth acceleration following unilateral nephrectomy, but not hepatectomy.[53] Consistent with these observations is the appearance during liver regeneration of factors in the peripheral blood that stimulate DNA synthesis in grafted hepatic parenchyma concomitant with DNA synthesis by the liver *in situ*.[52] Thus, liver regeneration in the nude mouse stimulated the growth of colon carcinoma cells. Additionally, Van Dale and Galand[54] inoculated rat colon adenocarcinoma cells intraportally and showed a dramatic increase in the incidence and growth of tumour colonies in the liver of partially hepatectomized rats compared with sham-operated controls.

Recently, TGF-α was described as a physiological regulator of liver regeneration by means of an autocrine mechanism.[51] TGF-α production by hepatocytes might also have a paracrine role, stimulating proliferation of adjacent non-parenchymal cells.[51,52] Furthermore, TGF-α may be a component of the paracrine regulatory loop, controlling hepatocyte replication at the late stages of liver regeneration.[52] Therefore, when normal tissues such as liver are damaged (possibly by invading tumour cells), growth factors are released to stimulate normal organ tissue repair, and these factors may also stimulate the proliferation of receptive malignant tumour cells (see below). Hence, tumour cells that either originate from or have affinities for growth in a particular organ can respond to appropriate organ-specific physiological signals.

Host–Tumour Cell Interactions Influencing the Biological Behaviour of Metastatic Cells

Insight into the molecular mechanisms regulating the different and distinct steps of the metastatic process as well as a better understanding of the interaction between the metastatic cell and the host microenvironment should provide a foundation for new therapeutic approaches. This section will review recent data from our laboratories and others supporting our contention that advances in the treatment of malignant tumours must involve strategies that exploit the malignant cell's interaction with specific organ microenvironments.

Regulation of the Multidrug Resistance Phenotype by the Organ Microenvironment

Several intrinsic properties of tumour cells can render them resistant to chemotherapeutic drugs, including increased expression of the multidrug resistance (MDR) genes, leading to overproduction of the transmembrane transport protein P-glycoprotein (P-gp).[55] Increased levels of P-gp can be induced by selecting tumour cells for resistance to natural product amphiphilic anticancer drugs.[54,55] Numerous reports have also described elevated expression of P-gp simultaneously with the development of the MDR phenotype in solid tumours of the colon, kidney and liver that had not been exposed to chemotherapy.[56,57] Since the development of MDR in tumour cells is a major barrier to therapy insight into the mechanisms by which the mediators affect this process is mandatory if successful treatments are to be designed. Present understandings have been derived from examining tumour cells growing in culture; the relevance of these findings to *in vivo* tumours is uncertain.[58]

P-glycoproteins are encoded by a small gene family, *mdr*, which in rodents consists of three members (*mdr*-1, *mdr*-2, *mdr*-3). Analysis of nucleotide and predicted amino acid sequences of full-length cDNA clones corresponding to the three mouse *mdr* genes has indicated that the encoded proteins are highly homologous.[59,60] Despite this homology, functional differences have been detected between the individual *mdr* genes: *mdr*-1

and *mdr*-3, but not *mdr*-2, are independently over-expressed in MDR cell lines of fibroblastic, lymphoid and reticuloendothelial origin. Both *mdr*-1 and *mdr*-3 confer drug resistance in transfection experiments, and the two encoded proteins appear to have overlapping but distinct substrate specificities.[61] In contrast, the transfection of mouse *mdr*-2 failed to confer drug resistance.[61]

Analysis of the mouse *mdr* gene transcripts in normal tissues has shown that the expression of the three genes is controlled in a tissue-specific manner.[60] Although selection of cells by exposure to various drugs may alter the normal pattern of *mdr* gene expression, organ-specific factors regulating *mdr*-1 and *mdr*-3 expression in normal tissues may determine which is over-expressed in an MDR derivative of a particular tissue type.[59]

Clinical observations have suggested that the organ environment influences the response of tumours to chemotherapy. For example, in women with breast cancer, lymph node and skin metastases respond better than lung or bone metastases.[62] Investigations of experimental systems have produced similar results:[2–5,63,64] a mouse fibrosarcoma growing subcutaneously in syngeneic mice was sensitive to systemic administration of doxorubicin (DOX), whereas lung metastases were not[4] and subcutaneous CT-26 murine colon tumours were sensitive to DOX, but metastases growing in the liver or lung were not.[64]

We initiated studies to determine how the organ microenvironment influences the response of tumour cells to chemotherapy. We found that murine CT-26 colon cancer cells growing in the lung (metastases) were relatively resistant to systemic therapy with DOX, whereas those in the subcutis were sensitive.[2] CT-26 cells harvested from lung metastases and treated *in vitro* exhibited more resistance to DOX than cells harvested from subcutaneous tumours or parental cells grown in culture .[2] Resistance was reversible by the addition of verapamil, and all CT-26 cells demonstrated similar sensitivities to 5-fluorouracil (5-FU). Hence, a direct correlation was observed between the increased resistance to DOX (*in vivo* and *in vitro*) of CT-26 cells and expression levels of *mdr*-1 mRNA transcripts and P-gp. The drug resistance and accompanying elevated expression of *mdr*-1 found for cells growing in the lung depended on interaction with the specific organ environment: once removed from the lung, the tumour cells

Table 3.1 *mdr* -1 gene expression in CT-26 murine colon carcinoma cells growing in culture for various times after solid tumour growth in the skin and lung

Tumour	Days in culture					
	3	7	14	21	28	35
Lung tumour	8.6*	2.0	0.8	2.2	n.d.	2.1
Subcutaneous tumour	1.7	0.6	0.6	0.8	1.4	1.4

*Densitometric quantitation of mRNA expression. The ratios of the areas between the 4.3-kb *mdr*-1 and the 1.3-kb GAPDH transcripts were compared in each case with the CT-26 P cells defined as 1.0. Liver metastases from CT-26 colon carcinoma cells showed patterns of *mdr*-1 gene expression similar to the lung metastases.

reverted to a sensitive phenotype similar to the parental cells, and *mdr*-1 mRNA and P-gp reverted to the baseline levels typical of CT-26 parental cells (Table 3.1).

The increased resistance to DOX in the CT-26 cells in lung metastases was not due to selection of resistant subpopulations. This conclusion is based on the results of a crossover experiment. Once implanted into the subcutis of syngeneic mice, CT-26 cells from lung metastases produced tumours that were sensitive to DOX. In parallel studies, DOX-sensitive CT-26 cells from subcutaneous tumours became resistant to the drug when they were inoculated intravenously and grew in the lung parenchyma as metastases. P-gp levels directly correlated with the drug resistance phenotype in these experiments.

An organ-specific response to DOX is not restricted to CT-26 cells. Previous reports with UV-2237 fibrosarcoma cells[4] and human KM12 colon carcinoma cells[5] also demonstrated significant differences in resistance to DOX (but not 5-FU) between subcutaneous tumours (sensitive) and lung or liver metastases (resistant). Similarly, in patients with colon carcinoma, high levels of P-gp expression were found on the invasive edge of the primary tumour (growing in the colon)[56,57] and in lymph node, lung and liver metastases.[57,65] The environmental regulation of the MDR phenotype may explain, in part, the polarized expression of *mdr*-1 in colon carcinomas[66] and the discrepancy between *in vitro* and *in vivo* expression levels of the MDR phenotype.[54,55,66] In any event, the models described here can be used to further investigate the molecular mechanisms that regulate the *in vivo* expression of the *mdr* genes. This has been reviewed.[3,67]

Organ-specific Modulation of the Metastatic Cell's Invasive Phenotype

As described thus far, the interaction of tumour cells with an organ environment can modulate their tumorigenic properties and metastatic behaviour. The implantation of HCC cells into the subcutis (ectopic site) or the wall of the cecum (orthotopic site) results in locally growing tumours.[31,32] Metastasis to distant organs, however, is produced only by tumours growing in the wall of the caecum.[31,32] This difference in production of distant metastasis directly correlated with the influence of the organ environment on the production of degradative enzymes by the colon cancer cells.[6–8]

The ability of tumour cells to degrade connective-tissue extracellular matrix (ECM) and basement-membrane components is an essential prerequisite for invasion and metastasis.[68–72] Among the enzymes involved in degradation of the ECM are the metalloproteinases, a family of metal-dependent endopeptidases.[71] These proteinases are produced by connective tissue cells as well as many tumour cells and include enzymes with degradative activity for interstitial collagen, type IV collagen, type V collagen, gelatin and proteoglycans. The M_r 72 000 type IV collagenase is a neutral metalloproteinase capable of degrading type IV collagen within the triple helical domain, resulting in one-fourth amino terminal and three-fourths carboxy terminal fragments from the intact molecule.[73] The enzyme is mostly secreted into an extracellular milieu in a proenzymatic form.[71]

Expression of the M_r 72 000 collagenase type IV is higher in colon carcinoma cells than in normal mucosa cells,[74] and the metastatic capacity of these tumour cells from orthotopic sites in nude mice directly correlates with the production of this enzyme activity:[6–8, 31,32] intracaecal tumours (in nude mice) of metastatic colon cancer secreted high levels of 92-kDa and 68-kDa gelatinase activities, whereas tumour cells growing subcutaneously (not metastatic) did not produce or secrete the 68-kDa gelatinase activity.[8,75] Moreover, histological examination of the colon carcinoma growing in the subcutis or caecum of nude mice revealed that mouse fibroblasts produced a thick pseudocapsule around the subcutaneous but not the caecal tumours.[75] These differences suggested that the organ environment profoundly influenced the ability of metastatic cells to produce ECM-degradative enzymes. Since recent analyses have demonstrated that the interaction of stromal fibroblasts can influence the tumorigenicity[76] and biological behaviour of tumour cells,[77,78] we investigated whether organ-specific fibroblasts could directly influence the invasive ability of the colon cancer cells. Coculturing fibroblasts from skin, lung, and colon of nude mice with highly invasive and metastatic KM12SM colon carcinoma cells[75] showed that these cells adhered to and invaded through mouse colon and lung, but not skin fibroblasts. Moreover, nude mouse skin fibroblasts (ectopic environment) but not colon or lung fibroblasts (orthotopic environments) inhibited the production of 72-kDa type IV collagenases (gelatinases) by highly invasive and metastatic KM12SM cells. This inhibition was due to a specific interaction between the colon carcinoma cells and skin fibroblasts. We based this conclusion on the data showing that nude mouse skin fibroblasts did not decrease the production of a 72-kDa type IV collagenase or the invasive capacity of human squamous cell carcinoma A431 cells. These data, therefore, directly correlated with our studies showing that the KM12SM colon cancer cells can grow in the wall of the caecum and the subcutis of nude mice, but are invasive only from the wall of the cecum.[8,32] Moreover, colon carcinoma growing in the subcutis did not produce type IV collagenase.[8] The present in vitro data directly correlate with the in vivo findings and suggest that fibroblasts populating the ectopic and orthotopic organs influence the invasive phenotype of these tumour cells.

There are several mechanisms by which stromal cells and tumour cells interact and influence each other. Both in vitro and in vivo studies have suggested that cell-to-cell contact is important and that, at the epithelial cell junction, both cancer cells and fibroblasts have an altered capacity to synthesize basement membrane molecules.[79] Epithelial cells produce a variety of growth factors that can influence fibroblast function, whereas fibroblasts produce ECM that can be tissue specific.[80,81] Growth factors can induce and alter ECM gene expression,[80,81] and the ECM can, in turn, influence the type and level of growth factor expressed and even their receptors in different cells.[82] Organ-specific ECM molecules influence clonal growth of tumours,[80,83] probably by regulating cell–cell adhesion and differentiation, maintenance of cell shape, response to hormones and growth factors, and expression of tissue-specific proteins.[80–83]

One possible regulator of metalloproteinase activity is the tissue inhibitor of metalloproteinases (TIMP) family, which can inhibit interstitial collagenase, stromelysin, and the 92-kDa type IV collagenase. TIMP-2 can also bind specifically to 72-kDa type IV collagenase.[84] Furthermore, transfection of 3T3 fibroblasts with antisense DNA of TIMP results in the production of tumorigenic and metastatic cells.[84] In our study using anti-TIMP monoclonal antibodies, TIMP was expressed similarly whether the colon carcinoma was growing in the subcutis or the caecum. Our data showed that the levels of type IV collagenolytic activity observed in the subcutaneous tumours were low because of low production of the 92-kDa and 72-kDa type IV collagenases, not TIMP inhibition of type IV collagenase.

The organ factors that modulate type IV collagenase production in the cecal wall and subcutis were also analysed. Various growth factors and cytokines have been shown to modulate the level of cell-secreted metalloproteinases and serine proteinases. Production of collagenases in normal fibroblasts can be induced by various tissue factors, e.g. interleukin-1 (IL-1), epidermal growth factor (EGF), TGF-α, platelet-derived growth factor (PDGF) and tumour-cell collagenase stimulatory factor. Similarly, TGF-α induces synthesis of urokinase-type plasminogen activator in lung carcinoma cells[85] and increases production of the 72-kDa type IV collagenase in fibroblasts.[86] Welch et al.[87] found that TGF-β, at a concentration as low as 50 μ/ml, can maximally enhance the production of 92-kDa and 72-kDa type IV collagenases and heparinase in rat 13762NF mammary adenocarcinoma MTLn3 cells. Pretreatment of MTLn3 cells with TGF-β significantly enhanced lung colonization after the cells were injected into the tail vein of a rat.[87] In different organs, the normal stroma surrounding primary tumours of KM12 HCC cells may contain different levels of these or other growth factors, and this difference may affect the production and secretion of type IV collagenases, heparinases and other tissue-degrading enzymes.

The exact mechanism by which nude mouse skin fibroblasts inhibit collagenase production by KM12SM cells was actively pursued by our laboratory. Since recombinant human interferon (IFN)-α and IFN-γ have been shown to modulate the invasive capacity of human melanoma cells under in vitro conditions,[88] we examined the effects of IFN-α, -β, and -γ on the production of gelatinase activity by KM12SM colon carcinoma cells. Whereas all the r-IFNs inhibited gelatinase production (68 kDa), only inhibition by IFN-β (fibroblast IFN) was significant.[75]

Improvement in the use of IFNs for treatment of HCC, HRCC or any other neoplasm is dependent on a better understanding of the mechanisms by which IFNs regulate different functions of tumour cells, perhaps through the invasive phenotype.

Regulation of Carcinoembryonic Antigen Expression in Colon Carcinoma Cells by the Organ Microenvironment

An essential step in the formation of hepatic metastasis is the adherence of tumour cells to the microvasculature of the liver. This process is both active and passive. Tumour cell emboli often circulate as a clump of cells adherent to other tumour cells or platelets. Mechanical trapping of these tumour cells occurs in the hepatic sinusoid, and yet <1% of cells survive even 5 days and only a percentage of these form metastases.[89] The mere trapping of cells in the hepatic circulation does not assure their survival; cell surface adhesion molecules specific for receptor molecules on the hepatic endothelial cells and/or ECM are necessary for attachment and subsequent growth in the liver. Tumour cells expressing specific adhesion molecules on their cell surface may show preferential metastasis to the liver. Examples of such adhesion molecules that may facilitate liver metastasis include the ganglioside GM_2,[90] oligosaccharides (sialyl Le structures), β_1 integrins[91] and CD44.[92] Interestingly, the tumour marker carcinoembryonic antigen (CEA) may play a role in cell adhesion in liver metastasis from colorectal cancer. Injection of CEA intravenously prior to injecting colon cancer cells in an experimental model of colon cancer increased the percentage of mice who developed liver metastases.[93] In other studies, transfection with the cDNA encoding CEA increased the metastatic potential of HCC cells.[94]

Carcinoembryonic antigen, first described in 1965 by Gold and Freedman,[95] is the most widely used clinical tumour marker for several neoplastic diseases, especially colorectal carcinomas.[96] It serves as a prognostic marker because, in most cases, an elevated preoperative serum CEA level is associated with a poor prognosis.[96] Recent studies have demonstrated that CEA is a member of an immunoglobulin supergene family functioning as an intercellular adhesion molecule.[97] Cells expressing CEA have been shown to aggregate under in vitro conditions, suggesting that CEA may promote the adhesion of tumour cells to each other (homo-

typic) or to host cells (heterotypic). Hence, tumour cells in circulating aggregates may have an increased capacity to arrest in distant capillary beds, resulting in an increased probability of metastasis.

Although the expression of CEA by HCC cells has been directly correlated with their metastatic potential,[98] its regulation is poorly understood.[99] Previous reports have demonstrated a positive relationship between the degree of differentiation of colorectal cancer and CEA production.[98] Several agents that alter the degree of cellular differentiation have also been shown to increase the level of CEA expression in these cell types.[100]

Recent results from our laboratories indicate that the expression of CEA is regulated by the organ microenvironment.[12] The orthotopic (caecal wall) implantation of colon carcinoma cells into nude mice yielded more-differentiated tumours, which then expressed high levels of steady-state CEA mRNA and protein. In contrast, ectopic (subcutaneous) tumours were less differentiated and produced low levels of steady-state CEA mRNA and protein. In the caecal wall of nude mice, KM20 cells (isolated from a moderately differentiated adenocarcinoma of the colon from a patient with high pre-operative serum CEA levels) produced differentiated lesions with higher levels of CEA mRNA and protein than lesions produced by KM12C cells (isolated from a poorly differentiated colon adenocarcinoma from a patient with a low preoperative serum CEA level). In culture, however, KM20 and KM12C cells produced similar levels of CEA mRNA and protein.

The level of CEA in the serum of patients with colorectal carcinoma is influenced by the balance between production of CEA by tumour cells and the ability of the liver to clear CEA from the blood.[96] Thus, elevated serum levels of CEA may be due to an increased tumour burden, especially metastatic lesions in the liver.[96] Our data do not address this possibility but show that CEA expression is indeed regulated by cell density. When cells enter quiescence, they can exhibit major alterations in cell surface receptors, expression of transcription factors, enzymes and cellular ultrastructure. The expression of basic fibroblast growth factor (bFGF), mdr-1 and type IV collagenases have been shown to be downregulated in confluent cultures,[101,102] and colon carcinoma cells have been shown to undergo polarization and differentiation when cultured to confluence.[103] The spontaneously differentiating Caco-2 cells and T84 cells were reported to express an increasing level of CEA when cultured to confluence.[104] In agreement with these data, we found that dense monolayer cultures or spheroids of the KM12 and KM20 colon cancer cell lines produced mucin after reaching confluence and showed increased expression of CEA. Incubation of KM12SM cells in serum-free medium decreased cell proliferation and enhanced CEA production. We also treated KM12SM cells (high production of CEA) with mitomycin-C and found that growth-arrested cells (under sparse conditions) produced higher levels of CEA. This finding suggested that CEA expression is influenced by cell proliferation. Moreover, medium taken from dense cultures increased the expression of CEA in tumour cells growing as sparse monolayers, indicating that CEA expression may be regulated by an autocrine mechanism.

Our data also indicate that CEA production does not always correlate with its mRNA level, agreeing with a recent report showing that treatment of colon carcinoma cell lines by relatively high concentrations of IFN-γ (1000 or 2000 U/ml) can disproportionately increase the CEA mRNA and protein.[104] Whether these results suggest that CEA expression by colon carcinoma cells is regulated by both transcriptional and post-transcriptional mechanisms needs further study. A recent report has identified the cis-acting elements involved in the transcriptional control of the *CEA* gene,[99] and treatment of colon carcinoma cells with TGF-β or IFN-γ has stimulated expression of *CEA*.[105,106] We cultured KM12SM cells with various concentrations of TGF-α, TGF-β, HGF, bFGF, vascular endothelial growth factor (VEGF), IL-1β and IFN-α, -β or -γ. Since none of the cytokines (at the concentrations used) affected cell division or influenced *CEA* expression, it remains unclear whether these or other cytokines can act as paracrine or autocrine factors that regulate *CEA* expression and production.

In conclusion, we have shown that the production of CEA by colon carcinoma cells can be modulated by specific organ microenvironments, cell density, and autocrine and paracrine factors. Because *CEA* expression levels and differentiation of tumour cells growing in the cecal wall of nude mice directly correlated with the pre-operative serum CEA level and pathological diagnosis of the original patient surgical specimens, we conclude that the orthotopic implantation of HCC xenografts provides a relevant model to study the regulation and role of CEA in the liver metastasis of HCC.

Host–Tumour Interactions in the Regulation of Angiogenesis

Although tumours 1–2 mm in diameter can receive all nutrients by diffusion, further growth depends on the development of an adequate blood supply through angiogenesis.[107] The induction of angiogenesis is mediated by several angiogenic molecules released by both tumour cells and host cells.[107,108] Prevascular tumours are often local benign tumours, whereas vascular tumours are malignant. Moreover, studies using light microscopy and immunohistochemistry concluded that the number and density of microvessels in different human cancers directly correlate with their potential to invade and produce metastasis.[109] Not all angiogenic tumours produce metastasis, but the inhibition of angiogenesis prevents the growth of tumour cells at both the primary and secondary sites.[108]

Inhibition of angiogenesis presents a novel and opportunity for treating metastases, that is by manipulation of the host microenvironment. Endothelial cells in tumour blood vessels divide rapidly, whereas those in normal tissues do not.[107,108] The division of endothelial cells is induced by a variety of mitogens, termed 'angiogenic factors', such as bFGF, IL-8 and VEGF. This has been reviewed.[6,107] Systemic administration of antibodies to bFGF,[110] VEGF[111] or angiogenin[112] has been shown to inhibit the *in vivo* (but not *in vitro*) growth of tumour cells, suggesting tumour growth may be inhibited indirectly by constraining angiogenesis. Treating neoplasms by targeting both the tumour cells (chemotherapy) and the organ environment (angiogenesis inhibitor) has been shown to produce additive or synergistic therapeutic effects in mice bearing the 3LL tumour.[113]

Recent studies have shown that the greater the vascularization of a tumour, the greater the chance of distant metastases.[109] This phenomenon may be due to two processes: (1) increased vascular proliferation in tumours is associated with a larger tumour mass, which would release more cells into the circulation, thus increasing the probability of metastasis; and (2) the increase in vasculature in highly angiogenic tumours increases the surface area through which tumour cells may enter the circulation.

The specific molecular determinants regulating angiogenesis in colon cancer metastasis are not yet defined, but some correlations have been made.

Immunohistochemical studies have demonstrated that blood vessel density in primary colon cancers was associated with the development of liver metastases.[114] Furthermore, VEGF expression in primary colon carcinomas correlated with the stage of disease as well as blood vessel counts.[114] This led to the hypothesis that VEGF may be an important angiogenic factor in HCC. Recent data supporting this premise showed high levels of VEGF mRNA transcripts in the liver metastases from patients with colon cancer, and the administration of anti-VEGF antibodies inhibited not only primary tumour growth but the number and size of experimental liver metastases.[115] Hence, VEGF may be one essential angiogenic factor mediating the development of HCC liver metastases.

Data from our laboratory have primarily concerned renal carcinoma, but is likely that the mechanisms are similar. We demonstrated that the organ microenvironment can directly contribute to the induction and maintenance of the angiogenic factors bFGF[9] and IL-8.[10] The production of these angiogenic factors by tumour cells or host cells (macrophages) or the release of bFGF from the ECM in the absence of angiogenesis inhibitors leads to growth of endothelial cells and hence vascularization.[107,108] Because the host microenvironment varies among different organs, we investigated whether bFGF expression (at the mRNA and protein levels) is influenced by the organ microenvironment. We implanted HRCC into the subcutis or the renal subcapsule of nude mice. The HRCC in the kidney were highly vascularized and produced a high incidence of systemic metastases. In contrast, the tumours in the subcutis were poorly vascularized and produced few metastases. We detected 10 to 20 times the amount of bFGF mRNA in HRCC growing in the kidney as compared with HRCC growing in the subcutis. These differences were confirmed at the protein level. These data therefore demonstrate an association between the production of bFGF by tumour cells and vascularization[107] and the influence of a specific organ's microenvironment on bFGF expression in HRCC.[9] Additionally, HRCC growing in the kidney produced lung metastases, whereas HRCC growing in the subcutis did not. The differential expression of bFGF could have contributed to the invasive-metastatic phenotype of the HRCC growing in the kidney since bFGF can stimulate the activity of proteolytic enzymes such as tissue type and urokinase type plasminogen activator[116] and

collagenase type IV,[117,118] all of which are produced by the HRCC (see previous section).

In patients, HRCCs produce various angiogenic factors including bFGF.[9-11] Reports indicate that the expression of bFGF in primary HRCC inversely correlates with survival,[119] as do elevated levels of bFGF in the urine of patients.[120] In adults, physiological angiogenesis (wound healing) is regulated by the balance of positive and negative molecules, which suggests the same might apply to treatment (or prevention) of metastasis. Several factors that downregulate or inhibit angiogenesis have already been incorporated into clinical trials, the most widely studied being IFN-α. Chronic daily administration of low-dose IFN-α has been shown to induce complete regression of life-threatening haemangiomas in infants[121] and highly vascular Kaposi's sarcoma.[122] The mechanisms responsible for this remarkable clinical outcome were not, however, identified at the time.

To identify the mechanisms, we tested the ability of IFN-α to downregulate bFGF mRNA expression and protein production in multiple carcinoma cell lines.[9-11] In fact, IFN-α or IFN-β downregulated the steady-state mRNA expression and protein production of bFGF in HRCC cells by mechanisms independent of their antiproliferative effects. The inhibition of bFGF mRNA and protein production required long-term exposure (>4 days) of cells to IFNs. Moreover, once IFN was withdrawn, cells resumed production of bFGF.[10] These observations were consistent with the clinical experience that IFN-α must be given for many months to bring about involution of haemangiomas.[121] The incubation of human bladder, prostate, colon and breast carcinoma cells with non-cytostatic concentrations of IFN-α or IFN-β also downregulated bFGF production.[10] Since IFN-α or IFN-β are constitutively produced by many host cells,[10] their physiological role in limiting angiogenesis should be further investigated. It is especially relevant in patients with renal cancer, since bFGF is a major angiogenic molecule in renal tumours and its level in the serum is inversely correlated with survival.[119] Whether this is true for other neoplasms remains to be elucidated.

These results link our work on invasive properties and angiogenic properties of human tumour cells as modulated by specific organ environments.[6,8,16,75,118] As described, the implantation of HRCC into the subcutis of nude mice yields not only localized non-invasive but also poorly vascularized tumours, whereas the implantation of the same cells into the kidney results in highly vascularized and invasive neoplasms.[9-11] These studies confirm the conclusion that cancer metastasis is highly selective and is regulated by a number of different mechanisms.[6] This conclusion is contrary to the once-accepted idea that metastasis represents the ultimate expression of cellular anarchy. The view that cancer metastasis is selective implies that understanding the mechanisms that regulate the process will lead to better therapeutic intervention. The control of invasive potential by primary tumours or angiogenesis in metastases by known inhibitors is an excellent example of exploiting this principle.

Growth Regulation of the Metastatic Cell at the Liver-specific Site

A mechanism that would explain the interaction between distinct colon carcinoma cells and the liver environment could involve the proliferation of tumour cells differentially expressing certain growth factor receptors and their response to liver-derived paracrine growth factors. Indeed, highly metastatic tumour cells from Dukes' stage D tumours or surgical specimens of liver metastases responded to mitogens associated with liver regeneration induced by hepatectomy in nude mice.[6,13,16,53] As described above, following partial hepatectomy the liver undergoes rapid cell division which involves quantitative changes in hepatocyte gene expression. TGF-α was recently shown to be one positive regulator of liver regeneration[51,52] as well as a mediator of the proliferation of normal colonic epithelial cells.[50] TGF-α exerts its effect through interaction with the epidermal growth factor receptor (EGF-R), a plasma membrane glycoprotein that contains a tyrosine-specific protein tyrosine kinase (PTK) in its cytoplasmic domain. The binding of TGF-α to the EGF-R stimulates a series of rapid responses, including phosphorylation of tyrosine residues within the EGF-R itself and within many other cellular proteins, hydrolysis of phosphatidyl inositol, release of Ca^{2+} from intracellular stores, elevation of cytoplasmic pH and morphological changes; after 12 h in the presence of TGF-α, cells synthesize DNA and ultimately divide.[123]

EGF-Rs are present on many normal and tumour cells.[123] Elevated levels and/or amplification of the EGF-R has been found in many human tumours and cell lines, including breast cancer,[124] gliomas,[125] lung

cancer,[126] bladder cancer,[127] tumours of the female genital tract,[128] the A431 epidermoid carcinoma,[129] prostate carcinoma[130] and colon carcinoma.[131] These results suggest the physiological significance of inappropriate expression of the EGF-R tyrosine kinase in abnormal cell growth control. Whether TGF-α is involved in the cellular proliferation of metastatic colon cancer in the liver is not known.

We therefore examined the expression and function of EGF-R in a series of HCC cell lines whose liver metastatic potential differed. Our results demonstrated that the expression of EGF-R at the mRNA and protein levels directly correlated with the ability of the HCC to grow in the liver parenchyma and hence produce hepatic metastases.[14] The EGF-Rs expressed on metastatic tumour cells were functional based on in vitro growth stimulation assays using picogram concentrations of TGF-α and specific as shown by neutralization with anti-EGF-R or anti-TGF-α antibodies. Moreover, EGF-R-associated PTK activity also paralleled the observed EGF-R levels. Immunohistochemical analysis of the low metastatic parental KM12C colon carcinoma cells demonstrated heterogeneity in the EGF-R-specific staining pattern, with <10% of the cells in the population staining intensely for EGF-R, whereas the in vivo selected highly metastatic KM12SM and KM12L4 cells exhibited uniform, intense staining. Western blotting confirmed the presence of higher EGF-R protein levels in the metastatic KM12L4 and KM12SM cells than in the low metastatic KM12C cells. Finally, isolation of the top and bottom 5% EGF-R-expressing KM12C cells by fluorescence-activated cell sorting confirmed the association between levels of EGF-R on the tumour cells and ability to produce metastatic nodules in the liver[14] (Table 3.2).

In our studies, we also observed a correlation between an increase in copy number of chromosome 7 (harboring the EGF-R gene), EGF-R expression and the ability of colon carcinoma cells to produce metastasis in the livers of nude mice. About 95% of KM12L4 cells had a chromosome 7/12 or 7/4 ratio >1.0 as compared with only 14% of KM12C cells, indicating a higher proportion of metastatic cells carried extra copies of chromosome 7. Gains of as many as 10 copies of particular chromosomes have been reported by fluorescence in situ hybridization (FISH) analyses in other solid tumours.[132] Dukes' stage C primary colon cancers often exhibit additions of chromosomes 8 and 12

Table 3.2 Experimental hepatic metastasis of FACS-sorted EGF-R expressing KM12C HCC cells

Cell line*	Spleen tumours**	Liver nodules		
		Incidence	Median	Range
KM12C	11/11	5/11	0	0–16
Bottom 5%	8/10	0/8	0	0
Top 5%	10/10	8/10	10	0–137
KM12L4	7/7	7/7	50	7–108

* 1×10^6 cells were injected into the spleens of nude mice. The animals were killed 30–40 days later.
** Number of mice with tumours/number of mice receiving injections.

and a loss of chromosome 17.[132] The correlation between chromosome copy number and the potential of colon cancer cells to produce liver metastasis may be direct or non-specific. Alternatively, the observed correlation may be a reflection of genomic instability, which can lead to any of a number of gene mutations or deletions on other chromosomes, which in turn may increase tumour cell proliferation and growth in the liver. Several independent reports have implicated gene sequences on chromosome 7 in the process of invasion and metastasis.[132] An increased copy number of chromosome 7, shown to be associated with high expression of the EGF-R, has been detected in advanced melanoma and in cancers of the breast, bladder, pancreas and brain. This has been reviewed by Radinsky.[15] These data suggest that increases in the copy number of chromosome 7, and thus in EGF-R expression, may provide a selective advantage during the metastatic process.

Our analyses indicated a direct correlation between EGF-R levels on cell lines isolated from HCC specimens and ability to produce liver metastases in nude mice. These findings are more generalized because in our analysis of formalin-fixed paraffin-embedded colon carcinoma surgical specimens for EGF-R transcripts using a rapid colorimetric in situ mRNA hybridization (ISH) technique,[133] we found that cell-surface hybridization with EGF-R-antisense hyperbiotinylated oligonucleotide probes in primary and metastatic colon carcinoma specimens directly correlated with immunohistochemistry and Northern blot analyses. Moreover, unlike Northern analyses, ISH showed intratumoral heterogeneity in EGF-R gene expression and identified particular cells expressing high levels of EGF-R in the tissues.[133]

Collectively, these data suggest that EGF-R is involved in tumour progression and dissemination and indicate that this receptor could be used as a target for therapy, as reviewed by Mendelsohn.[134] Anti-EGF-R monoclonal antibodies (mAb), which block ligand binding, prevent the growth in culture of cells that are stimulated by EGF or TGF-α as well as the growth of human tumour xenografts bearing high levels of EGF-R.[134] Recent studies have also indicated that anti-EGF-R mAb substantially enhance the cytotoxic effects of doxorubicin or cis-diamminedichloroplatinum on well-established xenografts.[135] Furthermore, clinical trials with squamous cell carcinoma of the lung have demonstrated the capacity of the anti-EGF-R mAb to localize in such tumours and to achieve saturating concentrations in the blood for >3 days without toxicity.[134,135] Other treatments targeting the EGF-R include inhibitors of receptor dimerization,[136] antisense RNA and EGF-R-specific PTK inhibitors[137] and overexpression of dominant-negative mutant receptors.[138,139]

Conclusions

A primary goal of cancer research is an increased understanding of the molecular mechanisms mediating the process of cancer metastasis. Analyses of cancer cells and the microenvironment has increased our understanding of the biological mechanisms mediating organ-specific metastasis. Insight into the molecular mechanisms regulating the pathobiology of cancer metastasis as well as a better understanding of the interaction between the metastatic cell and the host environment should produce a foundation for new therapeutic approaches. As reviewed here, the liver microenvironment can profoundly influence the pattern of gene expression and the biological phenotype of metastatic tumour cells, including resistance to chemotherapy, induction of CEA, modulation of the invasive phenotype, regulation of angiogenesis and proliferation of the metastatic cell at the organ-specific metastatic site. Each of these studies indicates that the production of clinically relevant metastases depends, in part, on the interaction of particular tumour cells with specific organ environments. Therefore, the successful metastatic cell whose complex phenotype helps make it the decathlon champion[59] must be viewed today as a cell receptive to its environment. The analyses presented herein add new evidence to support the concept that cancer metastasis is not a random process; it is a regulated process that can be analysed on the molecular level in the context of the relevant organ environment. This new knowledge should eventually lead to the design and implementation of more effective therapies for this dreaded disease.

References

1. Pickren JW, Tsukada Y, Lane WW. Liver metastasis: Analysis of autopsy data, In *Liver Metastasis*, Weiss L, Gilbert HA (eds) 1982, vol. 5, pp. 2–18. Boston, GK Hall Medical Publishers.
2. Dong Z, Radinsky R, Fan D, Tsan R, Bucana CD, Wilmanns C, Fidler IJ. Organ specific modulation of steady-state *mdr* gene expression and drug resistance in murine colon cancer cells. *J Natl Cancer Inst* 1994; **86**:913–920.
3. Fidler IJ, Wilmanns C, Staroselsky A, Radinsky R, Dong Z, Fan D. Modulation of tumor cell response to chemotherapy by the organ environment. *Cancer Metastasis Rev* 1994; **13**:209–222.
4. Staroselsky A, Fan D, O'Brian CA, Bucana CD, Gupta KP, Fidler IJ. Site-dependent differences in response of the UV-2237 murine fibrosarcoma to systemic therapy with Adriamycin. *Cancer Res* 1990; **40**:7775–7780.
5. Wilmanns C, Fan D, O'Brian CA, RAdinsky R, Bucana CD, Tsan R, Fidler IJ. Modulation of doxorubicin sensitivity and level of P-glycoprotein expression in human colon carcinoma cells by ectopic and orthotopic environments in nude mice. *Int J Oncol* 1993; **3**:413–422.
6. Fidler IJ. Modulation of the organ microenvironment for treatment of cancer metastasis. *J Natl Cancer Inst* 1995; **87**:1588–1592.
7. Gohji K, Fidler IJ Tsan R, Radinsky R, von Eschenbach AC, Tsuruo T, Nakajima M. Human recombinant interferons-beta and gamma decrease gelatinase production and invasion by human KG-2 renal carcinoma cells. *Int J Cancer* 1994; **58**:380–384.
8. Nakajima M, Morikawa K, Fabra A, Bucana CD, Fidler IJ. Influence of organ environment on extracellular matrix degradative activity and metastasis of human colon carcinoma cells. *J Natl Cancer Inst* 1990; **82**:1890–1898.
9. Singh RK, Bucana CD, Gutman M, Fan D, Wilson MR, Fidler IJ. Organ site-dependent expression of basic fibroblast growth factor in human renal cell carcinoma cells. *Am J Pathol* 1994; **145**:365–374.
10. Singh RK, Gutman M, Bucana CD, Sanchez R, Llansa N, Fidler IJ. Interferons alpha and beta downregulate the expression of basic fibroblast growth factor in human carcinomas. *Proc Natl Acad Sci USA* 1995; **92**:4562–4566.
11. Singh RK, Gutman M, Radinsky R, Bucana CD, Fidler IJ. Expression of interleukin 8 correlates with the metastatic potential of human melanoma cells in nude mice. *Cancer Res* 1994; **54**:3242–3247.
12. Kitadai Y, Radinsky R, Bucana CD, Takahashi Y, Xie K, Tahara E, Fidler IJ. Regulation of carcinoembryonic antigen expression in human colon carcinoma cells by the organ environment. *Am J Pathol* 1996; **149**:1157–1166.
13. Radinsky R. Paracrine growth regulation of human colon carcinoma organ-specific metastases. *Cancer Metastasis Rev* 1993; **12**:345–361.
14. Radinsky R, Risin S, Fan D, Dong Z, Bielenberg D, Bucana CD, Fidler IJ. Level and function of epidermal growth factor receptor predict the metastatic potential of human colon carcinoma cells. *Clin Cancer Res* 1995; **1**:19–31.
15. Radinsky R. Modulation of tumor cell gene expression and phenotype by the organ-specific metasatic environment. *Cancer Metastasis Rev* 1995; **14**:323–338.
16. Fidler IJ. Special Lecture: Critical factors in the biology of human cancer metastasis: Twenty-eighth GHA Clowes Memorial Award Lecture. *Cancer Res* 1990; **50**:6130–6138.
17. Fidler IJ, Radinsky R. Editorial: Genetic control of cancer metastasis. *J Natl Cancer Inst* 1990; **82**:166–168.
18. Kerbel RS. Growth dominance of the metastatic cancer cell: Cellular and molecular aspects. *Adv Cancer Res* 1990; **55**:87–132.
19. Hart IR. 'Seed and soil' revisited: mechanisms of site specific metastasis. *Cancer Metastasis Rev* 1982; **1**:5–17.
20. Nicolson GL. Cancer metastasis: Tumor cell and host organ properties important in metastasis to specific secondary sites. *Biochim Biophys Acta* 1988; **948**:175–224.
21. Paget S. The distribution of secondary growths in cancer of the breast. *Lancet* 1889; **1**:571–573.
22. Tarin D, Price JE., Kettlewell MGW *et al.* Mechanisms of human tumor metastasis studied in patients with peritoneovenous shunts. *Cancer Res* 1984; **44**:3584–3592.
23. Ewing J. *Neoplastic Diseases*, 1928, 6th edn Philadelphia, W.B. Saunders.
24. Boring CC, Squires TS, Tong, T. *Cancer Statistics 1993. CA* 1993; **41**:7–26.
25. Russell AH, Tong D, Dawson LE, Wisbeck W. Adenocarcinoma of the proximal colon: Sites of initial dissemination and patterns of recurrence following surgery alone. *Cancer* 1984; **53**:360–367.
26. Benotti P, Steele G. Patterns of recurrent colorectal cancer and recovery surgery. *Cancer* 1992; **70**:1409–1413.
27. Buyse M, Zelenuick-Jacquotte A, Chalmers TC. Adjuvant therapy of colorectal cancer: Why we still don't know. *JAMA* 1988; **259**:3571–3578.
28. Pestana C, Reitemeier RJ, Moertel CG *et al.* The natural history of carcinoma of the colon and rectum. *Am J Surg* 1964; **108**:826–829.
29. Jessup JM, Gallick GE. The biology of colorectal carcinoma. *Curr Probl Cancer* 1992; **5**:264–328.
30. Giavazzi R, Campbell DE, Jessup JM, Cleary K, Fidler IJ. Metastatic behavior of tumor cells isolated from primary and metastatic human colorectal carcinomas implanted into different sites of nude mice. *Cancer Res* 1986; **46**:1928–1933.
31. Morikawa K, Walker SM, Jessup JM, Fidler IJ. *In vivo* selection of highly metastatic cells from surgical specimens of different colon carcinomas implanted into nude mice. *Cancer Res* 1988; **48**:1943–1948.
32. Morikawa K, Walker SM, Nakajima M, Pathak S, Jessup JM, Fidler IJ. Influence of organ environment on the growth, selection, and metastasis of human colon carcinoma cells in nude mice. *Cancer Res* 1988; **48**:6863–6871.
33. Giavazzi R, Jessup JM, Campbell DE, Walker SM, Fidler IJ. Experimental nude mouse model of human colorectal cancer liver metastasis. *J Natl Cancer Inst* 1986; **77**:1303–1308.
34. August DA, Ottow RT and Sugarbaker EV. Clinical perspectives of human colorectal cancer metastasis. *Cancer Metastasis Rev* 1984; **3**:303–325.
35. Jessup JM, Giavazzi R, Campbell D, Cleary KR, Morikawa K, Hostetter R, Atkinson EN, Fidler IJ. Metastatic potential of human colorectal carcinomas implanted into nude mice:

Prediction of clinical outcome in patients operated upon for cure. *Cancer Res* 1989; **49**:6906–6910.

36. Jessup JM, Giavazzi R, Campbell D, Cleary KR, Morikawa K, Fidler IJ. Growth potential of human colorectal carcinomas in nude mice: association with preoperative serum concentration of carcinoembryonic antigen. *Cancer Res* 1988; **48**:1689–1692.

37. Singh RK, Tsan R, Radinsky R. Influence of the host microenvironment on the clonal selection of human colon carcinoma cells during primary tumor growth and metastasis. *Clin Expt Metastasis* 1997; **15**:140–150.

38. Cornil T, Man MS, Fernandez B, Kerbel RS. Enhanced tumorigenicity, melanogenesis and metastasis of a human malignant melanoma observed after subdermal implantation in nude mice. *J Natl Cancer Inst* 1989; **81**:938–944.

39. Shafie SM, Liotta LA. Formation of metastasis by human breast carcinoma cells (MCF-7) in nude mice. *Cancer Lett* 1980; **11**:81–87.

40. Tan MH and Chu TM: Characterization of the tumorigenic and metastatic properties of a human pancreatic tumor cell line (ASPC-1) implanted orthotopically into nude mice. *Tumour Biol* 1985; **6**:89–98.

41. McLemore TL, Liu MC, Blacker PC, Gregg M, Alley MC, Abbott BJ, Shoemaker RH *et al.* Novel intrapulmonary model for orthotopic propagation of human lung cancers in athymic nude mice. *Cancer Res* 1987; **47**:5132–5140.

42. Deuel TF. Polypeptide growth factors: Roles in normal and abnormal cell growth. *Annu Rev Cell Biol* 1987; **3**:443–492.

43. Zarrilli R, Bruni CB, Riccio A. Multiple levels of control of insulin-like growth factor gene expression. *Mol Cell Endocrinol* 1994; **101**:R1–R14.

44. Stiles CD, Capone GT, Scher CD, Antoniades HN, Van Wyk JJ, Pledger WJ. Dual control of cell growth by somatomedins and platelet-derived growth factor. *Proc Natl Acad Sci USA* 1979; **76**:1279–1283.

45. Long L, Nip J, Brodt P. Paracrine growth stimulation by hepatocyte-derived insulin-like growth factor-1: A regulatory mechanism for carcinoma cells metastatic to the liver. *Cancer Res* 1994; **54**:3732–3737.

46. Roberts AB, Thompson NL, Heine U, Flanders C, Sporn MB. Transforming growth factor β: Possible roles in carcinogenesis. *Br J Cancer* 1988; **57**:594–600.

47. Schwarz LC, Gingras MC, Goldberg G, Greenberg AH, Wright JA. Loss of growth factor dependence and conversion of transforming growth factor-β1 inhibition to stimulation in metastatic H-ras-transformed murine fibroblasts. *Cancer Res* 1988; **48**:6999–7003.

48. Fan D, Chakrabarty S, Seid C, Bell CW, Schackert H, Morikawa K, Fidler IJ. Clonal stimulation or inhibition of human colon carcinomas and human renal carcinoma mediated by transforming growth factor-β1. *Cancer Commun* 1989; **1**:117–125.

49. Malden L, Novak U, Burgess A. Expression of transforming growth factor alpha messenger RNA in normal and neoplastic gastrointestinal tract. *Int J Cancer* 1989; **43**:380–384.

50. Markowitz SD, Molkentin K, Gerbic C, Jackson J, Stellato T, Willson JKV. Growth stimulation by coexpression of transforming growth factor-α and epidermal growth factor receptor in normal an adenomatous human colon epithelium. *J Clin Invest* 1990; **86**:356–362.

51. Mead JE, Fausto N. Transforming growth factor α may be a physiological regulator of liver regeneration by means of an autocrine mechanism. *Proc Natl Acad Sci USA* 1989; **86**:1558–1562.

52. Michalopoulos GK. Liver regeneration: Molecular mechanisms of growth control. *FASEB J* 1990; **4**:176–187.

53. Gutman M, Singh RK, Price JE, Fan D, Fidler IJ. Accelerated growth of human colon cancer cells in nude mice undergoing liver regeneration. *Invasion Metastasis* 1994–95; **14**:362–371.

54. Van Dale P, Galand P. Effect of partial hepatectomy on experimental liver invasion by intraportally injected colon carcinoma cells in rats. *Invasion Metastasis* 1988; **8**:217–227.

55. Rothenberg M, Ling V: Multidrug resistance: Molecular biology and clinical relevance. *J Natl Cancer Inst* 1989; **81**:907–910.

56. Goldstein LJ, Galski H, Fojo A, Willingham M, Lai SL, Gazdar A, Pinker R, Green A, Grist W, Brodeur GM, Lieber M, Cossman J, Gottesman MM, Pastan I. Expression of a multidrug resistance gene in human tumors. *J Natl Cancer Inst* 1989; **81**:116–124.

57. Weinstein RS, Shriram JM, Dominguez JM, Lebovitz MD, Koukoulis GK, Kuszak JR *et al.* Relationship of the expression of the multidrug resistance gene product (P-glycoprotein) in human colon carcinoma to local tumor aggressiveness and lymph node metastasis. *Cancer Res* 1991; **51**:2720–2726.

58. Morrow CS, Cowan KH. Mechanisms and clinical significance of multidrug resistance. *Oncology* 1988; **2**:55–63.

59. Raymond M, Rose E, Housman DE, Gros P. Physical mapping, amplification, and overexpression of the mouse *mdr* gene family in multidrug-resistant cells. *Molec Cell Biol* 1990; **10**:1642–1651.

60. Croop JM, Raymond M, Haber D, Devault A, Arceci RJ, Gros P, Housman DE. The three mouse multidrug resistance (*mdr*) genes are expressed in a tissue-specific manner in normal mouse tissues. *Molec Cell Biol* 1989; **9**:1346–1350.

61. Devault A, Gros P. Two members of the mouse *mdr* gene family confer multidrug resistance with overlapping but distinct drug specificities. *Molec Cell Biol* 1990; **10**:1652–1663.

62. Slack NH, Bross JDJ. The influence of site of metastasis on tumor growth and response to chemotherapy. *Br J Cancer* 1975; **32**:78–86.

63. Teicher BA, Herman TS, Holden SA, Wang Y, Pfeffer MR, Crawford JW, Frei E. Tumor resistance to alkylating agents conferred by mechanisms operative only *in vivo*. *Science* 1990; **247**:1457–1461.

64. Wilmanns C, Fan D, O'Brian CA, Bucana CD, Fidler IJ. Orthotopic and ectopic organ environments differentially influence the sensitivity of murine colon carcinoma cells to doxorubicin and 5-fluorouracil. *Int J Cancer* 1992; **52**:98–104.

65. Bradley G, Sharma R, Rajalakshmi S, Ling V. P-glycoprotein expression during tumor progression in the rat liver. *Cancer Res* 1992; **52**:5154–5161.

66. Herzog CE, Tsokos M, Bates SE, Fojo AT. Increased mdr-1/P-glycoprotein expression after treatment of human colon carcinoma cells with P-glycoprotein antagonists. *J Biol Chem* 1993; **268**:2946–2952.

67. Kerbel RS, Kobayashi H, Graham CH. Intrinsic or acquired drug resistance and metastasis: Are they linked phenotypes? *J Cell Biochem* 1994; **56**:37–47.

68. Liotta LA, Thorgeirsson UP, Garbisa S. Role of collagenases in tumor cell invasion. *Cancer Metastasis Rev* 1982; **1**:277–288.

69. McDonnell S, Matrisian LM. Stromelysin in tumor progression and metastasis. *Cancer Metastasis Rev* 1990; **9**:305–319.

70. Sloane BF. Cathepsin B and cystatins: Evidence for a role in cancer progression. *Semin Cancer Biol* 1990; **1**:137–152.

71. Stetler-Stevenson WG. Type IV collagenases in tumor invasion and metastasis. *Cancer Metastasis Rev* 1990; **9**:289–303.

72. Testa JE, Quigley JP. The role of urokinase-type plasminogen activator in aggressive tumor cell behavior. *Cancer Metastasis Rev* 1990; **9**:353–367.

73. Liotta LA, Tryggvason K, Garbissa S, Hart I, Foltz CM, Shafie S. Metastatic potential correlates with enzymatic degradation of basement membrane collagen. *Nature* 1980; **284**:67–68.

74. Levy A, Cioce V, Sobel ME, Garbisa S, Grigioni WF, Liotta LA, Stetler-Stevenson WG. Increased expression of the 72 kDa type IV collagenase in human colonic adenocarcinoma. *Cancer Res* 1991; 51:439–444.

75. Fabra A, Nakajima M, Bucana CD, Fidler IJ. Modulation of the invasive phenotype of human colon carcinoma cells by fibroblasts from orthotopic or ectopic organs of nude mice. *Differentiation* 1992; 52:101–110.

76. Chung LWK. Fibroblasts are critical determinants in prostatic cancer growth and dissemination. *Cancer Metastasis Rev* 1991; 10:263–275.

77. Cornil I, Theodorescu D, Man S, Herlyn M, Jambmrosie J, Kerbel RS. Fibroblast cell interactions with human melanoma cells affecting tumor cell growth are a function of tumor progression. *Proc Natl Acad Sci USA* 1991; 88:6028–6032.

78. Schor SL, Schor AM. Clonal heterogeneity in fibroblast phenotype: Implications for the control of epithelial--mesenchymal interactions. *BioEssays* 198; 7:200–204.

79. Bouziges F, Simo P, Simon-Assman P, Haffen K, Kedinger M. Altered deposition of basement-membrane molecules in co-cultures of colonic cancer cells and fibroblasts. *Int J Cancer* 1991; 48:101–108.

80. Reid LM, Abreu SL, Montgomery K. Extracellular matrix and hormonal regulation of synthesis and abundance ofmessenger RNAs in cultured liver cells. In: *The Liver: Biology and Pathobiology*, 2nd edn, Arias IM, Jakoby WB, Popper H, Schachter D, Shafritz DA, (eds). 1988; 717–737. New York, Raven Press.

81. Roberts AB, Sporn MB, Assoian RK, Smith JM, Roche NS, Wakefield LM, Heine VI, Liotta LA, Falanga V, Kehr LJM. Transforming growth factor type B: Rapid induction of fibrosis and angiogenesis *in vivo* and stimulation of collagen formation *in vitro*. *Proc Natl Acad Sci USA* 1986; 83:4167–4171.

82. Gordon PB, Choi HU, Conn G, Ahmed A, Ehrmann B, Rosenberg L, Hatcher VB. Extracellular matrix heparan sulfate proteoglycans modulate the mitogenic capacity of acidic fibroblast growth factor. *J Cell Physiol* 1988; 140:584–592.

83. Zvibel I, Halay E, Reid LM. Heparin and hormonal regulation of mRNA synthesis and abundance of autocrine growth factors: Relevance to clonal growth of tumours. *Molec Cell Biol* 1991; 11:108–116.

84. Goldberg GI, Marmer BL, Grant GA, Eisen AZ, Wilhelm S, He CS. Human 72-kilodalton type IV collagenase forms a complex with a tissue inhibitor of metalloproteinases designated TIMP-2. *Proc Natl Acad Sci USA* 1989; 86:8207–8211.

85. Keski-Oja J, Blasi F, Leof EB, Moses HL. Regulation of the synthesis and activity of urokinase plasminogen activator in A549 human lung carcinoma cells by transforming growth factor-beta. *J Cell Biol* 1988; 106:451–459.

86. Overall CM, Wrana JL, Sodek J. Independent regulation of collagenase, 72-kDa progelatinase, and metalloendoproteinase inhibitor expression in human fibroblasts by transforming growth factor-beta. *J Biol Chem* 1989; 25:1860–1869.

87. Welch DR, Fabra A, Nakajima M. Transforming growth factor-beta stimulates mammary adenocarcinoma cell invasion and metastatic potential. *Proc Natl Acad Sci USA* 1990; 87:7678–7682.

88. Hujanen ES, Turpeenniemi-Hujanen T. Recombinant interferon alpha and gamma modulate the invasive potential of human melanoma *in vitro*. *Int J Cancer* 1991; 47:576–581.

89. Barbera-Guillem E, Smith I, Weiss L. Cancer-cell traffic in the liver. I. Growth kinetics of cancer cells after portal-vein delivery. *Int J Cancer* 1992; 52:974–977.

90. Coulombe J, Pelletier G. Gangliosides and organ-specific metastatic colonization. *Int J Cancer* 1993; 53:104–109.

91. Fujita S, Suzuki H, Kinoshita M, Hirohashi S. Inhibition of cell attachment, invasion and metastasis of human carcinoma cells by anti-integrin beta-1 subunit antibody. *Jpn J Cancer Res* 1992; 83:1317–1326.

92. Tanabe KK, Ellis LM, Saya H. Expression of the CD44R1 adhesion molecule is increased in human colon carcinomas and metastases. *Lancet* 1993; 341:725–726.

93. Jessup JM, Thomas P. Carcinoembryonic antigen: function in metastasis by human colorectal carcinoma. *Cancer Metastasis Rev* 1989; 8:263–280.

94. Hashino J, Fukuda Y, Oikawa S, Nakazato H, Nakanishi T. Metastatic potential of human colorectal carcinoma SW1222 cells transfected with cDNA encoding carcinoembryonic antigen. *Clin Exp Metastasis* 1994; 12:324–328.

95. Gold P, Freedman SO. Demonstration of tumor-specific antigen in human colonic carcinoma by immunological tolerance and absorption techniques. *J Exp Med* 1965; 121:439–462.

96. Steele G Jr, Zamcheck N. The use of carcinoembryonic antigen in the clinical management of patients with colorectal cancer. *Cancer Detection Prevention* 1985; 8:421–427.

97. Benchimol S, Fuks A, Jothy S, Beauchemin N, Shirota K, Stanners CP. Carcinoembryonic antigen, a human tumor marker, functions as an intercellular adhesion molecule. *Cell* 1989; 57:327–334.

98. Tibbetts LM, Doremus CM, Tzanakakis GN, Vezeridis MP. Liver metastasis with 10 human colon carcinoma cell lines in nude mice and association with carcinoembryonic antigen production. *Cancer* 1993; 71:315–321.

99. Hauck W, Stanners CP. Transcriptional regulation of the carcinoembryonic antigen gene. *J Biol Chem* 1995; 270:3602–3610.

100. Toribara NW, Sack TL, Gum JR, Ho SB, Shively JE, Willson JKV, Kim YS. Heterogeneity in the induction and expression of carcinoembryonic antigen-related antigens in human colon cancer cell lines. *Cancer Res* 1989; 49:3321–3327.

101. Murphy PR, Sato R, Sato Y, Friesen HG. Fibroblast growth factor messenger ribonucleic acid expression in a human astrocytoma cell line: regulation of serum and cell density. *Molec Endonucl* 1988; 2:591–598.

102. Xie B, Bucana CD, Fidler IJ. Density-dependent induction of 92-kD type IV collagenase activity in cultures of A431 human epidermoid carcinoma cells. *Am J Pathol* 1994; 144:1058–1067.

103. Pinto M, Robine-Leon S, Appay M-D *et al.* Enterocyte-like differentiation and polarization of the human colon carcinoma cell line Caco-2 in culture. *Biol Cell* 1983; 47:323–330.

104. Hauck W, Stanners CP. Control of carcinoembryonic antigen gene family expression in a differentiating colon carcinoma cell line, Caco-2. *Cancer Res* 1991; 51:3526–3533.

105. Chakrabarty S, Jan Y, Brattain MG, Tobon A, Varani J. Diverse cellular response elicited from human colon carcinoma cells by transforming growth factor-β. *Cancer Res* 1989; 49:2112–2117.

106. Kanai T, Hibi T, Hayashi A, Takashima J, Shiozawa M, Aiso S, Toda K, Iwao Y, Watanabe M, Tsuchiya M: Carcinoembryonic antigen mediates *in vitro* cell aggregation induced by interferon-γ in a human colon cancer cell line: requirement for active metabolism and intact cytoskeleton. *Cancer Lett* 1993; 71:109–117.

107. Folkman J. The role of angiogenesis in tumor growths. *Semin Cancer Biol* 1992; 3:65–67.

108. Fidler IJ, Ellis LM. The implications of angiogenesis for the biology and therapy of cancer metastasis. *Cell* 1994; 79:185–188.

109. Weidner N, Carroll PR, Flax J, Blumenfeld W, Folkman J. Tumor angiogenesis correlates with metastasis in invasive prostate carcinoma. *Am J Pathol* 1993; 143:401–409.

110. Hori A, Sasada R, Matsutani E, Naito K, Sakura Y, Fujita T, Kozai Y. Suppression of solid tumor growth by immunoneutralizing monoclonal antibody against human basic fibroblast growth factor. *Cancer Res* 1991; **51**:6189–6194.

111. Kim KJ, Olson K, French T, Vallee B, Fett J. A monoclonal antibody to human angiogenin suppresses tumor growth in athymic mice. *Cancer Res* 1994; **54**:4576–4579.

112. Olsson L. Phenotypic diversity of malignant cell populations: Molecular mechanisms and biological significance. *Cancer Res* 1986; **3**:91–114.

113. Teicher BA, Alvarez-Sotomayor E, Huang ZD. Antiangiogenic agents potentiate cytotoxic cancer therapies against primary and metastatic disease. *Cancer Res* 1992; **52**:6702–6704.

114. Takahashi Y, Kitadai Y, Bucana CD, Cleary K, Ellis LM. Expression of vascular endothelial growth factor and its receptor, *flk-l*, correlates with vascularity, metastasis, and proliferation of human colon cancer. *Cancer Res* 1995; **55**:3964–3968.

115. Warren RS, Yuan H, Matli M, Gillett NA, Ferrara N. Regulation by vascular endothelial growth factor of human colon cancer tumorigenesis in a mouse model of experimental liver metastasis. *J Clin Invest* 1995; **95**:1789–1797.

116. Presta M, Maier JA, Ragnotti GJ. The mitogenic signaling pathway but not the plasminogen activator-inducing pathway of basic fibroblast growth factor is mediated through protein kinase C in fetal bovine aortic endothelial cells. *Cell Biol* 1989; **109**:1877–1884.

117. Buckley-Sturrock A, Woodward SC, Senior RM, Grimm GL, Klagsbrun M, Davidson JM. Differential stimulation of collagenase and chemotactic activity in fibroblasts derived from rat wound repair tissue and human skin by growth factors. *J Cell Physiol* 1989; **138**:70–78.

118. Gohji K, Fidler IJ Tsan R, Radinsky R, von Eschenbach AC, Tsuruo T, Nakajima M. Human recombinant interferons-beta and -gamma decrease gelatinase production and invasion by human KG-2 renal carcinoma cells. *Int J Cancer* 1994; **58**:380–384.

119. Nanus DM, Schmitz-Drager BJ, Motzer RJ, Lee AC, Vlamis V, Cordon-Cardo C, Albino AP, Reuter VE. Expression of basic fibroblast growth factor in primary human renal tumors: Correlation with poor survival. *J Natl Cancer Inst* 1994; **85**:1597–1599.

120. Nguyen M, Watanabe H, Budson AE, Richie JP, Hayes DF, Folkman J. Elevated levels of an angiogenic peptide, basic fibroblast growth factor, in the urine of patients with a wide spectrum of cancers. *J Natl Cancer Inst* 1994; **86**:356–361.

121. Ezekowitz RAB, Mulliken JB, Folkman J. Interferon alfa-2α therapy for life-threatening hemangiomas of infancy. *N Engl J Med* 1992; **326**:1456–1463.

122. Real FX, Oettgen HF, Krown SE. Kaposi's sarcoma and the acquired immunodeficiency syndrome: Treatment with high and low doses of recombinant leukocyte interferon. *J Clin Oncol* 1986; **4**:544–551.

123. van der Geer P, Hunter T, Lindberg RA. Receptor protein-tyrosine kinases and their signal transduction pathways. *Annu Rev Cell Biol* 1994; **10**:251–337.

124. Sainsbury JRC, Sherbert GV, Farndon JR, Harris AL. Epidermal growth factor receptors and oestrogen receptors in human breast cancer. *Lancet* 1986; **i**:364–366.

125. Bigner SH, Humphrey PA, Wong AJ, Vogelstein B, Mark J, Friedman HS, Bigner DD. Characterization of the epidermal growth factor receptor in human glioma cell lines and xenografts. *Cancer Res* 1990; **50**:8017–8022.

126. Harris AL, Neal DE: Epidermal growth factor and its receptor in human cancer. In: *Growth Factors and Oncogenes in Breast Cancer*, Sluyser M (ed.) 1987; pp. 60–90. Chichester, UK: Ellis Horwood, Ltd.

127. Neal DE, Marsh C, Bennet MK, Abel PD, Hall RR, Sainsbury JRC, Harris AL. Epidermal growth factor receptor in human bladder cancer: Comparison of invasive and superficial tumours. *Lancet* 1985; **i**:366–368.

128. Gullick WJ, Marsden JJ, Whittle N, Ward B, Bobrow L, Waterfield MD. Expression of epidermal growth factor receptors on human cervical, ovarian, and vulvar carcinomas. *Cancer Res* 1986; **46**:285–292.

129. Ullrich AL, Coussens L, Hayflick JS, Dull TJ, Gray A, Tam AW, Lee J, Yarden Y, Libermann TA, Schlessinger J, Downward J, Whittle ELV, Waterfield MD, Seeburg PH. Human epidermal growth factor receptor cDNA sequence and aberrant expression of the amplified gene in A431 epidermoid carcinoma cells. *Nature (London)* 1984; **309**:418–425.

130. Scher HI, Sarkis A, Reuter V, Cohen D, Netto G, Petrylak D, Lianes P, Fuks Z, Mendelsohn J, Cordon-Cardo C. Changing patterns of expression of the epidermal growth factor receptor and transforming growth factor α in the progression of prostatic neoplasms. *Clin Cancer Res* 1995; **1**:545–550.

131. Gross ME, Zorbas MA, Daniels YJ, Garcia R, Gallick GE, Olive M, Brattain MG, Boman BM, Yeoman LC. Cellular growth response to epidermal growth factor in colon carcinoma cells with an amplified epidermal growth factor receptor derived from a familial adenomatous polyposis patient. *Cancer Res* 1991; **51**:1452–1459.

132. Waldman FM, Carroll PR, Kerschmann R, Cohen MB, Field FG, Mayall BH. Centromeric copy number of chromosome 7 is strongly correlated with tumor grade and labeling index in human bladder cancer. *Cancer Res* 1991; **51**:3807–3813.

133. Radinsky R, Bucana CD, Ellis LE, Sanchez R, Cleary KR, Brigati DJ, Fidler IJ. A rapid colorimetric *in situ* messenger RNA hybridization technique for analysis of epidermal growth factor receptor in paraffin-embedded surgical specimens of human colon carcinomas. *Cancer Res* 1993; **53**:937–943.

134. Mendelsohn J. The epidermal growth factor receptor as a target for therapy with antireceptor monoclonal antibodies. *Semin Cancer Biol* 1990; **1**:339–344.

135. Baselga J, Norton L, Masui H, Pandiella A, Coplan K, Miller Jr WH, Mendelsohn J. Antitumor effects of doxorubicin in combination with anti-epidermal growth factor receptor monoclonal antibodies. *J Natl Cancer Inst* 1993; **85**:1327–1333.

136. Lofts FJ, Hurst HC, Sterberg MJE, Gullick WJ. Specific short transmembrane sequences can inhibit transformation by the mutant *neu* growth factor receptor *in vitro* and *in vivo*. *Oncogene* 1993; **8**:2813–2820.

137. Fry DW, Kraker AJ, McMichael A, Ambroso LA, Nelson JM, Leopold WR, Connors RW, Bridges AJ. A specific inhibitor of the epidermal growth factor receptor tyrosine kinase. *Science* 1994; **265**:1093–1095.

138. Kashles O, Yarden Y, Fischer R, Ullrich A, Schlessinger J. A dominant negative mutation suppresses the function of normal epidermal growth factor receptors by heterodimerization. *Mol Cell Biol* 1991; **11**:1454–1463.

139. Selva E, Raden DL, Davis RJ: Mitogen-activated protein kinase stimulation by a tyrosine kinase-negative epidermal growth factor receptor. *J Biol Chem* 1993; **268**:2250–2254.

Staging and Prognostic Factors

Leandro Gennari, Roberto Doci and Paola Bignami

Introduction

Autopsy series report that the incidence of liver metastases ranges from 10% to 50% in cancer patients. All malignant tumours can develop synchronous or metachronous liver metastases, for which multiple therapeutic options are available. In the past, several attempts have been made to tract liver metastases using different schedules of anti-cancer drugs. Over the last decade, new approaches such as liver resection, percutaneous ethanol injection (PEI), transarterial chemoembolization (TACE), and cryosurgery amongst others have been used. Although encouraging results have been reported after almost every type of therapy, the choice of treatment is difficult and often depends on the specialisation of the clinician performing the diagnosis. One of the most important considerations concerning the choice of treatment is the stage of the disease and the prognostic factors which can influence survival.

Staging

The staging of cancer is the evaluation of anatomical stage of disease in terms of extent, progression and severity. Since the extent of the disease plays an important role in choosing the type of treatment, and the progression and severity influence prognosis, accurate pre-treatment staging becomes mandatory. Such staging will allow the identification of homogeneous groups of patients for whom an appropriate therapy should be given.

An accurate staging is drawn mainly from histological, anatomical and biological factors. Biopsy performed preoperatively will indicate the histological type of cancer and its grading. Imaging will give information concerning the extent of the disease within the invaded organ, detect lymphadenopathy and detect distant metastases.

Advances in cellular and molecular biology offer additional information which better define the biological characteristics of the tumour and can consequently influence prognosis as well as management. There is therefore much information to be assimilated by accurately stage the patient.

After carrying out all the examinations necessary to exclude any extrahepatic relapse the key issue concerns the extent of liver involvement and related prognostic factors. The grouping of patients in well-defined stages can be done using a classification which defines the anatomic distribution of the disease and permits the creation of homogeneous groups of patients with different prognosis (staging system). A knowledge of the disease stage allows the rationalisation of the therapeutic options and the objective evaluation of the obtained results. Until recently, the lack of an accepted classification of liver metastases has been considered responsible for the present difficulty in assessing the efficacy of differing treatment options.

This is particularly true with the recent trend towards aggressive multi-modal therapies for hepatic metastases which emphasises the need for a common language among oncologists.

Hermanek has emphasised the necessity for a uniform classification system to assist treatment planning, to estimate prognosis and to evaluate results of clinical studies.[1] Since 1970 several classifications have been proposed. Some of these were based on the extent of liver involvement or

Table 4.1   Mean survival of patients with hepatic metastases, according to their number. Modified from Nielsen *et al.*[3]

Metastases	Number of cases	Mean survival time (months)
Few	24	18
Several	14	9
Numerous	27	5

Table 4.2   Classification of hepatic metastases according to the general rules of the TNM classification. From Gennari *et al.*[5]

H	Synchronous hepatic metastases
rH	Metachronous hepatic metastases
(r)H1	Liver involvement equal to or less than 25%
(r)H2	Liver involvement between 25–50%
(r)H3	Liver involvement more than 50%
s	Single metastasis
m	Multiple monolateral metastases
b	Bilateral metastases (both surgical lobes)
i	Infiltration of contiguous structures or organs
F	Impairment of liver function
C	Presence of cirrhosis

took into account one parameter only while the site of metastases was rarely considered as a factor in staging. Pettavel *et al.*[2] proposed in 1967 a classification in four stages which included the size of metastases, liver function and clinical hepatomegaly. In 1970 Nielsen *et al.*[3] added another factor – the number of liver deposits (Table 4.1). Pettavel's classification suffered from the fact that hepatomegaly can be due to non-neoplastic disease and that the evaluation of numerous or several metastases is often subjective. Although Pettavel amongst others considered the site as a factor in staging this was not included in a new classification proposed by this group in 1983[4] because, in agreement with Fortner, it was felt that treatment options were not necessarily dependent on the number of metastases.

In the definition of a proper classification and staging system, it would appear that three important considerations should be taken into account:

● rational therapeutic planning;
● objective and correct evaluation of the treatment according to different stages of the disease;
● the use of a common language among the different clinical components.

In 1982 we made a new proposal[5] in which details concerning percentage of liver involvement, site and number of metastases are reported (Table 4.2). Its prognostic validity was described both in reports from Italy and from other international centres.[8,9] Our experience on liver resection for metastases has shown that there is a clear difference in survival between patients in stage III and I–II (Figure 4.1). As a consequence, surgical treatment for patients classified H3s and H3m becomes questionable if the aim is to increase survival, whereas it may sometimes be acceptable if the target is to increase the quality of remnant life. The classification and the staging system seem to be very useful in the analysis of phase III studies, inasmuch as they allow an analysis among groups of patients truly homoge-

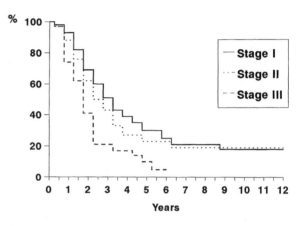

Figure 4.1.   Actuarial survival of patients after radical resection of hepatic metastases according to Gennari's staging system.

neous for prognostic factors. In general, the classification and staging systems permit a more critical analysis of published series and allow more accurate conclusions to be drawn. It is clear that, in evaluating results, other elements must be taken into account. These include the therapeutic index of pharmacological agents and biological markers such as the ploidy, cell kinetics, expression of *p53*, etc.

Known classifications are questionable because they do not include all factors. In the future, it is likely that a more general classification will be necessary for grouping patients. Such a classification should include macroscopic and topographic factors as well as the biologic characteristics of the tumour. With such a system it may be possible to treat patients in a more clearly defined manner and to analyse comparative data in a more accurate manner.

Prognostic Factors

Clinico-pathologic Factors in Patients with Unresected Metastases

Most studies devoted to the natural history of hepatic metastases have analysed series of patients observed in an era when modern diagnostic technologies were not available.[3,4,10–16] However, even if the assessment of several characteristics was approximate, they clearly indicated that the most important prognostic factor was tumour burden. Heavy burden had a mean survival of a few months, while solitary metastasis of limited extent was compatible with a mean survival of about two years.[12,15,16] All reports had no survivors longer than five years.

During recent years three important studies have been reported on patients with hepatic metastases, where modern imaging and sophisticated statistical analyses have been carried out. Stangl et al.[17] reported an analysis on 484 untreated patients whose overall median survival was 7.5 months; 21 variables were evaluated and 17 of them had statistical significance, but only six emerged after multivariate analysis as independent prognostic indicators – extent of liver involvement, grading and stage of primary, extrahepatic disease, carcinoembryonic antigen level and patient age. Among these, the most important was the extent of parenchymal invasion. The median survival of patients with favourable factors was 21.3 months, while that of patients with adverse factors was 3.8 months. Finan et al.[18] analysed a series of 90 patients, with synchronous hepatic metastases, 70% of whom had resection of the primary tumour. Overall median survival was 10.3 months. Thirteen variables were significant prognostic indicators using univariate analysis, but only six of these remained significant using multivariate analysis – the percentage of liver replacement, the stage and grade of primary, weight loss, albuminaemia and alkaline phosphatase. The authors constructed a clinical scoring index and a computer survival model that allowed the identification of patients who would survive more than 12 months. Chang et al.[19] reported an analysis carried out on 67 patients with unresectable hepatic metastasis and no extrahepatic spread treated with systemic or locoregional chemotherapy. The median survival observed was 15 months; only two out of 22

Table 4.3 Multivariate analysis of prognostic factors in patients with unresected hepatic metastases.

Parameter	Stangl et al.[17]	Finan et al.[18]	Chang et al.[19]
Patients (n)	484	90	67
Age	+	–	–
Stage of primary	+	+	–
Grade	+	+	–
PHI*	+	+	+
Extrahepatic disease	+		
CEA	+		
Albumin	–	+	–
Alkaline phosphatase	–	+	+
Weight loss		+	

+ independent prognosticator
* PHI = percentage hepatic involvement.

variables considered were significant using multivariate analysis: alkaline phosphatase and extent of liver involvement. The median survival of patients with favourable factors was 35.6 months and 7.9 months for those with unfavourable ones.

All studies, despite differing statistical analysis and type of treatment performed, stress the importance of the percentage of hepatic replacement, while the grading and stage of primary and the alkaline phosphatase level were significant prognostic factors in two out of three reported studies (Table 4.3). Reported data allow to conclude that median survival is highly variable, ranging from four months to three years and is conditioned by patient and disease characteristics; it is also evident the importance of bearing in mind such characteristics that can heavily interfere with the results of treatments.

Clinico-pathologic Factors in Patients with Resected Metastases

The role of prognostic factors is of great importance should surgery be the treatment of choice. Since liver surgery involves more risks (and cost) than other types of therapy, our end point must be to treat only those patients for whom there is a good probability of success. As far as the five year survival of resected patients is concerned, data from literature reports a range of 27–32%, with 20% being the median value. Many prognostic factors have been analysed in the series reported in literature, and those recognised as important at univariate analysis are as follows:

Univariate Analysis

Age and Sex
In almost all reported series the age and sex had no prognostic importance.

Site of Primary
Site of the primary in the colon or in the rectum did not influence prognosis.

Stage of Primary
This is one of the most important prognostic factors. In our experience[20] the five-year survival for Dukes A–B has been about 40%, whereas that for Dukes C was approximately 25%. Similar data were reported by other authors.[6,21–30] Scheele et al.[31] reported that the stage of the primary tumour had prognostic value only when metastases were detected synchronously.

Time of Diagnosis
The impact of the interval between primary diagnosis and detection of liver metastases differs within the reported studies. Some authors[20,23,30,32] did not find any difference, while others have shown a statistical difference when the interval between diagnosis of primary disease and metastases is more than one[26] to two[28,33] years. This behaviour might be related to a different speed in growth of primary and metastatic cells, as suggested by studies with thymidine-labelling index.

Extent of Parenchymal Replacement
The diameter of the largest metastasis has been found to be prognostic at cut-off points of 5 cm[28,31] or 8 cm[26]; we preferred to consider the percentage of liver involvement: the classification we proposed in 1982 distinguished three situations: a replacement less than 25%, between 25 and 50% and more than 50%. In our experience this variable has been highly predictive, the five-year survival in the three groups being 27, 16 and 8% respectively. Similar results are reported by other authors.[29,32]

Number of Metastases
It is generally believed[20,22,32,28,2–4] that prognosis is better if the number of metastases are less than four. In our experience all patients with more than three metastases developed recurrences within five years. The five-year survival was 29% for a single metastasis, 21% for two or three and 17% for four or more. Sometimes satellitosis may be detected and in this case the prognosis is worse.[31]

Site of Metastases
According to reported data[20,26,28–31] there is no statistical difference in prognosis between metastases located in one lobe or both lobes concurrently. This fact is important as it justifies an aggressive approach even if metastases are bilateral.

Carcinoembryonic Antigen (CEA)
The prognostic value of CEA has not been frequently used, but some authors report a correlation between circulating levels and the probability of relapse.[26,28,29,31,34] Nordlinger and Jaeck[28] reported a five-year survival of 30% for resected patients with CEA value less than 5 ng/ml and 18% for those with CEA values more than 30 ng/ml.

Resection Margin
A safe margin of resection is an essential prerequisite for prolonged survival.[26,28,31,32,35,36] Liver resection is commonly considered radical when the margin of resection is at least 1 cm from the tumour edge. Nordlinger and Jaeck[28] reported a 30% five-year survival for resections with a margin of resection greater than 1 cm from the tumour, a figure which drops to 15% when resection is performed with a lesser margin. Scheele et al.[31] confirmed these findings but did not report any difference between resection margins of less than 0.5 cm or between 0.5 and 1 cm. Sometimes a metastasis located near an important vascular structure does not allow a safe margin of 1 cm, but this factor should not exclude resection.

Type of Resection
If a radical resection is performed, results are equivalent between major resection and segmentectomy. In our experience, five-year survival figures are 28% and 18% after minor and major hepatic resection respectively. This difference in survival is due to the extent of liver involvement, and implicit locally advanced stage of disease, for patients undergoing major resection compared to segmentectomy. These data support the concept of performing limited but radical liver resection,[33,37–42] and justify an aggressive surgical approach even for bilateral metastases,[43,44] reduce postoperative morbidity and mortality and also increase the possibility of re-resection should local relapse occur.

Extrahepatic Disease
The detection of extra-hepatic disease is an important prognostic factor which excludes surgical treatment. Although many reports show no five-year

Table 4.4 Multivariate analysis of prognostic factors in patients with resected hepatic metastases

Parameter	Fortner et al.[23]	Ekberg et al.[32]	Registry[26]	Nordlinger and Jaeck[28]	Hoenberger et al.[29]	Doci et al.[20]	Scheele et al.[27]	Jatzko et al.[30]
Patients (n)	75	72	789	1681	166	219	350	66
Sex	–	–	–	–	+	–	–	–
T stage	+	–	+	+	–	+	+	+
T grade		–			–	–	+	+
Diagnosis time	–	–	+	+	+	–	+	–
Preop. CEA	–		–	+	–	–	–	
Metastases (n < 4)	–	+	+	+	–	–	–	–
Satellitosis							+	
Size or PHI*		–	+	+	+	+	–	–
Type of surgery	–	–	–	–		–	+	+
Resection margin		+	–	+		–	–	–
Extrahepatic disease	+	+		–			–	
Stage of metastases	+			+		+		–

* Percentage of hepatic involvement.
+ independent prognosticator

survivors,[26,28,34] a recent report by Scheele and co-workers[31] demonstrated a five-year survival of 34% when an aggressive surgical approach for lung metastases or local recurrence of the primary was adopted. Metastases to hepatic lymph-nodes are a poor prognostic factor also and are a contraindication to hepatic resection,[26] even if one study demonstrated a five-year survival of 12% after radical resection of metastatic lymph nodes.[28]

Multivariate Analysis

Modern studies on prognosis of metastatic disease have employed multifactorial analyses to clarify which factors are independent prognosticators. In Table 4.4, eight studies are reported: 15 variables were examined in 3427 patients and, of these, three resulted as being the most important:

1. Stage of primary according to Dukes classification was an independent variable related to prognosis in six out of eight analyses;
2. In four out of seven studies, the volume of metastases or the extent of liver involvement were independent indications of survival;
3. Extrahepatic disease was considered in four studies only because its presence was not included in the analysis of the other studies. As might be expected, this factor was a strong independent variable of outcome. In one study only[31] did extrahepatic disease not prove to be a prognostic factor when all the recurrences were radically removed.

The time interval between the primary diagnosis and development of metastases, the grading and the number of metastatic deposits resulted as being independent variables in 50% of the analyses; the distance of the resection margin from the tumour edge and the type of surgery performed were quoted as variables in one-third of the studies.

In conclusion, the results of the multivariate analysis can be summarised as follows:

1. Extrahepatic disease must be carefully looked for. Although an unfavourable factor, if completely resected with low operative risk, ablation can sometimes offer unexpected results.
2. Even in Dukes C rectal cancer or locally advanced disease (more than 50% of liver involvement or maximum diameter larger than 5–8 cm), the possibility to obtain good results after radical surgery cannot be excluded.
3. The main goal should be a safe margin of resection defined as a parenchymal cut at least 1 cm from the tumour edge.
4. The prognostic significance related to the type of liver resection is not clear. It is common opinion that whenever possible, anatomical resection should be preferable and that in all cases intra-operative ultrasonography must be carried out to detect subclinical metastases.
5. Liver resection is questionable when more than four metastases are diagnosed, while in general the number of hepatic metastases should be considered in relation to the other prognostic factors.

Biological Factors in Patients with Resected Metastases

In recent years different biological markers have been investigated in relation to the prognosis of different human tumours, but only a few reports have been devoted to hepatic metastases from colorectal cancer. Only single biological variables have been evaluated, in particular DNA ploidy,[26,30] cell kinetics,[31] k-ras status[28] and p53 mutations.[33]

In 104 patients submitted to radical hepatic resection, we[45] investigated the prognostic importance of the following biomarkers: 3H-dT labelling index (LI); p53 protein expression; Bcl-2 expression and DNA ploidy. Clinical parameters were also considered – stage of primary tumour, percentage of hepatic replacement (PHR) and number of metastases. At univariate analysis 3H-dT LI showed a significant correlation with disease-free survival: patients with rapidly proliferating liver lesions had 100% recurrence rate within four years as compared with the 76% recurrence rate of patients with slowly proliferating lesions ($P = 0.01$). Aneuploid and p53-positive lesions relapsed more frequently than diploid and p53-negative ones, but the difference was not significant ($P = 0.09$). Both Dukes' stage of primary and PHR were highly significant prognostic variables. Using multivariate analysis, 3H-dT LI and Dukes' stage emerged as significant independent factors. In the group of patients with Dukes' B tumour and slowly proliferating lesions the crude cumulative recurrence rate at four years was 70% as compared with 95% in Dukes C patients with a high proliferative index ($P = 0.002$).

The conclusion from studies on prognostic factors demonstrates that some characteristics of the primary and metastatic tumour emerge and are related to outcome of patients following treatment. The study of some biological markers may open new ways of interpreting standard prognostic variables.

References

1. Hermanek P. Liver metastases: classification and staging system in malignancies of the liver. *Eur Clin Digest Dis* 1992; Suppl. **1**:15–22.
2. Pettavel J, Morgenthaler F. Natural history of cancer metastatic to the liver and protracted arterial infusions. *5th International Congress of Chemotherapy, Vienna, 1967.* (Abstract)
3. Nielsen J, Balslev I, Jensen HE. Carcinoma of the colon with liver metastases. *Acta Chir Scand* 1971; **137**:463–465.
4. Pettavel J, Leyvraz S, Douglas P. The necessity for staging liver metastases and standardizing treatment–response criteria. The case of secondaries of colo-rectal origin. In: *Liver Metastases.* van de Velde CJH, Sugarbaker PH (eds), 1984: 154–168. Dordrecht, Martinus Nijhoff Publishers.
5. Gennari L, Doci R, Bozzetti F, Veronesi U. Proposal for a clinical classification of liver metastases. *Tumori* 1982; **68**:443–449.
6. Doci R, Gennari L, Bignami P, et al. One hundred patients with hepatic metastases from colorectal cancer treated by resection: analysis of prognostic determinants. *Br J Surg* 1991; **78**:797–801.
7. Gennari L, Bozzetti F, Doci R et al. Patterns of failure after surgical resection of liver metastases from colorectal cancer. In: *Current Topics in Surgical Oncology.* Fegiz G, Ramacciato G, Vitelli C, De Angelis R. (eds), 1991:327–332. Masson.
8. Holm A, Bradly E, Aldrete JS. Hepatic resection of metastases from colorectal carcinoma. Morbidity, mortality and pattern of recurrence. *Ann Surg* 1989; **209**:428–434.
9. Hughes KS, Sugarbaker PH. Resection of the liver for metastatic solid tumors. In: Surgical treatment of metastatic cancer. SA Rosenberg (ed), 1987:125–164.
10. Jaffe BM, Donegan WI, Warson F et al. Factors influencing survival in patients with untreated hepatic metastases. *Surg Gynecol Obstet* 1968; **127**:1–11.
11. Bengmark S, Hafstrom I. The natural history of primary and secondary malignant tumors of the liver. The prognosis for patients with hepatic metastases from colonic and rectal carcinoma by laparotomy. *Cancer* 1969; **23**:198–202.
12. Wood CB, Gillis CR, Blumgart LH. A retrospective study of the natural history of patients with liver metastases from colorectal cancer. *Clin Oncol* 1976; **2**:285–288.
13. Bengtsson G, Carlson G, Hafstrom L, Jonsson PE. Natural history of patients with untreated liver metastases from colorectal cancer. *Am J Surg* 1976; **141**:586–589.
14. Goslin R, Steele G, Zamcheck N et al. Factors influencing survival in patients with hepatic metastases from adenocarcinoma of the colon or rectum. *Dis Colon Rectum* 1982; **25**:749–753.
15. Lahr CJ, Soong SJ, Cloud G et al. A multifactorial analysis of prognostic factors in patients with liver metastases from colorectal carcinoma. *J Clin Oncol* 1983; **1**:720–726.
16. Wagner JS, Adson MA, van Herden JA et al. The natural history of hepatic metastases from colorectal cancer. *Ann Surg* 1984; **199**:502–507.
17. Stangl R, Altendorf-Hofmann A, Carnley RM, Scheele J. Factors influencing the natural history of colorectal liver metastases. *Lancet* 1995; **343**:1405–1410.
18. Finan PJ, Marchal RJ, Cooper EH, Giles GR. Factors affecting survival in patients presenting synchronous hepatic metastases from colorectal cancer: A clinical and computer analysis. *Br J Surg* 1985; **72**:373–377.
19. Chang AE, Steinberg SM, Culnane M, White ED. Determinants of survival in patients with unresectable colorectal liver metastases. *J Surg Oncol* 1989; **40**:243–251.
20. Doci R, Bignami P, Montalto F, Gennari L. Prognostic factors for survival and disease-free survival in hepatic metastases from colorectal cancer treated by resection. *Tumori* (Suppl) 1995; **81**:143–146.
21. Attiyeh FF, Wanebo HJ, Stearns MW. Hepatic resection for metastasis from colorectal cancer. *Dis Colon Rectum* 1978; **21**:160–162.
22. Iwatsuki S, Byers WS, Jr, Starzl TE. Experience with 150 liver sections. *Ann Surg* 1983; **197**:247–253.
23. Fortner Jg, Silva JS, Golbey RB et al. Multivariate analysis of a personal series of 242 consecutive patients with liver metastases from colorectal cancer. Treatment by hepatic resection. *Ann Surg* 1984; **198**:306–316.

24. Adson MA, Van Heerden JA, Adson MH *et al.* Resection of hepatic metastases from colorectal cancer. *Arch Surg* 1984; **119**:647–651.

25. Butler J, Attiyeh FF, Daly JM *et al.* Hepatic resection for metastases of the colon and rectum. *Surg Gynecol Obstet* 1986; **162**:109–113.

26. Registry of Hepatic Metastases. Resection of the liver for colorectal carcinoma metastases. A multi-institutional study of indication for resection. *Surgery* 1988; **103**:278–288.

27. Scheele J, Stangl R, Altendorf-Hofmann A, Gall FP. Indicators of prognosis after hepatic resection for colorectal secondaries. *Surgery* 1991; **110**:13–29.

28. Nordlinger B, Jaeck D. *Traitement des Mètastases Hèpatiques des Cancers Colorectaux*, 1992. Paris, Springer-Verlag.

29. Hohenberger P, Schlag PM, Gerneth T, Herfarth C. Pre- and post-operative carcinoembryonic antigen determination in hepatic resection for colorectal metastases. Predictive value and implications for adjuvant treatment based on multivariate analysis. *Ann Surg* 1994; **2**:135–143.

30. Jatzko GR, Lisborg PH, Stettner HM, Klimpfinger MH. Hepatic resection for metastases from colorectal carcinoma. A survival analysis. *Eur J Cancer* 1995; **31**:41–46.

31. Scheele J, Stangl R, Altendorf-Hofmann A, Paul M. Resection of colorectal liver metastases. *World J Surg* 1995; **19**:59–71.

32. Ekberg M, Tranberg KG, Andersson R *et al.* Determinants of survival in liver resection for colorectal secondaries. *Br J Surg* 1986; **73**:727–731.

33. Logan SE, Meier SJ, Ramming KP *et al.* Hepatic resection for metastatic colorectal carcinoma: A ten year experience. *Arch Surg* 1982; **117**:25–28.

34. Cady B, McDermott WV Jr. Major hepatic resections for metachronous metastases from colon cancer. *Ann Surg* 1985; **201**:204–209.

35. August Da, Sugarbaker Ph, Ottow RT *et al.* Hepatic resection of colorectal metastases: influence of clinical factors and adjuvant intraperitoneal 5-fluorouracil via Tenckoff catheter on survival. *Ann Surg* 1985; **201**:210–218.

36. Holm A, Bradley E, Joaquim S, Aldrek S. Hepatic resection of metastases from colrorectal carcinoma. *Ann Surg* 1990; **209**:428–433.

37. Cox DR. Regression models and life tables (with discussion). *J R Statist Soc* 1972; **34**:187–220.

38. Petrelli NJ, Nambisa RN, Herrera L, Mittelman A. Hepatic resection for isolated metastasis from colorectal carcinoma. *Am J Surg* 1985; **149**:205–209.

39. Stehlin JS, De Ipolyi PD, Greeff PJ *et al.* Treatment of cancer of the liver. *Ann Surg* 1988; **208**:23–25.

40. Flanagan L, Foster JH. Hepatic resection for metastatic cancer. *Am J Surg* 1967; **113**:551–557.

41. Rajpal S, Dasmahapatra KS, Ledesma ET *et al.* Extensive resection of isolated metastases from carcinoma of the colon and rectum. *Surg Gynecol Obstet* 1982; **155**:813–816.

42. Bozzetti F, Bignami P, Morabito A *et al.* Patterns of failure following surgical resection of colorectal cancer liver metastases. *Ann Surg* 1987; **205**:264–270.

43. Doci R, Gennari L, Bignami P *et al.* Morbidity and mortality after hepatic resection of metastases from colorectal cancer. *Br J Surg* 1995; **82**:377–381.

44. Nordlinger B, Vaillant JC, Guiguet M *et al.* Survival benefit of repeat liver resections for recurrent colorectal metastases: 143 cases. *J Clin Oncol* 1994; **12**:1491–1496.

45. Costa A, Doci R, Mochen C, Bignami P *et al.* Cell proliferation-related markers in colorectal liver metastases: Correlation with patient prognosis. *J Clin Oncol* 1997; **15**:2008–2014.

Diagnosis of Liver Metastasis

Doris N. Redhead and Edward Leen

5

Introduction

Focal liver disease may be detected incidentally during cross-sectional imaging studies, at the time of cancer screening or follow-up and during laparotomy. Where surgery is being undertaken for colorectal cancer, for example, 26% of patients may be expected to have liver metastases and while a metastasis is the most common liver tumour detected and the majority arise from a colorectal primary cancer, some of the lesions found will represent benign disease of no clinical significance. A number of benign processes, such as haemangiomas and cysts, can mimic metastatic disease closely and in order that the most appropriate management is applied, it is clearly of paramount importance that an accurate distinction is made between significant and insignificant disease. Accurate characterization of a focal liver lesion, e.g. a simple cyst, may be possible using conventional ultrasound alone while other more complex pathologies may require multiple imaging studies and biopsy before a confident diagnosis can be made.

While biopsy might allow a rapid and accurate diagnosis, there is increasing recognition that seeding of tumour cells can occur as a result of percutaneous needling procedures and this may have an adverse effect on outcome. In addition, biopsy of a vascular lesion, e.g. a hepatoma, adenoma or haemangioma is not without risk of haemorrhage. Furthermore biopsy results may be misleading as tumour tissue may not be obtained from the area sampled and so giving false reassurance.

There is now a disparate array of sophisticated imaging technologies available for the evaluation of hepatic lesions and an accurate diagnosis can be made in most cases without biopsy.

Since the presence of liver metastatic deposits from primary breast, lung or pancreatic carcinoma reflects widespread disease, surgery is rarely applicable in these patients. However, where the primary lesion is a colorectal cancer or an apudoma (carcinoid or pancreatic islet cell tumour), the survival following hepatic resection is significantly improved. The five year survival of those who have surgical resection for colorectal metastases, for example, is 33% while for those who are not surgical candidates the survival is 10–35% at six months. Early detection and accurate staging of the disease is clearly important. To allow curative resection to be undertaken, there should be no evidence of extrahepatic disease and removal of all the tumour with clear resection margins must be possible while at the same time leaving sufficient well-vascularized tissue to sustain liver function. Imaging studies, therefore, require to exclude extrahepatic disease and to document the number and size of the lesions present. Since most hepatic resections are based on the segmental anatomy described by Couinaud and Bismuth, the imaging studies should allow visualisation of the hepatic vasculature and demonstration of the liver lesions in relation to these major vascular structures. An assessment of the volume of the proposed liver remnant may be important when an extensive resection is proposed and particularly where there is cirrhosis present. Should the remaining liver prove too small to support liver function, postoperative liver failure will result. It is known that liver affected by cirrhosis will not hypertrophy to the same extent as normal tissue and consequently particular attention has to be paid to the volume of liver left in the patient with cirrhosis.

Unfortunately only 12% patients will have metastatic disease confined to the liver and only 5–10% will be considered suitable candidates for hepatic resection.

Where the disease is confined to the liver but is not suitable for surgical resection, alternative local techniques designed to destroy liver tumours may be used. These include: cryosurgery, interstitial therapies, percutaneous alcohol, focussed ultrasound, insertion of radiofrequency electrodes and hepatic artery perfusion therapy. These procedures are mainly performed under imaging guidance. The changes induced in the liver by these various maneouvres can be confusing on imaging studies and differentiation from residual or recurrent tumour is required.

The choice of strategy employed in the detection, characterization, staging and follow-up of liver lesions will depend on the particular skills and facilities in each unit. There is, however, a general consensus with regard to the sensitivity and specificity of the various techniques used and these will be alluded to throughout the text.

Conventional Ultrasound

The traditional method of diagnosing hepatic metastases has been laparotomy. It is now well recognized that this technique is limited with an overall accuracy of 76%, a sensitivity and specificity of 60 and 88% respectively.[1] The poor sensitivity of surgical exploration became more evident with the emergence of ultrasonography (US) into routine clinical practice in the late seventies.

Recent technological innovations have led to higher definition imaging and the advent of improved duplex/colour Doppler imaging has simplified the non-invasive assessment of hepatic vascular structures as well as tumour vascularization. As liver imaging is being recognized as having clinically distinct tasks and as different imaging strategies are required for particular settings, the role of ultrasonography has become more clearly defined in the various stages of patient management.

Screening for Liver Tumours

In many centres ultrasonography is used routinely in the initial assessment to detect the presence of liver tumours, because of its non-invasiveness, low cost and availability. Results of studies evaluating the role of ultrasound as a screening tool for liver tumours vary depending on the clinical context. In a screening program of 100 patients with chronic liver disease, Takayasu and colleagues have shown that the sensitivity of ultrasonography in detecting small hepatocellular carcinomas (1–3 cm in diameter) was as high as 92% compared with 91% and 98% for computed tomography (CT) and intraoperative ultrasound (IOUS) respectively.[2] However in a recent comparative study of 161 patients with colorectal cancer, the sensitivity of ultrasound in the global detection of liver metastases was only 34% compared with 54% for CT.[3] The poor performance of both ultrasound and CT in this study can be explained by the fact that follow-up and postmortem were used as the gold standard. This in contrast to other comparative studies which use IOUS or CT arterioportography (CTAP) as the gold standard These studies do not take into account the presence of 'occult' metastases.[4]

Detection and Assessment of Tumour Burden

Studies of resected livers evaluating accurate assessment of tumour burden (i.e. total number of lesions present) using lesion by lesion analysis, have confirmed the limitation of ultrasonography. In a study comparing US, CT and CT angiography, Soyer et al. reported that US has the lowest sensitivity rate, missing 33% of the metastatic lesions.[5] In another comparative study, Machi and colleagues have demonstrated that the overall accuracy of ultrasound was 71% with a sensitivity and specificity of 38% and 97% respectively.[1] In an earlier report the same group had shown the sensitivity of US was 41%.[6] According to Ferrucci, false negative rates for ultrasonography exceed 50%.[7]

Characterization

Although the sensitivity of conventional ultrasonography is poor, specificity as high as 97% has been reported.[1] It is particularly useful in differentiating solid lesions and cysts. There has been scepticism regarding the usefulness of ultrasonography in the differentiation between benign and malignant lesions, as they share the same acoustic features. However within a given clinical context, in experi-

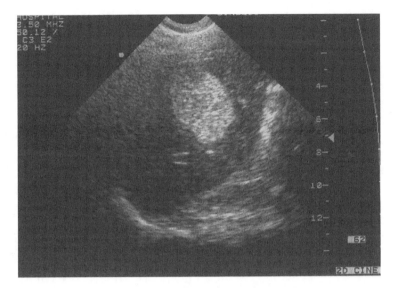

Figure 5.1.   Liver ultrasound showing the classical hyperechoity of a haemangioma.

enced hands the diagnosis can be accurate. Haemangiomas and metastases are the two commonest tumours which may be either hypoechoic or hyperechoic (Figure 5.1). In contrast to haemangiomas, metastases are often surrounded by a hypoechoic halo. In a retrospective study of 100 patients with liver tumours, 50% of which have histological proof of malignancy, Wernecke and colleagues assessed the diagnostic value of the sonographic halo sign in differentiating benign and malignant lesions.[8] The halo sign could be detected in 88% of malignant tumours (sensitivity of 88% and specificity of 86%, positive and negative predictive value of 86% and 88% respectively). Differentiation is most difficult when the lesions are less than 1.5 cm in diameter as they are too small to have any characteristic features. However, there is now evidence to suggest that contrast enhanced conventional or Doppler ultrasonography may be particularly useful in these cases.[9,10] In contrast CT remains limited in the differentiation between haemangiomas and metastases. Only 54% of haemangiomas have the typical pattern of contrast enhancement with the remaining 46% sharing the same pattern of enhancement as 77% of metastases.[11]

Localization of Hepatic Tumours

For accurate localization of lesions to specific segments, visualization of the lesion with respect to the hepatic vasculature is required through scanning in transverse and sagittal planes. Transverse scanning enables the visualization of the three main hepatic veins thereby defining the segments II, IV, VIII and VII. The combination of transverse and sagittal images enable precise localisation of the lesions within them, for example segment II versus, III, VIII versus V and VII versus VI. However compared with CT and magnetic resonance (MRI), localization with ultrasonography is more difficult in practice and may not provide all the detailed anatomical information required for segmental resections. Furthermore it may be impossible when the lesions are large. The addition of colour Doppler imaging may be useful in clearly defining any tumour involvement of major vessels in cases where MRI and CT are equivocal.

Assessment of Extrahepatic Disease

With regard to extrahepatic disease, examination is limited with poor detection rates for retroperitoneal lymphadenopathy and local recurrence as these areas are often compromised by overlying bowel gas. Furthermore dissemination beyond the abdomen is not assessable by ultrasound.

The relatively poor performance of ultrasonography is not surprising as there are inherent performance limits on the hardware; the inverse relationship between the frequency of the ultrasound transducer and depth of penetration through the tissues at the expense of resolution is a

Table 5.1 Sensitivity of IOUS vs US vs CT in the detection of liver metastases

Study	US	Bolus-CT	IOUS
Machi et al. (1987)[6]	41.3%	47.8%	97.8%
Machi et al. (1991)[1]	38%	43%	82%
Charnley et al. (1991)[12]	35%	69%	93%
Soyer et al. (1992)[5]	68%	71%	96%

significant factor with respect to imaging a relatively large organ such as the liver; accessibility to the posterior aspects of the liver is therefore limited; poor penetration through fat in general is problematic especially in fatty/cirrhotic livers and obese patients. In addition it is very operator dependent and the sonographic images are not easily reproducible for comparative purposes. All of these factors lead to higher false negatives and/or underestimation of the tumour burden.

Intraoperative Ultrasound

Intraoperative ultrasound (IOUS) is generally regarded as being very useful in the detection of small hepatic metastases (0.5 cm in diameter) as well as an adjunct in liver resection by demonstrating the anatomical relationship of the tumours to major vessels and bile ducts. Machi and colleagues have shown that IOUS has an overall accuracy, sensitivity and specificity of 87, 82 and 92%, respectively, in the detection of hepatic metastases (Table 5.1).[1]

In Charnley's study[12] of 99 patients undergoing surgery for colorectal cancer, metastases were identified by palpation in 18 patients, by abdominal ultrasound in 9 patients, by CT scan in 18 patients and by IOUS in 24 patients. Of all patients, 26 had metastases detected at the time of surgery by one or more of the investigations.

More recently, Soyer et al. compared IOUS and pre-operative CTAP scans in the detection of colorectal hepatic metastases.[5] Fifty-six metastases were pathologically proven. CTAP depicted 51 of the 56 metastases (91%) whilst IOUS depicted three metastases not detected by CTAP scan (96%). There was no statistical significance in sensitivity between the two techniques. The authors concluded that IOUS does not increase the number of detected liver metastases when CTAP is considered as the pre-operative standard of reference. They suggested that both techniques are complementary.

Contrast Enhanced Ultrasonography

Carbon dioxide

With the current limits of ultrasound performance, there is a need to develop ultrasound agents for liver imaging. Early research has been focused mainly on a contrast agent which was suitable for echocardiography. As a result the contrast agents which were developed initially were of limited use in imaging the liver, as the large size and instability of the bubbles precluded their passage through the pulmonary circulation after intravenous injection.

In a study of 184 patients with proven liver tumours, Kudo and colleagues assessed the use of carbon dioxide enhanced sonographic examination to characterize the tumours.[9] The carbon dioxide microbubbles were prepared by vigorously mixing 10 ml of carbon dioxide, 10 ml of heparinized normal saline and 5 ml of the patient's own blood. The advantage of such a combination was that blood increases the viscosity and surface tension of the solution thereby producing smaller microbubbles with improved stability, and carbon dioxide is readily cleared from the lungs. Sonographic 'angiography' was performed by injecting 5–20 ml of carbon dioxide microbubbles (at a rate of 1–2 ml/s) through a catheter placed within the hepatic artery (proper, left and right) using the same technique as conventional selective hepatic angiography. It was reported that the technique allowed the characterization of the hepatic tumours based on their vascular anatomy and was useful in differential diagnosis of the lesions. Hepatocellular carcinomas displayed a homogeneous or mosaic hypervascular pattern with peripheral arterial blood supply (sensitivity 90%; specificity 89%). In contrast focal nodular hyperplastic nodules were characterized by an early central hypervascular supply to give a uniform or lobulated enhancement (sensitivity and specificity 100%). Adenomatous hyperplasia, haemangioma and metastasis displayed 'spotty pooling' and peripheral hypervascularity patterns, respectively. However haemangiomas could be differentiated by the peripheral enhancement gradually infiltrating to the centre and lasting up to 30–60 min after injection (sensitivity and specificity 100%).

Using the same technique, the same group of workers confirmed its ability to detect small hepatocellular carcinomas measuring <1 cm in diameter which had been missed by the more conventional techniques. In addition, it was reported that the precise evaluation of tumour vascularity also enabled the determination of appropriate therapeutic strategy for these tumours.[13]

In a more recent study, the use of carbon dioxide alone in the sonographic examination of 45 patients with hepatocellular carcinomas was compared with digital subtraction angiography (DSA), conventional ultrasound, CT and CT arterioportography.[14] Sonographic examination was performed during the injection of 10–20 cc of carbon dioxide (at a rate of 1 cc per second) via a catheter placed within the proper hepatic artery. This technique described as 'echocarbography' allowed the detection of more lesions than any of the other modalities and no side effects had been reported.

Kubo and colleagues described an alternative pre-operative technique for the localization of hepatomas using carbon dioxide enhanced ultrasonography in cases where CT and MRI were equivocal.[15] Percutaneous transhepatic carbon dioxide enhanced US portography was performed through a 5.5Fr catheter introduced via a puncture of a portal branch in the non-cancerous area under sonographic guidance using a Seldinger method. The technique was found useful in segmental localisation of the tumours in all 12 cases undergoing segmentectomy or subsegmentectomy. Intra-operative use of this technique is also possible.

The use of carbon dioxide requires the catheterization of the hepatic artery or portal vein which is invasive and the agent itself is unstable, being readily diffusible into the carrier fluid thereby shortening its lifetime and contributing to some of the problems of reproducibility and efficacy.

Saccharide-Based Microbubbles: Echovist and Levovist

Echovist (Schering AG Berlin, Germany) consists of monosaccharide galactose crystalline microparticles which form a matrix of air bubbles of uniform size. A series of animal studies and clinical trials have confirmed its safety and efficacy in enhancing venous vessels and right heart cavities following injection of the aqueous galactose solution via a peripheral vein. However it does not have transpulmonary stability. Therefore it has to be administered via other routes in order to enhance the liver.

El Mouaaouy et al. assessed the intraoperative use of Echovist using a rat liver model. Homogeneous contrast enhancement of the entire liver parenchyma was achieved following injection of either 0.3 ml at a concentration of 200 mg/ml via the bile duct, or at least 0.3 ml at a concentration of 300 mg/ml via the hepatic artery or portal vein.[16] The enhancement lasted for at least 10 min with the three routes of administration. Improved detection of liver tumours as small as 3 mm in diameter was reported. Preliminary results of an ongoing clinical study suggest that Echovist may be used to enhance intraoperative sonography to detect occult liver metastases.

The invasive nature of the method of administration of carbon dioxide or Echovist to image the liver is a major drawback in clinical practice. Levovist (Schering AG Berlin, Germany) a derivative of Echovist with minor galenic modification of the microparticles, was developed and it contains 99.9% D-galactose and 0.1% palmitic acid. Some 99% of the microparticles are 8 μm in diameter and 99% of the microbubbles are <4 μm in size. The palmitic acid improves the intravascular stability and reproducibility of the microbubbles. The microbubbles can survive pulmonary transit to increase blood echogenicity and Doppler signal intensity in the arterial system by 10–20 dB. To prepare Levovist, sterile water is added to the galactose microparticles contained in a vial (10 ml water gives a concentration of 300 mg/ml) which is then shaken vigorously for 5–10 s. A proportion of the microparticles will dissolve until solubility equilibrium is reached, whilst the remaining microparticles are stabilized. Gas saturation within the liquid compartment takes place and the solid surfaces of the microparticles act as origins and stabilizing sites for the formation of new microbubbles of certain diameter range, whilst larger bubbles rapidly disappear.

Unlike Echovist, the transpulmonary agent Levovist can be administered via a peripheral vein for Doppler imaging of the hepatic vascular structures and tumour vascularity. Although there is no enhancement of the liver parenchyma itself on B mode imaging, there is increased echogenicity of the portal and hepatic venous blood. A recent European phase III multicentre trial assessed the diagnostic efficacy and safety of Levovist in over 1200 patients with diagnostically suboptimal Doppler scans for indications ranging from cardiovascular disease to tumour vascularity. The trial confirmed the safety and efficacy of the agent with over 50% increase in diagnostic confidence.[17]

Another study evaluating the use of the agent in the Doppler imaging of hepatic vessels confirmed the effective enhancement of the Doppler signals and it was suggested that the agent may be useful in the assessment of critically ill or obese patients.[18]

There are several studies evaluating the use of Levovist in Doppler imaging of hepatic tumours. In a study of 28 patients with histologically proven liver tumours (2 hepatocellular carcinomas, 2 carcinoid and 24 colorectal cancer metastases), highly significant enhancement of the colour Doppler signals was observed in 25 cases, lasting for a mean period of 180 s (s.d. 45).[19] No enhancement was observed in three colorectal cancer patients undergoing regional chemotherapy. In colorectal hepatic metastases a characteristic pattern, with predominantly increased tumour rim enhancement, was demonstrated with colour Doppler scans. In the hepatocellular carcinomas an infiltrating enhanced 'basket-like' pattern of hypervascularity was observed. Increased homogeneous colour Doppler signals (which had been absent on baseline scans) were observed throughout the carcinoid lesions after the injection of Levovist.

In another study of 38 patients with hepatocellular carcinomas, a similar enhanced pattern of hypervascularity was also demonstrated following the injection of Levovist.[20] The characteristic hypervascular nature of focal nodular hyperplasia and adenomas was clearly demonstrated following Levovist administration. In contrast, there was little or no enhancement of Doppler signals in the case of haemangiomas.[10] Further studies are still required to assess whether these findings are specific enough to be of any diagnostic value in clinical practice.

There are currently several other agents in various phases of clinical trials. The use of these agents in combination with 'harmonic' imaging, as well as 'power' or 'energy' Doppler imaging, clearly holds out great prospects for both diagnostic and therapeutic purposes. Preliminary studies of agents specifically targetted to the cells of the reticuloendothelial system (RES), such as SHU 563A (Cavisomes from Schering AG, Berlin) and NUS

(Nycomed, Oslo) suggest that the detection and characterization of liver lesions with little or no RES activity may be improved. However whether this type of enhanced ultrasonography in clinical practice will be more sensitive than enhanced CT or magnetic resonance imaging (MRI) for detection of small tumours, remains to be seen. Furthermore it is logical to assume that the use of these RES agents would be of great value to enhance intraoperative ultrasonography in the detection of small liver tumours as previously demonstrated in animal models even with the use of blood pool agents.[16]

Detection of Occult Metastases

Conventional imaging techniques such as US, CT and MRI are limited in the diagnosis of small liver metastases because there is a threshold size and contrast below which discrimination between normal and abnormal tissue is impossible. There is therefore a need to explore alternative techniques to identify those patients with occult liver tumours.

It has long been known that the presence of even small liver tumours is associated with subtle changes in the liver blood flow. Whereas the normal liver receives approximately 25% of its blood supply via the hepatic artery and about 75% via the portal vein, liver metastases derive a much greater proportion of their blood supply from the hepatic arterial flow and a lesser proportion from the portal venous flow.

There is also evidence to suggest that a circulating vasoconstrictor agent is implicated in the hepatic haemodynamic changes associated with the presence of microscopic intrahepatic metastases. Carter and colleagues isolated a segment of small bowel in a normal rat and alternately cross-perfused it with arterial blood from a tumour-bearing animal (HSN sarcoma model) and a control animal.[21] A significant reduction in the portal blood flow with a corresponding increase in the vascular resistance through the isolated segment was demonstrated. The authors suggested that the increase in the vascular resistance was due to a circulating humoral vasoconstrictor present in the blood of tumour-bearing animals. Using a different model, Warren and colleagues confirmed these results using plasma of patients with proven overt and occult liver metastases.[22] These findings are consistent with the earlier results of studies evaluating changes in liver blood flow in patients with liver metastases. They support the view that measurement of the relative hepatic arterial contribution to total liver blood flow may provide an alternative method of detecting small liver tumours.

A Doppler US study of 50 control subjects and 135 colorectal cancer patients (67 with histologically proven liver metastases and 68 with an apparently disease-free liver on the basis of laparotomy and CT scan) showed that there was clear separation of the Doppler perfusion index (DPI) between controls and patients with overt liver metastases (DPI = ratio of hepatic arterial to total liver blood flow).[23] Thirty-eight of the 68 patients with an apparently disease-free liver also had an abnormally elevated DPI value at the time of presentation. After one year follow-up, 21 of the 38 patients with an abnormally high DPI had developed liver metastases and a further 4 patients had died with no postmortem. The 30 patients with normal DPI remained disease-free. The authors suggested that the measurement of DPI may be of value in the early detection of occult liver metastases.

In a further study of 90 patients with colorectal cancer undergoing apparently curative surgery on the basis of laparotomy and CT scan, DPI was shown to be more sensitive than IOUS in the detection of occult liver metastases.[24] Of the 23 patients who subsequently developed liver metastases at one year follow-up, only 4 had been detected by IOUS whilst all had been predicted by an abnormally high DPI at time of presentation.

Analysis of the two-year outcome data of 80 colorectal cancer patients who had undergone apparently curative resection of the primary tumour, clearly showed that DPI was an independent predictor of survival.[25] At two years, the overall survival of patients with an abnormal DPI was 37% compared with 97% for those with a normal DPI value. In contrast Dukes staging failed to clearly identify those at high risk of early death with the overall two-year survival being 73% and 49% for Duke B and C, respectively. Taking into account the combined Dukes and DPI data, the two-year survival of patients with Dukes B disease with an abnormal DPI value was 44% compared with 95% for those with a normal DPI value. The two-year survival of patients with Dukes C stage disease with an abnormal DPI value was 23% compared with 100% for those with a normal DPI.

Multicentre trials are still needed to confirm these data as the technique would enable the earlier identification of patients at high risk of recurrence from occult metastases. These patients may be suitable for adjuvant portal vein infusion or systemic chemotherapy. In addition, DPI may be used to decide whether to offer extensive resection to achieve cure in the very old or high surgical risk patients. Moreover, DPI may offer better low cost surveillance of patients who have undergone primary resection.

Ultrasound Guided Biopsy

The common indications for ultrasound guided hepatic biopsy are as follows:

- to establish the diagnosis of a focal lesion in a patient who has no known primary
- to confirm the diagnosis of metastases or a second primary hepatic tumour in a patient with known primary tumour; and
- to confirm whether the residual hepatic mass represents viable malignancy in a patient who has received antitumour therapy.

To minimize biopsy complications there are several precautions to be taken. Any coagulopathy needs to be corrected prior to the procedure, by administration of appropriate elements (vitamin K, platelets and/or fresh frozen plasma). The presence of ascites alone is not a contraindication to biopsy. However combined coagulopathy and ascites is very risky even after embolisation of the biopsy tract.

The use of thin biopsy needle (20 gauge or less) is advised in the presence of obstructive jaundice to reduce the risk of biliary peritonitis or if a bowel loop is in the proposed needle tract.

The choice of modality used to guide the liver biopsy depends mainly on the skill of the operator and whether the lesion is adequately visualised. In contrast to US, CT has the advantage of precise localization of the needle tip especially for small lesions, visualization of the necrotic tissue within the lesion and of the vital structures to be avoided in the trajectory (bowel and vascular structures). However ultrasound is cheaper, readily available and does not involve radiation.

CT Scanning

Computed tomography is recognized as the most accurate and most widely available technique for detecting and characterising liver lesions. It is more sensitive than US in tumour detection, particularly small tumours (<1 cm) (see Table 5.1).

Requirements for an optimal examination include:

- the administration of intravenous contrast delivered rapidly[26,27];
- the acquisition of images during peak liver enhancement before contrast equilibrium (within 2–3 min of an intravenous injection); and
- with sufficient speed to minimize respiratory artefacts.

The peak enhancement time will vary depending on the patient's weight, cardiovascular status and other factors such as the state of hydration, renal function and the presence of underlying disease.[28]

Smartprep is a facility now available on some scanners, which removes the guesswork when choosing the optimal temporal window. It ensures that scanning occurs during peak enhancement. It is an automated contrast monitoring system, designed by General Electric Systems, Milwaukee, WI.[29]

Precontrast Scans

Identification of liver lesions on CT scanning depends on the lesion having a different density from the surrounding liver parenchyma. Metastases usually appear as hypodense and are round or oval. They may have a clearly defined or ill-defined margin. Scans taken prior to intravenous contrast administration are useful when:

- the liver lesion is hypervascular and may become isodense on portal venous imaging;
- to visualize calcification and haemorrhage. Calcification may be seen in metastases from a variety of sites including mucinous carcinoma of the colon, stomach and pancreas and may follow chemotherapy or radiotherapy. Haemorrhage may be a feature of hepatic adenoma, hepatocellular carcinoma, haemangioma and cysts. It is rare in metastases, although it has been reported in melanoma metastases, but may be seen following biopsy,

- to identify steatosis which can be mistaken for tumour infiltration. The presence of fat also changes the appearance of metastases as they may appear isodense or hyperdense on CT. Metastases within a fatty liver may also exhibit posterior echo enhancement on ultrasound, which is normally a feature of cysts. This appears to be due to the increased attenuation of the ultrasound beam by the fat and the greater transmittance posterior to the lesion relative to that of the surrounding tissue. On CT scanning, diffuse infiltrative metastatic disease may be difficult to evaluate particularly where there is steatosis. This type of pattern may be seen with metastases from breast, colon and pancreatic primary lesions and is also seen with lymphoma. Fatty infiltration is seen particularly in relation to alcohol abuse, diabetes, and obesity. It may affect a focal area of the liver or the entire organ.
- The preliminary scans also allow an estimation of the size of the liver and the subsequent contrast study can be tailored accordingly.

Multiplicity of lesions favours a diagnosis of metastatic disease but multiple cysts and abscesses can give a similar appearance. The Hounsfield attenuation values (0–10 in cysts) may help in differentiation but hypodense metastases have a range of attenuation from 0–75 HU and this may not be conclusive. Infected cysts may have higher attenuation. Cystic metastases, however, may also occur and may have an attenuation of <20 HU. Cystic metastases may arise from colorectal, carcinoid, ovarian or other primary lesions. On ultrasound scanning, a posterior echo enhancement is characteristic of a fluid-filled lesion but where the metastasis contains a cystic component, posterior enhancement may also be present. Necrotic or cystic metastases may become secondarily infected and the differentiation from abscesses with CT attenuation values of 0–45 HU, may be impossible on imaging studies. Biopsy may also be unhelpful as pus may be obtained from both types of lesion. Observation over a period may show resolution of the changes but resection may be the best management option. Abscesses may be pyogenic, hydatid or amoebic. A full abdominal and pelvic scan should be undertaken in these patients to search for a source of infection, e.g. appendicitis or diverticulitis.

Unenhanced scans are insensitive in the detection of small lesions and in order to improve the conspicuity of liver lesions and the detection rate, techniques have been devised which increase the contrast difference between the lesion and the liver.

Secondary deposits in the liver receive their blood supply predominantly from the hepatic arterial blood and the majority are hypovascular appearing on unenhanced scans as areas of low attenuation. During angiography, most metastases receive so little arterial blood that they are not identified unless they are of sufficient size or so numerous that they displace vascular structures. Similarly when intravenous contrast is administered during CT, because there is a paucity of vessels delivering contrast to the lesion, they do not enhance. The portal venous blood contributes 75% of the hepatic blood flow and this supplies normal liver tissue. As this enhances, the difference in attenuation values between the tumour and the surrounding liver is increased, improving conspicuity of the lesion. A number of studies have shown that the lesion detection rate is improved when intravenous contrast is used.

Liver Screening Protocol

Using a spiral scanner:

- Precontrast 10 mm scans are taken from the diaphragm through the liver. These may be axial or helical.
- 100 ml i.v. non-ionic contrast medium are injected at 2–3 ml/s using a power injector.
- Using a scan delay of 40–45 s 7 mm × 7 mm scans are performed craniocaudally through the liver.

Using a non-spiral scanner, the delay should be less, since the scanning time will be greater than it is for the spiral scanner.

Postcontrast, metastases do not enhance but they may exhibit peripheral ring enhancement around the low attenuation lesion. This reflects peripheral vascularity around an avascular lesion and is particularly evident on CT angiography (CTA) examinations (see below).

Protocol for Hypervascular Lesion

Precontrast 10 mm scans are obtained through the liver. The most superior and inferior limits of scanning are chosen. An estimate of the liver size and time of each phase is provided. It is our practice to

perform the biphasic examination by scanning through the liver using 7-mm intervals in a caudocranial direction from the most inferior level chosen, introducing a 10–20 s delay (depending on the time taken to complete the initial phase) at the most superior level, followed by craniocaudal scanning during the portal venous phase, again using 7-mm intervals. The initiation of scanning is triggered by means of the Smartprep facility, and placing the 'region of interest' icon on the abdominal aorta.

Delayed Scanning

CT scanning 4–6 hours after contrast injection may be helpful in differentiating tumours from perfusion defects. After this period of time the hepatocytes will have excreted approximately 1–2% of the contrast load administered. Where there is a perfusion defect, particularly after CTAP (see below) this will appear isoattenuating with normal liver.

Detection of Extrahepatic Disease

In the case of patients with a history of a colorectal primary lesion, a full abdominal and pelvic scan is performed to evaluate the presence of extrahepatic disease, particularly the recognized sites of nodal spread and to look for recurrence of tumour at the primary site. Following the contrast liver study, scanning is continued from the inferior aspect of the liver to the symphysis pubis at 10-mm intervals. A chest radiograph is included in the initial assessment. Some centres would routinely perform CT examination of the thorax in addition, where resection is being considered. CT will detect more lesions than are demonstrated by chest radiography.

CT scanning does, however, underestimate the extent of extrahepatic tumour. Large peritoneal or capsular deposits can be detected but subtle neoplastic infiltration to the peritoneum cannot be identified by cross-sectional imaging and identification of metastatic spread to normal-sized lymph nodes is a further area where CT imaging is deficient, identifying between only 22–73% involved nodes.

The dual blood supply of the liver together with the fact that the predominant blood supply to both primary and secondary liver tumours is arterial and the predominant blood supply to normal liver is derived from the portal vein, has stimulated the development of techniques which either selectively increase the density of either hepatic arterial or portal venous blood.

CT Arterial Portography (CTAP)

The patient is initially brought to the vascular suite where, under local anaesthesia and using a percutaneous transfemoral access, a catheter is placed in either the superior mesenteric or the splenic artery. A 6Fr superior mesenteric catheter or sidewinder configuration is used. It is adviseable to use a catheter with multiple sideholes as impaction of an end-hole catheter tip into a small branch will lead to extravasation of contrast and a non-uniform delivery of the agent resulting in a degradation of the images. Catheter placement in the splenic artery produces greater parenchymal enhancement and fewer nontumoural perfusion defects. With the catheter tip well sited in the splenic artery, no contrast can enter the hepatic arterial system prior to the delivery of portal venous contrast to the liver parenchyma. Using the superior mesenteric artery, preliminary angiography is required to ascertain whether there is a replaced or right hepatic artery arising from this vessel and if so, to advance the catheter tip more distally to avoid contrast entering this vessel early and degrading the examination. It is our experience that even when there is no aberrant hepatic artery, contrast can pass via the pancreatico-duodenal arcades to the hepatic artery during contrast injection. The less contrast used during catheter placement the better as that used will equilibrate prior to CT scanning and some lesion to liver contrast will be lost. In general, an experienced angiographer can site a splenic artery catheter without preliminary angiography and only a small volume of contrast (5–10 ml) is required to check that a branch artery has not been inadvertently selected.

Following catheter placement, the patient is transferred to the CT scanning suite. Preliminary low-dose 10-mm unenhanced scans are carried out. An average volume of 100 cc of contrast is injected at 3–4 ml/s using a pump injector and 7 mm × 7 mm or 10 mm × 10 mm scans obtained after a 20–25 s delay. Depending on the patient or liver size, the volume of contrast is modified. It is our practice to use a biphasic examination, beginning to scan at around 30 s after initiation of injection (or using Smartprep

localized on the spleen, with a splenic artery injection) and scanning in a caudocranial direction to the diaphragm After a 18–20 s delay, a second spiral is performed in a craniocaudal direction. The first spiral allows excellent visualization of the portal veins before parenchymal opacification and the hepatic veins have opacified by the time the cranial sections are obtained (Figure 5.2). The second spiral provides good parenchymal enhancement.

The examination is associated with tumorous and artefactual defects in around 20% patients. Large tumours may compress or occlude portal branches giving rise to diminished flow in the tumour-bearing area. The most common non-tumourous defects occur in the left lobe immediately anterior to the porta or adjacent to the intersegmental fissure. These 'pseudolesions' appears to be the result of aberrant portal venous drainage and have been well described. They appear as low density lesions with a rounded or flat configuration. Delayed scanning will show that these areas will become isodense with adjacent liver tissue later. CTAP is unreliable in patients when there is portal hypertension and is not accurate in assessing extrahepatic disease. Nevertheless it is currently recognized as the best modality for detecting focal liver lesions, particularly those <1 cm in diameter and is routinely employed prior to surgical resection in many hepatobiliary centres. Soyer reported a 94% detection rate for hepatic metastases from colorectal cancer using CTAP.[30]

A study by Seneterre showed that ferumoxide-enhanced MRI was more accurate that nonenhanced MRI and equivalent to CTAP in sensitivity and specificity for the detection of hepatic metastases.[31] However in this study, limited angiography was performed prior to catheter placement for CTAP and a non-spiral scanner was used, factors which may have affected the CTAP results. Nevertheless CTAP is an invasive examination which is currently reserved for those patients under consideration for hepatic resection. MR is noninvasive and can be used as a screening tool.

Soyer examined 11 patients using both CTAP and MRI-AP (MRI-during arterial portography).[32] In the MRI study he injected 4 ml of a 0.5 mmol/kg solution of gadolinium tetraazacyclododecane tetaacetic acid (DOTA) into the superior mesenteric artery during multisection gradient echo imaging. The MRI examination depicted 29 of 31 masses (sensitivity 94%) while the CTAP detected 27 of the 31 masses (87% sensitivity) Neither examination had a false positive

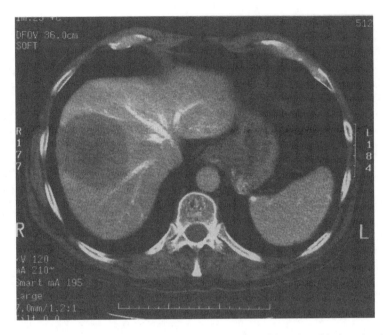

Figure 5.2. CTAP showing a large metastasis in segment 8. Good delineation of the hepatic veins.

(specificity 100%). It is likely, however, that MRI-AP would suffer from the same perfusion defects as CTAP since these are the result of aberrant venous drainage. This study also did not use spiral scanning. The numbers are small and although the results with MRI-AP were comparable to those of CTAP, larger numbers would be required before any definite conclusion could be reached.

Intraoperative ultrasound (IOUS) rivals CTAP in sensitivity and in addition can provide information with regard to peritoneal and nodal spread which is not obtainable by other means of pre-operative imaging. CTAP, however, can provide a detailed map of the hepatic vascular structures and the relationship of tumours to these vessels. It can prevent unnecessary laparotomies in some cases by demonstrating the extent of disease.

Because spiral scanning allows a fast and continuous volumetric data acquisition, three-dimensional reconstruction of the hepatic vascular structures can be used to demonstrate segmental anatomy with CTA and CTAP studies. Depiction of the hepatic arteries and the portal venous system, comparable or even better than conventional angiograms can be achieved. Maximum intensity projection images (MIPs) (Figure 5.3) can be obtained and a surface rendering of the liver (Figure 5.4) may provide additional information.

MRI angiography can also display the vascular structures without an arterial catheter or contrast injection but at present this is not as accurate as CT reconstructions. However as technological improvements develop, pre-operative hepatic angiography may be replaced by CT or MRI three-dimensional reconstructions.

Volumetric analysis using three-dimensional CTAP can be used to assess the volume of the proposed liver remnant when a major resection is planned. Where this is estimated to be too small (<35%) of the total liver volume, portal vein embolization may be employed to induce atrophy in the tumour-bearing area and compensatory hypertrophy in the non-diseased lobe, thus enabling safe resection to be undertaken (see below).

CT Angiography (CTA)

This technique is less frequently used than CTAP. The technique is similar, in that the patient is initially brought to the vascular suite, where, under local anaesthesia, and using a transfemoral approach, a catheter is placed in the proper hepatic artery prior to transfer to CT scanning. Initial digital

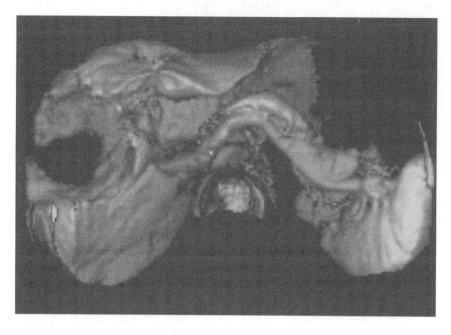

Figure 5.3. Three-dimensional surface rendered CTAP image in a patients with a right lobe metastasis.

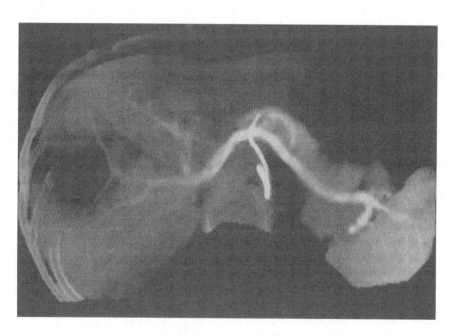

Figure 5.4. MIP reconstruction of portal veins in patient with right lobe metastasis.

angiography is required to evaluate the arterial anatomy.

Since only 50% patients have standard hepatic arterial anatomy (the entire hepatic arterial supply arising via the coeliac axis and common hepatic artery), there will be areas of liver parenchyma which will not be perfused during the CT study.

A volume of approximately 10 ml of contrast, with concentration of 300 mg iodine per ml, is diluted with 20 ml of saline and the mixture is introduced by pump injector at a rate of 2–3 mls.

In a study of 100 patients, who had contrast enhanced CT, CTA and MRI prior to laparotomy, CTA detected 94% of all the lesions, MRI only 70%

and CT 66%. CTA had a sensitivity of 82% in detecting lesions of <1 cm compared with 20% during MRI and 5% on CT. MRI provided the best definition of the hepatic vasculature and was most accurate in assessing vascular involvement. None of the techniques was accurate in defining extrahepatic disease.[33]

With CTA, the hypovascular lesions do not enhance but may show a marked peripheral rim enhancement. Hypervascular lesions show the feeding arteries to the lesions and focal enhancement against the unenhanced liver parenchyma.

CT Biopsy Technique

Most percutaneous biopsy procedures are performed using ultrasound guidance but in certain specific situations, CT is better, e.g. if the lesion is not easily seen by ultrasound and better visualized by CT or where a safe track to the lesion, without passing through bowel for example, is difficult to see on ultrasound. As with other biopsy techniques, correction of any clotting derangement is carried out prior to the procedure. A preliminary scan is performed to localize the lesion. A metal marker is applied to the skin surface. This can be seen on the subsequent scans and aids localization. Spiral CT has helped to speed up biopsy procedures. The scans are examined to determine the safest route to the lesion and if necessary the gantry can be tilted to enable the optimal route to be accessed. The distance to the lesion is measured on the scan. The laser light on the scanner is used to mark the skin level. The skin surface is cleansed in a sterile fashion and local anaesthesia is introduced. The needle is advanced to the required distance and a scan performed to assess the accuracy of the puncture. Adjustments can be made with repeated scans until the optimum biopsy is obtained. Stereotaxic CT guidance devices can be helpful when the target lesion is small and deeply located.

Magnetic Resonance Imaging

The search for the optimal MRI pulse sequences in the detection and characterisation of liver metas-

tases is still continuing. The general trend is to shorten the duration of the examination time for practical purposes, without degradation of the image quality. But there is as yet little consensus among investigators as to which set of parameters is best because of the large number of permutations. Technical details of the physics of MRI and the sequence variations available are not included in this text. Interested readers are referred to major Radiology and MRI textbooks.

Contrast Agents

The use of contrast agents in the detection of liver tumours requires optimisation of the pulse sequences according to the type of agents used (e.g. Gadolinium DTPA, Superparamagnetic Iron Oxides (SPIO), Ultrasmall SPIO (USPIO) or Manganese DpDp).

Gadolinium DTPA is an extracellular agent with pharmacokinetics similar to that of intravenous contrast agents used in conjunction with CT scanning and similar rapid imaging strategies are therefore required.

The SPIOs target the reticuloendothelial system (RES). The timing of the scans is less critical with these agents compared with gadolinium DTPA. With their use, there is loss of signal intensity of the liver and spleen when used in comjunction with the T2 weighted sequences (Figure 5.5). There is no uptake by tumours devoid of Kupffer cells and they maintain their baseline signal intensity. The lesion to liver contrast-to-noise ratio is therefore markedly increased with resulting improvement in the detection and characterisation of liver tumours. However a recent study comparing SPIO-enhanced MRI (using Endorem) with IOUS and histology as the gold standard, showed that the sensitivity of Endorem-enhanced MRI in the detection of liver metastases was only 56% compared with 80% for IOUS.[34]

The rapid pace of technological developments in MRI and to some extent in CT, has led to numerous studies comparing the two modalities in the detection and characterisation of hepatic tumours. Many of these studies are not comparable due to the use of different MRI and CT techniques and hardware. However there is now some consensus that MRI is as sensitive as CT (if not more so) in the detection of

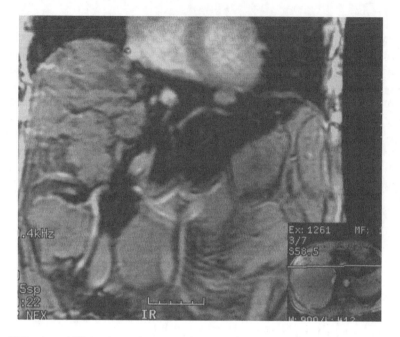

Figure 5.5. SPIO-enhanced MR showing total tumour replacement of the right lobe and a small metastasis in segment 2.

liver tumours. In the characterisation and differentiation between benign and malignant hepatic tumours, MRI is now well recognised to be superior to CT. MRI is still a relatively new modality and most of the current techniques are likely to undergo further refinement before their ultimate clinical role is clear.

Follow-up Post-therapy

Follow-up of patients who have undergone surgery or other interventional therapies for metastatic liver disease involves, in addition to clinical evaluation and assessment of serum tumour markers, a regular imaging survey of the liver itself. For the most part, US or contrast-enhanced CT are used for this purpose. In certain situations, MRI imaging may be more accurate. Following lipoidol chemoembolization of liver metastases, for example, successful destruction of the lesions or recurrent growth is difficult to evaluate using US and CT. MRI has been shown to be more accurate in assessing the results of these therapies.

MRI-guided Biopsy

In order to perform MRI-guided intervention, the scanner used must have an open configuration to allow operator access and in addition a variety of MRI-compatible tools must be available. Research is underway into the design of an appropriate scanner with the specific performance of interventional procedures in mind. Real-time MRI capabilities are required in order to target and guide needle position. This is a development which will be available in the foreseeable future.

Angiography and Venography

Angiography is not used in the detection of liver tumours but can demonstrate hypervascular tumours, e.g. hepatic adenomas, focal nodular hyperplasia and hypervascular metastases. Abscesses can mimic hypervascular metastases on angiographic studies and biopsy should be carried out when the clinical picture warrants further clarification. With improvements in CT and MRI, there is less need for conventional angiographic examinations.

Angiography still has a role, however:

- It provides a roadmap prior to hepatic resection, or for palliative therapy such as hepatic arterial or portal venous chemotherapy infusion, devascularization procedures or chemoembolization. Anatomical variations are common: a right or replaced hepatic artery may arise from the superior mesentric artery in up to 25% cases while a left or accessory left hepatic artery may arise from the left gastric artery in approximately 18% cases. Pre-operative identification of variations of normal anatomy is useful in surgical planning and in the patient for whom regional infusion therapy is to be undertaken and so appropriate measures are planned to ensure optimum liver perfusion.
- It allows identifying the source of bleeding in patients with spontaneous haemorrhage from a liver tumour and directing embolization.
- It can be used in characterization problems, e.g. 'haemangioma or metastasis', where cross-sectional imaging results are equivocal. On angiographic studies, haemangiomas have a classical peripheral enhancement which gradually fills in centripetally. The contrast is retained in the lesion well after the contrast has cleared from the surrounding parenchyma and vessels. Hypervascular metastases do not generally have this 'filling-in' feature and do not retain the contrast in the same way as contrast clears from the lesion fairly rapidly. There is frequently a central area of non-vascularity in large lesions, where there is fibrosis, necrosis or thrombosis. If the characteristic features are present, the diagnosis by angiography is evident as with CT and MRI. However a thrombosed haemangioma may not have the classical appearance and may appear avascular.

Haemangiomas are common, occurring in 1–20%, mainly in women of the postmenopausal age group. In general they appear as solitary lesions but in >10% they are multiple. They may occur in association with focal nodular hyperplasia and have been described in association with cysts. For the most part they are asymptomatic but they can enlarge in pregnancy and there is a small risk of spontaneous rupture. Biopsy of the lesion can add to the risk of rupture. They may thrombose when the patient is on oestrogen therapy. Using MRI, cysts and haemangiomas can usually be differentiated. Where the lesions are discovered incidentally on US, CT or MRI and have a typical appearance, no further action is required. In the patient who has a known history of primary malignant disease, where the findings are atypical, where the liver function tests are abnormal or the patient has symptoms, such as right upper quadrant pain, further tests should be considered. Angiography is safer than biopsy. SPECT (single photon emission computerized tomography, see below) may be considered and if the results remain inconclusive, follow-up studies or biopsy may be required.

The technique of hepatic arteriography involves the selective examination of the coeliac axis and superior mesenteric artery. Superselective catheterization of all the hepatic arteries may be required. In some cases, there may be blood supply from extrahepatic arteries such as the adrenal or the phrenic artery and these vessels may require selective studies also. Selective splenic artery or superior mesenteric studies should include films taken during the portal venous phase in those patients considered for hepatic resection. Up to 15% patients with liver metastases will have tumour thrombus within the portal or the hepatic veins. Ascites and varices may be evident.

In patients being considered for surgical resection and in whom there is doubt about the size of the potential liver remnant (especially in a cirrhotic patient), angiography can provide useful information to delineate clearly the hepatic vascular structures. In a small percentage of patients in whom the proposed disease-free liver remnant is small, contralateral portal vein embolization may be considered. The nutrients within the portal vein are hepatotrophic and occlusion of the portal vein branches leads to atrophy of the non-perfused area. The redirecting of all the portal flow to a small area stimulates hypertrophy of the normal tissue and in some cases this will render the patient suitable for curative surgery.

The technique of portal vein embolization involves gaining access to the right or left portal branch percutaneously. Preliminary sedation and analgesia is administered. Using local anaesthesia and a technique similar to that used for right or left transhepatic cholangiography, a peripheral branch of the portal vein is selected. Either fluoroscopic or US guidance may be used. A 5Fr catheter is advanced into the main portal vein. Contrast is injected and films obtained in order to map out the portal venous anatomy. The branch (or branches) supplying the diseased area is selected and embolized with gelfoam, detachable balloon or coils. The transhepatic track is embolised as the catheter is withdrawn to avoid bleeding from the track. Follow-up volumetric studies are carried out using CT or MRI. Hypertrophy of the disease-free liver may take several weeks or months.

Small hypovascular tumours will not be identified during angiography unless they cause displacement of the vascular structures. Large masses will show mass effect. Metastases can invade the portal vein although not as frequently as hepatocellular carcinoma. Focal atrophy of the liver may result from portal vein invasion. Atrophy may also be evident following chemoembolization procedures. This may be the result of fibrosis around the portal vein branches or reduced blood supply to the area.

The role of angiography has changed, having been superseded by other modalities in the demonstration of vascular structures. Angiographic techniques remain important in characterization of a few select lesions and in the planning and delivery of the interventional therapies.

Hepatic Scintigraphy

Planar Scintigraphy and SPECT (single photon emission computerized tomography)

Since US, CT and MRI studies may all fail to characterise a small percentage of haemangiomas, radionuclide studies using ^{99m}Tc-radiolabelled red blood cells have also been used to resolve problems. A small volume of the patient's blood is labelled with ^{99m}Tc pertechnetate and re-injected when the patient is positioned in a tomographic gamma camera. A dynamic study is performed followed by the acquisition of a static image. After a further 90–120 min, a SPECT scan is obtained. The introduction of SPECT, a single slice tomographic technique, improves the evaluation of small lesions due to better spatial resolution. By a data reconstruction process, images of body sections can be obtained. This can be useful in separating background activity from lesion activity. An uncomplicated peripheral haemangioma of $\geq$ 1 cm can be accurately diagnosed by demonstrating slow uptake during the

arterial phase and delayed blood pool activity. In contrast, hypervascular metastases or hepatocellular carcinomas should show increased activity during the arterial phase as well as delayed blood pool activity. However false-negative scans can occur when the haemangiomas are affected by thrombosis or fibrosis and where the lesion is adjacent to a large blood vessel.

PET (position emission tomography)

Positron emission tomography also provides information displayed in tomographic sections. This technique employs positron emitters, e.g. ^{15}O, ^{11}C, ^{13}N, ^{18}F and ^{68}Ga to label naturally occurring biomolecules and pharmaceutical agents. In the context of liver tumour detection, IF-2-fluoro-2-deoxy-D-glucose (FDG), which shows an increased uptake in tumour tissue, has been used. It is useful not only in the detection of tumour but in monitoring its response to treatment. The agent 5-fluorouracil may be used in the systemic chemotherapy of colorectal malignancy. However, the overall response rate is low (10–15%) Those tumours exhibiting a high uptake of FDG should show a good response to this treatment. FDG SPECT is feasible, cheaper and more accessible than PET. It has a lower sensitivity than PET in the detection of lesions <3 cm. PET, however, is very expensive and there is limited access to it.

Radioimmunodetection

The development of radioimmunodetection techniques may in the future allow more accurate staging of metastatic disease. Although labelled antibody techniques for tumour scanning dates back to the mid seventies, monoclonal antibody (mAb) imaging has been available for clinical application only in the last few years. The concept is similar to nuclear medicine studies. A monospecific antibody to a tumour-associated antigen is tagged with a radioactive moiety and injected into the patient. Distribution of the antibody can then be imaged to identify focal areas of uptake. A number of different antibody carriers and radionuclide tags are under investigation. The antibody component of the complex is designed to attach selectively to antigen receptors on the tumour cell surface. Aggregates of the complex then appear as areas of increased uptake or 'hot spots' on the photoscans, outlining tumour deposits.

At the present time mAb is more likely to be used as a complementary technique to improve tumour detection in areas where CT and MRI are still less than optimal. It appears to be more sensitive than CT scanning in the detection of colorectal cancer and may be useful in depicting small peritoneal deposits. However it is still limited in the detection of hepatic metastases because of the background uptake in the liver. Using ^{111}In-labelled mAb CCR086, sensitivity in the detection of colorectal liver metastases was only 68%.[35] The same group of workers have also shown that the sensitivity in colorectal hepatic metastases detection was only 20% when using ^{111}In-labelled mAb CYT-103.[36] However this technique was reported to be particularly useful in identifying sites of disease not visualised with CT.[37] Metastatic disease in the lungs, bones, extra-abdominal lymph nodes and brain have also been identified by mAb imaging. Results of a multicentre trial assessing OncoScint Cr 103 suggest that the technique is more sensitive than CT in the detection of extrahepatic disease whilst CT is superior in the detection of liver metastases. The combination of the two techniques can provide complementary information and greater overall accuracy than either test alone.[38] A more recent study evaluating the use of SPECT and CT/MRI image registration in radiolabelled mAb ^{131}I-CC49 studies of colorectal carcinoma suggest that the technique would allow more accurate anatomic assessment of sites of abnormal uptake.[39] Further studies are still required to improve the technique.

Radiolabelled monoclonal antibodies to carcinoembryonic antigen or tumour-associated glycoprotein can be used to detect liver metastases in colorectal cancer and have a higher sensitivity than CT scanning in the detection of extrahepatic metastases.[40] False positives do occur with this technique and further refinements are required. Immunoscintigraphy may be helpful in locating metastases when the serum carcinoembryonic antigen concentrations rise.

Radiolabelled antibodies can detect the primary disease but are of greater value in tumour staging, in detecting recurrent tumour and occult metastatic disease. A single injection of the radiotracer allows the whole body to be imaged. Five per cent of patients with colorectal carcinoma will have lung or bone secondaries at the time of presentation. Routine chest radiography is generally performed but it is not considered cost-effective to perform routine bone scanning in these patients. This is gen-erally reserved for the investigation of symptomatic lesions. Immunoscintography may have a future role in the preliminary staging assessment.

It is currently considered that the most important role for immunoscintigraphy is in the follow-up of patients with colorectal cancers for detection of recurrent disease.

Radioimmunoguided surgery has also been described. In this technique, the patient is given an intravenous injection of colorectal cancer antigens labelled with ^{125}I and during laparotomy, a hand held gamma detecting probe is used to locate tumour tissue and guide biopsy.[41]

Conclusion

It is recognized that, even with the use of state-of-the art pre-operative imaging facilities, some patients classified as 'resectable' will not be considered suitable candidates at the time of surgery. Currently available imaging studies understage metastatic disease. Extrahepatic disease, particularly peritoneal spread and metastatic disease within small lymph nodes, will not be identified. Early detection of liver metastases measuring only a few millimetres in size is desirable in order that more patients can benefit from curative surgery. Spiral CT arterial portography is considered to be in the lead in detection of small liver lesions but SPIO contrast-enhanced MRI scanning is set to challenge its lead. Both of these techniques now regularly identify sub-centimetre lesions. MRI is judged best in characterizing liver lesions but characterization of these small nodules is a problem since classical features associated with specific lesions have not developed at this early stage and serum tumour markers will not be evident. None of the preoperative techniques allows the detection of microscopic metastases. Neither CTAP nor SPIO-enhanced MRI is accurate in the assessment of extrahepatic disease. This is best evaluated by laparoscopic and intra-operative examination, which provide complementary information to the imaging studies. The growing development of radioimmunodetection may hold the key to further progress in this area.

There have been tremendous advances in technology in the last ten years particularly in relation to ultrasound, CT and MRI with the development of new contrast agents for all of these modalities. The application of multiplanar reformatting in CT and MRI adds a further dimension to these studies. Indeed, the capability of the integral computerized facilities of modern scanners is by no means fully exploited. Hepatic surgeons and radiologists are interactive in the drive to achieve a 100% diagnostic accuracy. Perhaps in the future the hepatobiliary specialist will have a single non-invasive tool available to provide all the required diagnostic information but that dream is not yet in our sights. As we are carried along enthusiastically on a tide of exciting innovations, we might be forgiven for believing that 'it is better to travel than to arrive'!

References

1. Machi J, Isomoto H, Kurhiji T et al. Accuracy of intraoperative ultrasound in diagnosing liver metastases from colorectal cancer: evaluation with post-operative follow-up results. World J Surg 1991; 15:551–557.
2. Takayasu K, Moriyama N, Muramatsu Y et al. The diagnosis of small hepatocellular carcinomas: Efficacy of various imaging procedures in 100 patients. AJR 1990; 155:49–54.
3. Leen E, Angerson WG, Wotherspoon H, Moule B, Cooke TG, McCardle CS Comparison of DPI and IOUS in diagnosing occult colorectal liver metastases. Radiology 1995; 195:113–116.
4. Soyer P, Levesque M, Elias D, Zeitoun G, Roche A. Preoperative assessment of resectability of hepatic metastases from colonic carcinoma: CT portography vs sonography and dynamic CT. AJR 1992; 159:741–744.
5. Soyer P, Levesque M, Elias D et al. Detection of liver metastases from colorectal cancer: comparison of intraoperative US and CT during arterial portography. Radiology 1992; 183:541–544.
6. Machi J, Isomoto H, Yamashita Y et al. Intraoperative ultrasonography in the screening for liver metastases from colorectal cancer: comparative accuracy with traditional procedures. Surgery 1987; 101(6):678–684.
7. Ferrucci JT. Liver tumour imaging: current concepts. AJR 1990; 150:473–484.
8. Wernecke K, Vassallo P, Bick U, Diederich S, Peters P. The distinction between benign and malignant liver tumours on sonography: value of a hypoechoic halo. AJR 1992; 159:1005–1009.
9. Kudo M, Tomita S, Tochio H et al. Sonographic angiography: value in differential diagnosis of hepatic tumours. AJR 1992; 158:65–74.
10. Maresca G, Barbaro B, Summaria V et al. Colour Doppler ultrasonography in the differential diagnosis of focal hepatic lesions. The SHU 508A experience. Radiol Med 1994; 87(Suppl 1 al n 5):41–49.
11. Freeny PC, Marks WM Hepatic haemangioma: dynamic bolus CT. AJR 1986; 147:711–719.
12. Charnley RM, Morris DL, Dennison AR et al. Detection of colorectal liver metastases using intraoperative ultrasonography. Br J Surg 1991; 78:45–48.
13. Kudo M, Tomita S, Tochio H et al. Small hepatocellular carcinoma: diagnosis with US angiography with intraarterial CO_2 microbubbles. Radiology 1992; 182:155–160.
14. Garbagnati F, Milella M, Spreafico C et al. US contrast enhancement with intraarterial CO_2 injection in staging hepatocellular carcinomas. Radiol Med 1994; 87:(Suppl. 1):65–
15. Kubo S, Kinoshita H, Hirohashi T et al. Preoperative localisation of hepatomas by sonography with microbubbles of carbon dioxide. AJR 1994; 1405–6.
16. El Mouaaouy A, Becker HD, Schlief R et al. Rat liver model for testing intraoperative echo contrast sonography. Surg Endosc 1990; 4:114–117.
17. Braunschweig R, Stern W, Dabidian A et al. Contrast enhanced colour Doppler studies of liver vessels. Abstract of Investigators meeting in Berlin. Echocardiography 1993; November issue.
18. Olliff S, Olliff J. Assessment of SHU 508A for enhancement of Doppler signals in liver and kidney vessels and renal tumours. Abstract of Investigators meeting in Berlin. Echocardiography 1993; November issue.
19. Leen E, Angerson WJ, Warren H et al. Improved colour Doppler flow imaging of colorectal hepatic metastases using galactose microparticles: a preliminary report. Br J Surg 1994; 220(5):663–667.
20. Angeli E, Carpanelli R, Crespi G et al. Efficacy of SHU 508 A in colour Doppler ultrasonography of hepatocellular carcinoma vascularisation. Radiol Med 1994; 87(Suppl. 1 al n.5):24–31.
21. Carter R, Anderson JH, Cooke TG et al. Is the change in the hepatic perfusion index in the presence of hepatic metastases due to a humoural agent? Br J Cancer 1992; 65:58.
22. Warren HW, Angerson WJ, Leen E et al. Haemodynamic changes associated with colorectal liver metastases: evidence of a humoural mediator. Br J Surg 1993; 80:1461.
23. Leen E, Angerson WJ, Wotherspoon H, Moule B, Cooke TG, McCardle CS 1993; Comparison of DPI and IOUS in diagnosing occult colorectal liver metastases. Ann Surg 1994; 220(5):663–667.
24. Leen E, Angerson WJ, Wotherspoon H, Moule B, Cooke TG, McCardle CS Comparison of laparotomy, CT, US and DPI in the detection of colorectal metastases. Radiology 1995; 195:113–116.
25. Leen E, Angerson WJ, Moule B, Cooke TG, McCardle CS Prognostic power of DPI in patients following curative resection for colorectal cancer: correlation with outcome at two years. Ann Surg 1996; 223(2):199–203.
26. PA Garcia, VM, Bonaldi, Bret PM et al. Effect of rate of contrast medium injection on hepatic enhancement at CT. Radiology 1996; 199:185–189.
27. Small WC, Nelson RC, Bernardino ME, Brummer LT Contrast-enhanced spiral CT of the liver: effect of different amounts and injection rates of contrast material on early contrast enhancement. AJR 1994; 163:87–92.
28. Dodd GD, Baron RL. Investigation of contrast enhancement in CT of the liver; the need for improved methods (commentary) AJR 1993; 160:643–646.
29. Silverman PM, Roberts S, Tefft MC et al. Helical CT of the liver; clinical application of an automated computer technique, Smartprep, for obtaining images with optimal contrast enhancement. AJR 1995; 165:73–78.
30. Soyer P, Bluemke DA, Hruban RH, Sitzmann JV, Fishman EK. Primary malignant neoplasms from colorectal cancer: detection and false positive findings with helical CT during arterial portography. Radiology 1994; 192:389–392.
31. Seneterre E, Taourel P, Bouvier Y et al. Detection of hepatic metastases: ferumoxide-enhanced MR imaging versus unenhanced MR imaging and CT during arterial portography Radiology 1996; 200:785–792.

32. Soyer P, J-P Laissy, A Sibert *et al.* Focal hepatic masses: comparison of detection during arterial portography with MR imaging and CT. *Radiology* 1994; 737–740.

33. Sitzmann JV, Coleman JA, Pitt HA, Zerhouni E, Fishman E, Kaufman SL. Preoperative assessment of malignant tumours. *Am J Surg* 1990; **159**:137–142.

34. Hagspiel KD, Neidl KFW, Eichenberger AC *et al.* Detection of liver metastases: comparison of SPIO enhanced and unenhanced MRI at 1.5T with dynamic CT, IOUS and percutaneous US. *Radiology* 1995; **196**:471–478.

35. Abdel-Nabi H, Levine G, Lamki L *et al.* Colorectal carcinoma metastases: Detection with [III]In-labelled monoclonal antibody CCRO86. *Radiology* 1990; **176**:117–122.

36. Abdel-Nabi H, Doerr RJ, Chan HW *et al.* [III]In-labelled monoclonal antibody immunoscintigraphy in colorectal carcinoma: safety, sensitivity and preliminary clinical results. *Radiology* 1992; **185**:179–186.

37. Collier BD, Abdel-Nabi H, Doerr RJ *et al.* Immunoscintigraphy performed with [III]In-labelled CYT-103 in the management of colorectal cancer: comparison with CT. *Radiology* 1992; **185**:179–186.

38. Doerr RJ, Abdel-Nabi H, Krag D *et al.* Radiolabeled antibody imaging in the management of colorectal cancer: results of a multicentre clinical study. *Ann Surg* 1991; **214**(2):118–124.

39. Scott AM, Macalpinlac HA, Divgi CR *et al.* Clinical validation of SPECT and CT/MRI image registration in radiolabeled monoclonal antibody studies of colorectal carcinoma. *J Nucl Med* 1994; **35**(12):1976–1984.

40. Lamki LM, Patt YZ, Rosenblum MG *et al.* Metastatic colorectal cancer: Radioimmunoscintigraphy with a stabilised [III]In-labeled F (ab')$_2$ fragment of an anti-CEA monoclonal antibody. *Radiology* 1990; **14**:370–374.

41. Aftab F, Stoldt HS, Testori A *et al.* Radioimmunoguided surgery and colorectal cancer (Review) *Eur J Surg Oncol* 1996 (Aug); 22(4): 381–388.

Surgical Resection

François Paye and Bernard Nordlinger

Introduction

The surgical resection of hepatic metastases from primary colorectal cancer remains today the only therapeutic modality able to ensure five-year survival rates of 25–30% and to ultimately cure some of these patients.[1,2] To achieve a curative resection of hepatic metastases, all the metastatic sites ideally should be resected with a margin of at least 1 cm of healthy parenchyma, while retaining enough liver parenchyma to ensure a normal liver function.[3] Careful patient selection to achieve complete resection is important. Resection should be performed with minimal blood losses in order to minimize postoperative morbidity and mortality and to minimize the recurrence rates.[4,5] To achieve these goals, a thorough knowledge of the liver anatomy is essential. The surgeon must be trained to this type of surgery.

Anatomical Considerations

The segmental structure of the liver was first described in France by Couinaud[6] and has since been adopted worldwide.[7] The liver is divided in two halves (left and right) by the main portal fissure, joining the gallbladder fossa to the anterior aspect of the inferior vena cava. The middle hepatic vein is included in this plane which does not correspond to a visible scissura on the liver surface. The 'right liver' is distinct from the right lobe separated from the left lobe by the umbilical fissure.

Each half of the liver, so defined, receives a portal branch and an arterial branch arising respectively from the division of the portal trunk and the hepatic artery. Each half of the liver is drained by a hepatic duct which joins with the other to form the main hepatic duct. This triad of portal, arterial and biliary elements is included in a dense connective tissue and constitutes the portal pedicle of each half liver. The further intraparenchymatous subdivisions of these portal pedicles determines the division of the liver parenchyma into eight functional entities called segments by Couinaud. Thus, the right liver includes four segments (V, VI, VII, VIII) and the left liver comprises three segments (II, III, IV). An additional segment, the caudate lobe, lies deeply posterior and encircles the inferior vena cava and usually receives its blood supply from the left Portal vein and left hepatic artery. Bile produced by segment I drains primarily through several small bile ducts joining the right and left main biliary ducts. Segments V and VIII form the right anterior sector receiving the corresponding portal pedicle. This sector is separated from the right posterior sector which is composed of segments VI and VII, by a transverse plane containing the right hepatic vein. In each right sector, the segments are separated by a virtual horizontal plane, located at the level of the portal division. The left liver is subdivided in two sectors by a transverse plane containing the left hepatic vein. The left anterior sector includes the segments IV (corresponding to the classical quadrate lobe) and III. The left posterior sector is constituted by the segment II only.

The three main hepatic veins (right, middle and left) delinate the sectors and ensure their venous drainage in the inferior vena cava. Short accessory hepatic veins drain segment I. Variations of the anatomy of the hepatic veins are now well identified

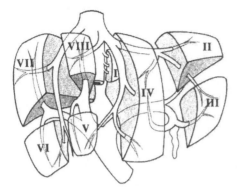

Figure 6.1. The 'exploded liver'. The main portal fissure divides the liver into the right and the left liver, each receiving a separate portal pedicule. Further subdivisions of these pedicules supply the differents sectors and their constitutive segments. The planes of the hepatic veins delineates the sectors.

by intra-operative ultrasound which can detect small accessory veins and atypical division of the main hepatic veins.

Some confusion can result from the American nomenclature in which the right anterior and posterior segments correspond respectively to the right anterior and posterior sectors named by Couinaud. According to this American nomenclature, the left lateral segment comprises the left lobe (Couinaud's segments II and III) and the left medial segment corresponds to the quadrate lobe (Couinaud's segment IV). The Couinaud's segments are named subsegments in this American nomenclature.[8,9]

Hepatic resections have to preserve the portal pedicles and the venous drainage of the remaining parenchyma. The image of the 'exploded liver' (Figure 6.1) should always be borne in mind by the surgeon performing a liver resection, whether segmental or non segmental.[10]

Determination of Resectability

Before undertaking resection of hepatic metastases, three questions must be answered. Are the hepatic lesions true liver metastases? Does the patient's condition allow their resection? Is the planned resection curative?

Diagnosis of Metastases

The diagnosis of liver metastases is developed elsewhere in this book and will therefore not be detailed here. In clinical practice, the surgeon faces two different situations:

- The primary tumour and the metastases are diagnosed synchronously, either before the operation through routine morphological scans, or intra-operatively by liver exploration. If a biopsy is necessary to confirm the diagnosis of the metastasis, it is best performed intra-operatively during the resection of the primary tumour.
- Metastases are discovered metachronously on scheduled repeated scans during the post-operative follow up. Changes on previously normal imaging examinations strongly suggest the diagnosis of hepatic metastases. If a resection is intended, percutaneous biopsy, which risks seeding tumorous deposits on the needle tract, should be avoided. If the diagnosis of hepatic metastasis is in doubt the diagnosis can be confirmed by intra-operative biopsy.

Condition of the Patient and Liver Function

The pre-operative assessment of the general health status of the patient establishes whether, the extent of the planned hepatic resection based on the available imaging data is permissable.

First, the anaesthesist determines whether the patient is able to support a long general anaesthetic procedure and potentially hemorrhagic surgery by standard clinical and anaesthetic criteria, briefly summarized in the ASA (American Society of Anesthiology) score. The cardiocirculatory status of the patient is carefully evaluated hemodynamic to ensure that the patient will tolerate the clamping manoeuvres used during the hepatic resection. Indeed, effects of clamping of the portal pedicle induces a small decrease of the cardiac output and a rise of the arterial pressure, whereas well-tolerated complete hepatic vascular exclusion induces a 50% decrease of the cardiac output with a stable arterial pressure.[11] These haemodynamic modifications are poorly tolerated in a patient treated by chronic adrenergic blockade or whose cardiac function is altered. An ultrasound preoperative assessment of cardiac function is often requested by the anaesthesiologist.

The hepatic functional reserve must be sufficient to allow the extent of the planned resection and to ensure both early recovery of postoperative liver function and subsequent liver regeneration. Metastases are rarely encountered in fibrotic or cirrhotic liver. The deleterious effect of previous chemotherapy on the liver parenchyma and the extent of the resection are therefore the only important considerations. Chemotherapy has reputedly caused liver steatosis and recent data have demonstrated that chemotherapy induces portal or periportal fibrosis and microvascular changes such as peliosis and sinusoidal congestion.[12] These vascular lesions could be responsible for the haemorrhagic difficulties frequently encountered by the surgeon during the parenchymatous section of the post-chemotherapy liver. In a healthy liver, resection of up to six of the eight anatomical segments or up to 75% of the liver volume can be undertaken without inducing postoperative hepatic failure. This resectable volume is reduced in situation where the non-tumorous parenchyma is diseased. The status of the non-tumorous liver is evaluated preoperatively by the hepatic biological blood tests – prothrombin time, albumin, AST, ALT, alkaline phosphatase, gammaGT, bilirubin. A biopsy of the non-tumorous liver is sometimes helpful. Dynamic tests of hepatic clearance such as the clearance of the indocyanine green can be used[13] but the maximum amount of (resectable) liver remains difficult to assess with certainty.

In some selected cases, selective portal embolization performed pre-operatively can induce hypertrophy of the segments which will be left in place. In some cases, this technique allows the surgeon to perform extensive resections, initially considered to be contraindicated because of the small volume of healthy parenchyma.[13,14]

Is the Resection Curative?

Control of Primary Site and Extrahepatic Sites

The primary tumour must be controlled by previous surgery, oncologically performed with adequate safety margins and lymphadenectomy. In patients with synchronous metastases, combined resection of the primary colorectal site and liver metastases is possible and have been reported without added morbidity.[15] Nevertheless, most surgeons prefer to delay the hepatic resection because of the need for a different incision to ensure good exposure for the colorectal and the liver resection. A delay of two or three months allows brief observation of the natural behaviour of the metastatic disease which could be important prognostically.[16] The role of adjuvant

chemotherapy during this delay remains unclear. Rarely, the presence of united extra-hepatic metastases involving lungs or adrenal glands do not necessarily contraindicate hepatic resection if these extrahepatic metastases are also resectable, by a simultaneous or planned staged resection.[17] Reported series of hepatic and lung metastases of colorectal origin favour of such an aggressive policy.[2,18,19]

Pre-operative investigations are therefore directed first to the primary site, including clinical examination, colonoscopy and pelvic ultrasound or MRI to dectect local recurrences of a primary rectal cancer. Chest X-rays and thoracic CT scan are systematically performed to look for pulmonary metastases. Brain CT scan and bone scintigraphy are performed only if symptoms are present, directing the clinician to possible extrahepatic metastases.

Pre-operative Assessment of the Hepatic Involvement

There is no place for palliative liver resections leaving behind known intra- or extrahepatic disease, because survival is not improved.[2,20] The planned resection has therefore to be curative, removing in one procedure all hepatic metastatic sites.[2,20] To delineate the hepatic involvement, a broad number of imaging techniques (detailed elsewhere in this book) is now available. For the follow-up of patients after the resection of their primary tumour, ultrasound is more widely used in Europe than in the United States, because of its general availability and its lower cost. Metastases of colorectal origin are therefore frequently detected on this examination. Doppler ultrasound can depict the arterial and portal vascular supply of the liver and identifies precisely the relationship between the lesion and the liver anatomy. However, its sensitivity is operator-related and is reported to be only 70%, often missing lesions of <2 cm.[21]

A CT scan is therefore usually performed with a bolus injection of intravenous iodine contrast (bolus dynamic computed tomography, CDTC). Sensitivities of 80% of CDTC have been reported.[21,22] It offers to the surgeon readily interpretable images of the metastases and an evaluation of the liver volumetry. This latter aspect is essential in the planning of major liver resection to appreciate the volume of liver parenchyma which will be left in place. In some centres, computed measurement of hepatic volumetry[23,24] is undertaken routinely. The portoscanner is currently the most sensitive technique used to detect hepatic metastases 1 cm in diameter.[25] They appear as small defects in the parenchyma at the portal phase of a superior mesenteric arterial injection, because of their exclusive arterial blood supply. CT angioportography (CTAP) should be systematically performed pre-operatively if a resection appears to be feasible on previous imaging modalities. However, its lack of specificity may mislead the surgeon, who should not deny the patient an exploratory operation on the sole basis of a questionable small defect on liver parenchymography.

MRI appears to be a less invasive and promising means of detecting small hepatic metastasis but its exact place in the detection strategy remains to be defined. variations in sequence and contrast injection[26] may improve its value and it was found to be less sensitive than the CTAP in a prospective comparative study.[27] We do not employ the technique in our daily practice.

With these various imaging procedures, it is possible to accurately define pre-operatively the appropriate type of liver resection in most cases. Some smaller lesions still remain undetected pre-operatively and will be discovered intra-operatively, contraindicating or modifying the resection initially planned. About two-thirds of the metastases judged pre-operatively to be resectable will be effectively resected.[28]

Intra-operative Assessment of the Lesions

The role of laparoscopy used alone or in combination with laparoscopic ultrasound is currently under evaluation. Early reports have shown some efficacy.[29] The results and indications of these new techniques which may avoid a useless larger abdominal incision in some patients are discussed elsewhere (See Chapters 5 and 7).

At laparotomy, a complete exploration of the abdominal cavity is mandatory. The entire gastrointestinal tract is explored and the diaphragm, the paracolic gutters and the pouch of Dougles are palpated for peritoneal deposits. The anatomical routes of lymphatic drainage of the primary tumour are exposed and palpated, as the origin of the inferior mesenteric artery for a primary rectal cancer. The coeliac area is palpated to exclude involvement of the lymphatics draining the liver. Any macroscopically suspect node or peritoneal deposit is biopsied for histological examination. The presence of metastatic lymph nodes in the porta hepatis and the coeliac region considerably worsens the prognosis but is not an absolute contraindication to resection, if they can be completely removed.[2] Several five-year recurrence free surviving patients have been reported.[2] The liver is thoroughly examined and palpated, before and after its mobilization.

Intra-operative ultrasound (US) should be systematically performed by a well-trained surgeon with assistance by a radiologist if required. Using high frequency probes, detection of small intrahepatic lesions can modify the extent of the initially planned operation.[30] US also guides fine needle biopsies necessary to define the precise nature of the detected lesions. Finally, it defines the anatomical relations of the metastases to the major intra-parenchymatous vessels[31] thereby determining the type of resection.

Technical Aspects of the Liver Resection

Methods of Dissection

Routes of Access and Exposure

Most commonly, a bilateral subcostal incison is used. The incision runs two or three fingers' breadths below each costal margin and had an upward extension to the xyphoid process. With the help of subcostal retractors, this incision gives a wide exposure of the liver and its afferent and efferent vascular pedicles. In some cases a more limited a supra-umbilical midline incision is sufficient to perform a left lobectomy or a simple anterior tumorectomy. However, in all cases, the whole liver has to be explorable by the chosen incision, by palpation and intra-operative ultrasound. The liver is mobilized by division of the ligament teres, the triangular ligaments and the lesser omentum.

The gallbladder is often removed. A small catheter can be left in place in the cystic duct for injection of diluted methylene blue and air in the biliary tree after the liver section, to detect small biliary leakage from the cut surface and check the integrity of the biliary tree of the remaining liver by visualization on intra-operative ultrasound of the small air bubbles which spread into the remaining hepatic segments.

If standard hepatic vascular exclusion is undertaken, the peritoneum is divided along the left side of the retrohepatic inferior vena cava (IVC). Slings are passed around the IVC above and below the liver. If there is venous invasion or a possible need for repair of the IVC or the hepatic veins, the retrohepatic IVC is completely freed along its posterior aspect and the right adrenal vein is electively ligated and divided.

The dissection of the portal pedicle is not always performed and depends on the type of hepatectomy and the surgeon's preference for clamping. The intrahilar dissection and the primary clamping or ligation of the segmental vascular elements can help to delineate precisely the plane of the parenchymatous section, by the visible margins of the induced ischaemia on the liver's surface. Alternatively control and division of the portal pedicles can be performed during the parenchymatous section.[32] This latter technique is probably easier and safer for a standard hepatectomy, if the plane of the section has been clearly established by anatomical landmarks and intra-operative ultrasound.

Vascular Clamping

Blood loss has correlated significantly with post-operative morbidity and early and late mortality[4,5,33]. To reduce the blood loss during the liver dissection, several methods of vascular clamping of afferent and efferent liver pedicles have been described.

Clamping of the Hepatic Pedicle (CHP)
The clamping of the hepatic pedicle (CHP) described by Pringle in 1908[34] is the simplest and the most widely used method. An atraumatic clamp is placed on the hepatic pedicle below the liver hilum, occluding both portal and arterial inflow. This is haemodinamically well tolerated with a rise of arterial pressure. The healthy liver can tolerate the induced normothermic ischaemia for >1 hour,[11,35] Although intermittent clamping with periods of liver reperfusion is used by some surgeons, there is yet no proven advantage of this technique on non-cirrhotic livers.

Standard Hepatic Vascular Exclusion (HVE)
To avoid blood loss by backflow from the main hepatic veins and their branches during the parenchymatous section, a complete vascular exclusion of the liver can be performed with complete isolation of the liver and the retrohepatic IVC. Separate vascular clamps are placed on the hepatic pedicle, the infrahepatic IVC and the suprahepatic IVC.[36,37] The adrenal vein should be occluded by the inferior caval clamp or otherwise be ligated before clamping (Figure 6.2). HVE induces a drop in cardiac output of nearly 50% by blood sequestration in the portal and peripheral venous circulation, but mean arterial pressure is usually maintained. The magnitude of these haemodynamic modifications and patient tolerance are variable. A preliminary test of 5 min of HVE should therefore be performed before starting the liver section. Good cooperation between the anaesthesiologist and the surgeon is of critical importance.[38]

Hepatic Vascular Exclusion with Preservation of Caval Flow
HVE is poorly tolerated or can not even be attempted because of impaired cardiac function in

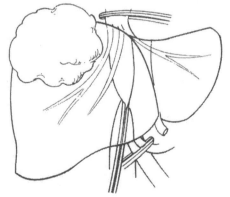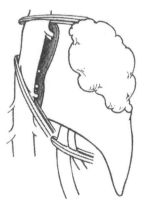

Figure 6.2. Standard hepatic vascular exclusion (HVE) by clamping of the hepatic pedicle, the infrahepatic vena cava and the suprahepatic vena cava (anterior and right sagittal views)

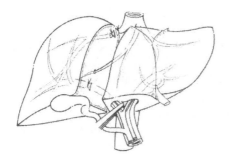

Figure 6.3. Selective vascular exclusion of the right liver. The right hepatic vein is either clamped or ligated in its short extraparenchymatous part. The clamping of the right portal pedicle induces a clear-cut ischaemic delineation of the portal scissural plane.

5–10% of patients.[11] More recently, HVE with preservation of caval blood flow has been used by some surgeons. The dissection requires ligation of the small hepatic veins between the anterior aspect of the retrohepatic IVC and the segment I. The main hepatic pedicle, and the origin of the main hepatic veins are clamped electively. A more selective exclusion of only the resected part of the liver can be performed by clamping only the afferent portal pedicle dissected in the liver hilum and the corresponding main hepatic vein (Figure 6.3). These types of selective HVE, though conceptually appealing, can be performed only by well-trained hepatic surgeons because of the risks involved in the dissection of the caval-hepatic venous confluence. We use it only if the standard HVE is not tolerated.

The choice between these different clamping procedures is guided primarily by the tumor location. Thus, a metastasis located near the caval-hepatic confluence can be resected safely under HVE, without risk of an incidental injury to a main hepatic vein, whereas an anteriorly located metastasis is resected easily under a clamping of the hepatic pedicle alone. Secondly, the respective competency and preference of the anaesthesic and surgical teams influence the final decision. In a few recent series, hepatic resections have been performed without any clamping procedure with no significant blood losses, because of the efficiency of the heaemostasis performed directly on the vascular pedicles encountered during the parenchymatous section.

Parenchymatous Section

Once the planes of section are defined, the liver capsule is incised with electric cautery. The parenchyma is divided using either a fine haemostat crushing the parenchyma or an ultrasound dissector. Small vacular and biliary pedicles are selectively clipped, tied, or cauterized before division. The main portal pedicles and hepatic veins encountered are secured by suture or automatic stapling device. After completion of section, the clamps are removed and haemostasis is completed by suture or cautery until a bloodless cut surface is obtained. The biliary leakages which are identified by injection of methylene blue through the cystic duct stump are suture ligated. Haemostasis of the cut surface can be completed by application of biological glue, haemostatic resorbable mesh, or superficial coagulation with an argon-beam coagulator. We usually drain the suphrenic and infrahepatic spaces, though the requirement for of such drainage is still debated.[39]

Segmental and Non-segmental Resections

The type and volume of liver resection depends on the number of metastases, their volume, their relationship to the hepatic veins and to the afferent portal pedicles, and is dependent on the need to remove a margin of at least 1 cm of healthy parenchyma.[1,2,40] To remove a larger volume of non-tumorous parenchyma does not decrease the risk of later recurrences,[2] but a formal resection with a reduced parenchymal cut surface is sometimes simpler and safer than a limited resection for a centrally located tumour. Furthermore, maximal sparing of liver parenchyma is often not mandatory for a metastatic liver which function and regeneration capacity are rarely impaired. Formal segmental and non-segmental resections can be undertaken in the same patient to treat multiple metastases (Figure 6.4).

Non-segmental Resections

Non-segmental resections, also called tumorectomies, metastasectomies or subsegmentectomies, are generally chosen for lesions of <3 cm, which are easily accessible and superficially located (Figure 6.5). More deeply located lesions, whatever their size, often require a more extended segmental resection.

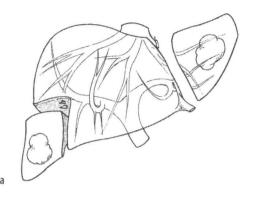
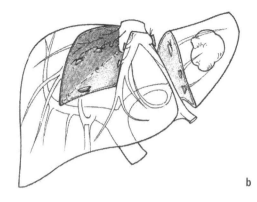
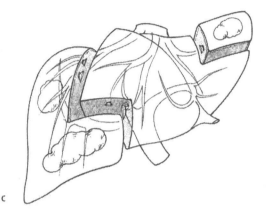

Figure 6.4. Various types of multi-bilobar segmentectomies.
(a) Segmentectomy VI + bisegmentectomy II–III (left lobectomy);
(b) Segmentectomy VIII + bisegmentectomy II–III (left lobectomy);
(c) Trisegmentectomy V + VI + VII + tumorectomy in the segment II.

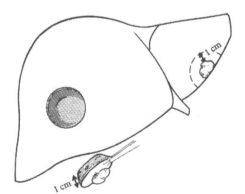

Figure 6.5. Non-segmental resection of superficial lesions is possible by a simple tumorectomy if the excision includes a rim of healthy parenchyma of at least 1 cm.

Segmental Resections

Uni- and Bisegmentectomies

All liver segments are theoretically resectable by uni- or multisegmentectomy.[32,41] However, in prac-

tice, only some of these resections are routinely performed, such as anterior segmentectomy IV (resection of the quadrate lobe), segmentectomy VI, bisegmentectomy anterior IV + V, and bisegmentectomies II and III (left lobectomy) and VI + VII (posterior sectoriectomy) (Figure 6.6). Other uni- or bisegmentectomies are more rarely used, such as the isolated segmentectomy I[42] or the bisegmentectomy V + VI.

To clearly delineate the limits of the parenchymatous section in these segmentectomies, and reduce blood losses, a balloon portal venous occlusion of the segment to be resected can be used[43] with intraoperative ultrasound guidance. But this complex procedure is often replaced by one which includes clamping of the whole liver pedicle.

Major Hepatectomies

An hepatic resection of three or more segments is considered as a major hepatectomy (Figure 6.7). Right hepatectomy is the most commonly per-

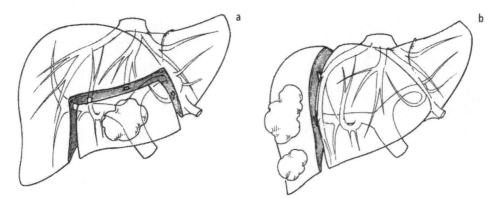

Figure 6.6.   (a) Bisegmentectomy of the anterior part of the segment IV and the segment V; (b) bisegmentectomy VI + VII (posterior right sectorectomy)

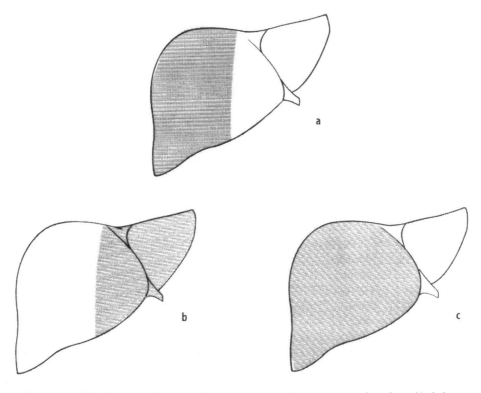

Figure 6.7.   Major hepatectomies resect at least three segments. The most commonly performed include:
(a)   the right hepatectomy (segments V, VI, VII, VIII);
(b)   the left hepatectomy (segments II, III, IV); and
(c)   the right lobectomy or extended right hepatectomy (segments IV, V, VI, VII, VIII).

formed with resection of segments V, VI, VII and VIII through a section plane along the main portal fissure to the right side of the middle hepatic vein. This operation was successfully performed in France for the first time by Lortat Jacob in 1952 for hepatic metastases. Left hepatectomy removes segments II, III and IV, running along the same plane but on the left side of the middle hepatic vein. The extended right hepatectomy adds the resection of segment IV to the right hepatectomy. The left extended hepatectomy adds the resection of segments V and VIII to the left hepatectomy. The resection of segment I can be associated to these extended major hepatectomies.

Table 6.1 Results of the resection of colorectal hepatic metastases

Authors	Year	Patients (n)	Operative mortality	Operative morbidity	3-year survival	5-year survival	10-year survival
Adson[44]	1984	141	2.8%	–	–	23%	–
August[3]	1985	33	0%	27%	53%	–	–
Bismuth[45]	1988	32	0%	–	33%	–	–
Bradpiece[7]	1987	24	8.3%	25%	30%	–	–
Butler[46]	1986	62	10%	20%	50%	34%	–
Cady[47]	1985	23	0%	–	–	–	–
Cobourn[48]	1987	41	0%	21%	–	25%	–
Doci[49]	1991	100	5%	39%	–	30%	–
Egeli[50]	1991	51	8%	–	34%	19%	–
Ekberg[51]	1986	72	5.6%	15%	30%	16%	–
Fortner[52]	1984	65	9%	27%	57%	30%	–
Gennari[53]	1986	48	2.1%	15%	53%	–	–
Holm[54]	1990	35	0%	–	31%	31%	–
Hughes[55*]	1986	859	–	–	–	33%	–
Iwatsuki[56]	1986	60	0%	13%	53%	45%	–
Lise[57]	1990	39	5%	–	55%	32%	–
Nordlinger[33]	1987	80	13%	51%	40%	25%	–
Sesto[58]	1987	61	7%	–	44%	28%	–
Scheele[20]	1991	207	5.5%	22%	41%	31%	21%
AFG[*†2]	1992	1818	2.4%	24%	41%	26%	12%

* Multicentric study. †Association of French Surgeons.
– unknown.

Postoperative Complications

The in-hospital mortality rate after the resection of hepatic metastases is currently <5%. A marked decrease has occurred in the last 15 years, mainly as a result of technical improvements of liver surgery (Table 6.1). This reduction in operative mortality rate is not only reported by specialized teams in liver surgery. In a recent large multicentric French study, the post-operative mortality rate was only 2.4% for 1895 resections.[2]

Postoperative Mortality

Death is related to the extent of liver resection. Postoperative death is more frequent after a major hepatectomy (3%) than after a minor resection, (1.2%).[2] Death can occur during the liver resection from massive intra-operative haemorrhage or gas embolism resulting generally from an accidental injury to the caval-hepatic confluence or an hepatic vein. Intraoperative deaths are now extremely rare, because of the wide use of the hepatic vascular exclusion techniques. Postoperatively, the early mortality related to the liver resection itself is mainly related to persistent or recurrent bleeding from the cut liver surface,[20] favouring the onset of hepatocellular failure. Hepatocellular failure led to death in 7% of cases in the French multicentric study.[2] Hepatocellular failure may be due to postoperative portal or arterial thrombosis and can occur also following extensive resection, performed on a liver the structure and function of which have been altered by previous systemic or intra-arterial chemotherapy. These latter deaths may be avoided by the precise assessment of hepatic function and volumetry prior to surgery.[13]

Postoperative death can be due to the anastomotic leakage of a colonic anastomosis if the resection of the primary colorectal tumor and metastasis has been undertaken. Scheele has reported two deaths due to anastomotic leakage among 90 simultaneous hepatic and colonic resections.[20] The operative mortality of such synchronous resections was significantly higher than when the two procedures were done on different occasions in the French multicentric study (6.1% versus 2.4% respectively).[2]

Non-surgical postoperative complications such as myocardial infarction, sudden cardiac arryhthmia, stroke, nosocomial pneumopathy and pulmonary embolism can also occur and may be fatal.[20] Their number is decreased by the careful pre-operative assessment of the patient's general condition and the systematic prophylaxis of postoperative deep vein thrombosis.

Postoperative morbidity

The postoperative outcome after hepatic resection for metastases is uneventful in 70–80% of patients in most recent series (Table 6.1). Postoperative morbidity should therefore no longer be considered as a main pitfall of surgical treatment. These low morbidity rates are responsible for the short duration of the mean postoperative stay, averaging 12–15 days in recent series.[2,59]

The morbidity directly related to the hepatic resection is mainly due to transient hepatocellular insufficiency and biliary fistula. The bile leakages encountered after major hepatectomies are often responsible for well circumscribed intra-abdominal collections which can be easily drained percutaneously under ultrasound or CT scan guidance. They can be responsible for a postoperative septic syndrome, but are rarely fatal if quickly treated. They usually resolve with drainage and antibiotic therapy, without the need for re-operation. A pleural effusion can occur, most often on the right side, if liver mobilization was performed by division of the right triangular hepatodiaphragmatic ligament.[60] However, a pleural effusion can also herald a subphrenic or biliary collection. If symptomatic, these pleural effusions are easily managed by placement of a chest drain.

Abdominal wound infection, gastrointestinal tract fistulas related to the dense adhesions from previous abdominal surgery, bleeding from extrahepatic dissection sites, and small bowel postoperative obstruction are rarely encountered in this supramesocolic non-contaminated surgery.

Results from Hepatic Metastases Resection

Colorectal Primary Tumours

The surgical resection is now a widely accepted treatment for hepatic metastases from colorectal primaries. Numerous series in the last decade have reported five year survival rates consistently between

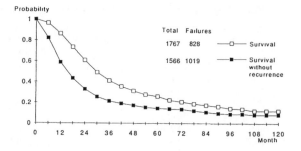

Figure 6.8. Overall survival and disease-free survival after complete resection of hepatic metastases (excluding operative deaths). Results of the multicentric study of the French Surgical Association. (Reproduced with permission from Nordlinger et al.[2])

20 to 35% (Table 6.1). Steele has stated that the flat part of the survival curve which begins at approximately five years implies expectedly that patients free of disease at this time are, in fact, permanently cured.[59] Ten year survival of 12–21% have been reported demonstrating clearly that some patients are definitely cured by surgery. The largest multicentric study, of the French Surgical Association has confirmed these findings (Figure 6.8).

Results of resection must be compared to the natural history of unresected hepatic metastases to ascertain the value of the surgical treatment. The surgical series of hepatic metastases are obviously biased by patient selection, whose general condition was considered fit enough to allow a resection. Patient performance status (as described by the Eastern Cooperative Oncology Group) and the extent of liver involvment are significant prognostic factors of natural history.[2,59] Due to the current acceptance of surgical treatment, there are no available prospective randomized comparative studies comparing observation to surgical resection. Factors associated with survival have been identified among non operated patients treated before widespread surgical treatment.[61-63] Patients who were asymptomatic at presentation with a solitary unresected metastasis had a median survival of 24 months[63], which was markedly longer than the 4–8 month survival of unselected non resected patients.[64,65] However, even patients with a nonresected solitary metastasis, did not survive to five years. Although recent improvements is palliative chemotherapy regimens have increased the survival of patients with unresectable disease by a few months, all patients ultimately die of progressive disease.[66]

Surgery remains the only treatment which ultimately provides cure to approximately 15–20% of the patients. Scheele[67] demonstrated clearly that patients developing tumour recurrence after an initially curative resection (complete resection of all hepatic lesions with microscopically negative margins and without extrahepatic disease) had a longer survival than patients whose resection was incomplete. This latter group, however has a similar survival rate to patients with resectable disease who had not undergo surgery. The forward shift of the survival curve of these curatively resected (but relapsing) patients averaged one year with some long term survivors at five and eight years. These observations demonstrate that a 'curative' resection can be a valuable palliative treatment, whereas a palliative resection is of no value. Recurrence after a curative resection occurs in 60–70% of patients.[2,59,67] The liver is involved in 50–70%, and the lungs in 50%. About 80% of these recurrences involve only one organ[2,55]. Whether all intra-hepatic recurrences result from occult metastases which were present but missed at the time of initial resection,[68] or whether they represent new metastases from occult extrahepatic disease is unknown. There is today no definite proof of the effectiveness of adjuvant chemotherapy in decreasing the recurrence rate after complete hepatic resection of metastases.[2] Two large retrospective studies[2,55] have suggested a significant survival advantage but prospective data are forthcoming.

Several prognostic factors have been studied to select more accurately in the preoperative period, the patients who will benefit from resection. They are discussed in detail in an other section of this book (Chap 4). Briefly, survival appeared to be affected in the largest available multicentric multivariate study,[2] by the stage of the primary tumour, the delay in appearance of metastases, the presence of extrahepatic spread, the number and the size of metastases, and the pre-operative carcinoembryonic antigen level. There is today no sufficient evidence to contraindicate complete resection of hepatic metastases on the sole basis of one of these prognostic factors. However, these factors have been used to establish a simple prognostic scoring system that could be useful to determine if surgical resection is worthwhile by comparison with the estimated operative risk.[69] This scoring system needs further prospective validation.

Repeat Hepatic Resections

The results of repeat resections of hepatic metastases have been evaluated for colorectal metastases. These resections are justified by the relatively low survival benefit of the various chemotherapy regimens in this setting.[66] Intrahepatic recurrence of colorectal metastases occur within the first two years in 60–70% of patients after the initial hepatic resection. Isolated hepatic recurrences have accounted for 25–30% of these cases.[82] Two recent large multicentric series[82,83] have assessed the results of repeat hepatic resections.

The resectability rate of these isolated liver recurrences was 24% in the French multicentric study.[83] Most repeat resections followed an initial limited minor hepatic resection. This finding had not resulted in a higher recurrence rate because of inadequate margins. Indeed, sufficient margins of normal parenchyma (<1 cm) were achieved,[83] but the greater feasability of a repeat resection after the first resection was related to the increased volume of residual liver parenchyma. This finding may supports the use of limited first resections rather than formal major hepatectomies, when both options are technically possible. The re-operation was macroscopically and histologically curative in 82% of patients in the American study[82] and about half of these patients underwent a major hepatectomy to resect these recurrences. However, in both sudies,[82,83] approximately 10% of patients underwent a simultaneous resection of an extrahepatic recurrence.

The operative mortality of these repeat resections is <2% and the postoperative morbidity affects 19–25% of patients. Thus, repeat liver resections do not appear to carry an operative risk greater than the first hepatectomy. Nevertheless, these repeat resections are frequently technically demanding, because of adhesions and modifications of the liver anatomy. They are therefore generally performed by specialized hepatic surgeons.

After such resection of recurrent isolated hepatic metastases, subsequent recurrent hepatic metastases occur in 50–60% of cases and a third resection is sometimes possible.[83] Three- and five-year survival rates of 35 and 17% have been reported for resections with some patients apparently cured.[82,83] The association of a synchronous resection of an extrahepatic recurrence worsens the prognosis[82] but does confer long term survival in some cases.[83]

Thus, recurrent resectable colorectal hepatic metastases carry an operative risk and a potential survival similar to that after resection of the first metastases. They should therefore always be considered for resection. Before attempting repeat resections, an interval of observation (whether a few weeks or month) followed by repeat imaging should be undertaken ensure that the hepatic recurrence does not herald diffuse rapidly growing metastatic disease. The role of adjuvant chemotherapy during this delay remains to be evaluated.

Non-Colorectal Primary Tumours

The indications for surgical resection of liver metastases originating from non-colorectal primaries remain controversial. Surgical series including large numbers of patients are lacking and there is no available randomized trial, comparing resection to chemotherapy alone.

Two types of liver metastases can be distinguished based on their different biological behavior: the neuroendocrine liver metastases and the non-colorectal non-endocrine metastases.

Neuroendocrine Metastases

In determining the indications for surgical treatment a number of factors must be considered. These would include the natural history of the neuroendocrine metastases to the liver, the presence of disabling or life-threatening neuroendocrine symptoms,[70] such as necrolytic migratory erythema due to glucagonoma or valvular heart disease due to carcinoid tumours, and the feasability of a surgical resection. Neuroendocrine metastases are slow-growing tumours and most often discovered when diffuse and non-resectable. Patients with unresectable hepatic neuroendocrine metastases have been reported to have median survival of 22–40 months only and a five-year survival rate of 28%,[71] modestly influenced by the various regimens of systemic chemotherapy.[71,72]

In some selected patients without prohibitive operative risk, complete resection of hepatic metastases with curative intent is feasible. This treatment is probably justified, despite the lack of any available prospective trial.[71] This policy could ultimately cure one-third of patients whose primary tumour has been curatively resected.[71,73] Resection may delay for several years the occurence of the carci-

noid syndrome and the symptoms related to the tumour volume itself. An actuarial five-year survival rate of 79%[71] and a five-year survival rate without recurrence of 52% after such resections has been recently reported and seems to justify this surgical attitude.[74] To allow the complete resection of numerous or large hepatic metastases, more complex procedures such as planned repeated hepatectomies or pre-operative liver hypertrophy induced by portal embolizations have been reported,[75] but their impact on long-term survival is difficult to assess.

Palliative resections of carcinoid hepatic metastases have been reported in patients suffering from carcinoid syndrome.[76] These debulking procedures offered alleviation of the disabling symptoms of the carcinoid syndrome such as diarrhoea and flushing episodes, if at least 90% of the functioning tumour was removed, but were less efficient for the cardiac symptoms. This aggressive palliative treatment is today challenged by the use of somatostatin analogues such as octreotide acetate and lanreotide and by the percutaneous hepatic repeated chemoembolization procedures which are able to alleviate, the carcinoid symptoms (for several months). A combination of these various non surgical therapies could provide both long term survival and control symptoms.[72] There is today no place for surgical liver devascularization which have been replaced by interventional radiological procedures.

Liver transplantation has been performed to cure non-resectable diffuse hepatic neuroendocrine metastases, but the results of the few reported cases are rather disappointing with frequent recurrences and high postoperative mortality.[74] Further studies are necessary to assess the role of liver transplantation in this still debated indication.

Non-colorectal, Non-neuroendocrine Metastases

The surgical indications in this heterogeneous group of hepatic metastases are dependent of their respective chemosensitivity. The results of surgical resection are difficult to assess with certainty because of the rarity of the reported cases. The group of tumours frequently resistant to chemotherapy comprises mainly gastrointestinal tract carcinoma other than those of colorectal origin, metastatic adenocarcinoma of unknown origin, renal cell carcinoma and melanoma. Several reports of resections of single isolated synchronous or metachronous hepatic metastases have shown some long-term survival and a probable definite cure is possible, but remains exceptional.[77]

Synchronous hepatic metastases discovered at operation have been resected by simple and limited hepatectomy. Nevertheless, for oesophagal or pancreatic carcinoma, these synchronous metastases are considered as a contraindication to the resection of the primary tumour, because of the poor results obtained by simultaneous resection.[77] A recent Japanese study reported three cases of five-year survival without evidence of recurrence after the resection of synchronous hepatic metastases of gastric origin, among 21 such resections performed. It was not precisely stated if these limited hepatic tumours were true metastases or contiguous involvment of the liver which might carry a better prognosis. The palliative value of such resections is sometimes evoked,[78] but remains controversial.

Curative resection of isolated intrahepatic adenocarcinoma of unknown origin can be justified for two reasons. Firstly chemotherapy will not confer a cure, and secondly primary intrahepatic cholangiocarcinoma are often undistinguishable from secondary lesions on pre-operative biopsy.

The resection of metachronous isolated liver metastases in this group of tumours has to be determined with each individual case, because of the lack of available valuable scientific data. A long delay separating the diagnosis of liver metastases from the resection of the primary favours an aggressive surgical policy.

For metastases originating from epidermoid lung or pharyngolaryngal carcinomas, and tumours arising from the anus, cervix, ovary and breast, chemotherapy induces an objective partial response in 50–70% of cases, but complete response occurs in <20% of cases and is frequently transient.[73] The question of surgical resection is usually raised following initial chemotherapy, if the metastases have not progressed. Few reports on the resection of these forms of isolated metastases are available, with five-year survival rates of 30%[79,80] being reported in selected cases. A recent report of 18 hepatectomies for breast cancer metastases combined with chemotherapy showed that only two patients had no evidence of recurrence at 29 and 46 months. It has been advocated for this group of tumours of intermediate chemosensitivity that only the metachronous completely resectable tumours should be considered for resection and only if these have occurred after a minimal delay of one to two years

from the resection of the primary, and if they have responded to chemotherapy. The role of this resection has still to be compared prospectively with maintenence chemotherapy or no treatment at all. The impact of the natural history of these tumours on survival could be in fact more important than surgical resection.

For tumours of high chemosensitivity such as lymphoma carcinoma of the testis and some pediatric tumours, the presence of hepatic metastases generally heralds generalized dissemination, and chemotherapy is the best treatment, able to cure a significant proportion of patients. Resection of residual hepatic and retroperitoneal masses after chemotherapy has been proposed for germ cell testicular carcinoma with two years survival rates of 60%, but long-term results of such aggressive policies are awaited.[81]

References

1. Scheele J. Hepatectomy for liver metastases. *Br J Surg* 1993; **80**:274–276.
2. Nordlinger B, Jaeck D, Guiguet M, Vaillant JC, Balladur P, Schaal JC. Surgical resection of hepatic metastases. Multicentric retrospective study by the French Association of Surgery. In: Nordlinger B, Jaeck D (eds) *Treatment of Hepatic Metastases of Colorectal Cancer*, 1992: 129–146. Paris, Springer-Verlag.
3. August DA, Sugarbaker PH, Ottow RT, Gianola FJ, Schneider PD. Hepatic resection of colorectal metastases: Influence of clinical factors and adjuvant intraperitoneal 5-fluorouracil via Tenckhoff catheter on survival. *Ann Surg* 1985; **201**:210–218.
4. Stephenson KR, Steinberg SM, Hughes KS, Vetto JT, Sugarbaker PH, Chang AE. Perioperative blood transfusions are associated with reduced time to recurrence and decreased survival after resection of colorectal liver metastases. *Ann Surg* 1988; **208**:679–687.
5. Weiden PL. Does perioperative blood transfusion increase the risk of cancer recurrence? *Eur J Cancer* 1990; **26**:987–989.
6. Couinaud C. *Le Foie: !Etudes Anatomiques et Chirurgicales*, 1957. Paris, Masson.
7. Bradpiece HA, Benjamin IS, Halevy A, Blumgart LH. Major hepatic resection for colorectal liver metastases. *Br J Surg* 1987; **74**:324–326.
8. Goldsmith NA, Woodburne RT. The surgical anatomy pertaining to liver resection. *Surg Gynecol Obst* 1957; **195**:310–315.
9. Starzl TL, Bell RH, Beart RW *et al.* Hepatic trisegmentectomy and other liver resections. *Surg Gynecol Obst* 1975; **114**:429–437.
10. Bismuth H. Surgical anatomy and anatomical surgery of the liver. *World J Surg* 1982; **6**:3–9.
11. Delva E, Camus Y, Nordlinger B *et al.* Vascular occlusions for liver resections. *Ann Surg* 1989; **209**:211–218.
12. Sebagh M, Adam R, Lemoine A *et al.* Evaluation histologique et biochimique de la toxicité hépatique de la

chimioththérapie systémique. *Gastroenterol Clin Biol* 1996; **20**:A1.

13. Elias D, Lasser P, Rougier P, Ducreux M, Bognel C, Roche A. Frequency, technical aspects, results and indications of major hepatectomy after prolonged intra-arterial hepatic chemotherapy for initially unresectable hepatic tumor. *J Am Coll Surg* 1995; **180**:213–219.

14. Kawasaki S, Maakushi M, Kasaku T *et al*. Resection for multiple metastatic liver tumors after portal embolization. *Surgery* 1994; **115**:674–677.

15. Elias D, Detroz B, Lasser P, Plaud B, Jerbi G. Is simultaneous hepatectomy and intestinal anastomisis safe? *Am J Surg* 1995; **169**:254–260.

16. Belghiti J. Synchronous and resectable hepatic metastases from colorectal cancer. Should a minimal interval be respected before performing hepatic resection? *Ann Chir* 1990; **44**:427–432.

17. Barr LC, Skene AI, Thomas JM. Metastasectomy: a review. *Br J Surg* 1992; **79**:1268–1274.

18. Smith JW, Fortner JG, Burt M. Resection of hepatic and pulmonary metastasis from colorectal cancer. *Surg Oncol* 1992; **1**:399–404.

19. Gough DB, Donohue JH, Trastek VA, Nagorney DM. Resection of hepatic and pulmonary metastases in patients with colorectal cancer. *Br J Surg* 1994; **81**:94–96.

20. Scheele J, Stangl R, Altendorf-Hofmann A, Gall FP. Indicators of prognosis after hepatic resection for colorectal secondaries. *Surgery* 1991; **110**:13–29.

21. Wernecke K, Rummenny E, Bongartz G. Comparative sensitivities of sonography, CT, and MRI imaging. *Am J Roentg* 1991; **157**:731–737.

22. Ferrucci JT. Liver tumor imaging, current concepts. *Am J Radiol* 1990; **155**:473–484.

23. Hashimoto D, Dohi T, Eng D *et al*. Development of a computer-aided surgery system: three dimensional graphic reconstruction for treatment of liver cancer. *Surgery* 1991; **109**:589–596.

24. Soyer P, Breittmayer F, Gad M, Levesque M, Roche A. Imagerie tridimensionelle de la segmentation hepatique: anatomie et volumétrie. *Rev Imag Med* 1991; **3**:741–745.

25. Sitzmann JV, Coleman JA. Preoperative assessment of malignant hepatic tumors. *Am J Surg* 1991; **159**:137–143.

26. Tubiana JM, Deutsch JP, Taboury J, Martin B. Imaging of hepatic colorectal metastases. Diagnosis and resectability. In: Nordlinger B, Jaeck D (eds) *Treatment of Hepatic Metastases of Colorectal Cancer*, 1992: 54–69. Paris, Springer-Verlag.

27. Soyer P, Levesque M, Caudron C, Elias D, Zeitoun G, Roche A. MRI of liver metastases from colorectal cancer vs. CT during arterial portography. *J Comp Ass Tomogr* 1993; **17**:67–74.

28. Elias D, Lasser P, Bognel C, Leclere J, Rougier P. Bilan de 242 laparotomies pour métastases hépatiques pratiquées en 5 ans à l'institut Gustave-Roussy. *J Chir* 1988; **125**:479–483.

29. John TG, Greig JD, Crosbie JL, Miles WFA, Garden OJ. Superior staging of liver tumors with laparoscopy and laparoscopic ultrasound. *Ann Surg* 1994; **6**:711–719.

30. Castaing D, Emond J, Kunstlinger F, Bismuth H. Utility of operative ultrasound in the surgery of liver tumors. *Ann Surg* 1986; **204**:600–605.

31. Castaing D, Kunstlinger F, Habib N, Bismuth H. Intraoperative ultrasonographic study of the liver. Methods and anatomic results. *Am J Surg* 1985; **149**:676–682.

32. Ton-That-Tung. *Les Résections Majeures et Mineures du Foie*, 1979. Paris, Masson.

33. Nordlinger B, Quilichini MA, Parc R, Hannoun L, Delva E, Huguet C. Hepatic resection for colorectal liver metastases – Influence on survival of preoperative factors and surgery for recurrences in 80 patients. *Ann Surg* 1987; **205**:256–263.

34. Pringle JH. Notes on the arrest of hepatic hemorrhage due to trauma. *Ann Surg* 1908; **48**:541–549.

35. Huguet C, Nordlinger B, Bloch P, Conard J. Tolerance of the human liver to prolonged normothermic ischemia. *Arch Surg* 1978; **113**:1448–1451.

36. Heaney JP, Stanton WK, Halbert DS, Seidel J, Vice T. An improved technique for vascular isolation of the liver. Experimental study and case reports. *Ann Surg* 1966; **163**:237–241.

37. Huguet C, Nordlinger B, Galopin JJ, Bloch P, Gallot D. Normothermic hepatic vascular exclusion for extensive hepatectomies. *Surg Gynecol Obstet* 1978; **147**:689–693.

38. Delva E, Barberousse JP, Nordlinger B *et al*. Hemodynamic and biochemical monitoring during major liver resection with use of hepatic vascular occlusion. *Surgery* 1984; **95**:309–317.

39. Franco D, Karaa A, Meakins JL, Borgonovo G, Smadja C, Grange D. Hepatectomy without abdominal drainage. Result of a prospective study in 61 patients. *Arch Surg* 1988; **210**:748–750.

40. Yamamoto J, Sugihara K, Kosuge T *et al*. Pathologic support for limited hepatectomy in the treatment of liver metastases from colorectal cancer. *Ann Surg* 1995; **221**:74–78.

41. Bismuth H, Houssin D, Castaing D. Major and major segmentectomies 'reglées' in liver surgery. *World J Surg* 1982; **6**:10–24.

42. Mizumoto R, Kawarada Y, Susuki H. Surgical treatment of hilar carcinoma of the bile duct. *Surg Gynecol Obstet* 1986; **192**:153–158.

43. Castaing D, Garden OJ, Bismuth H. Segmental liver resection using ultrasound guided selective portal occlusion. *Ann Surg* 1989; **210**:13–19.

44. Adson MA, van Heerden JA, Adson MH, Wagner JS, Ilstrup DM. Resection of hepatic metastases from colorectal cancer. *Arch Surg* 1984; **119**:647–651.

45. Bismuth H, Castaing D, Traynor O. Surgery for synchronous hepatic metastases of colorectal cancer. *Scand J Gastroenterol* 1988; **23**:144–149.

46. Butler J, Attiyeh FF, Daly JM. Hepatic resection for metastases of the colon and rectum. *Surg Gynecol Obstet* 1986; **162**:109–113.

47. Cady B, McDermott WV. Major hepatic resection for metachronous metastases from colon cancer. *Ann Surg* 1985; **201**:204–209.

48. Cobourn CS, Makowka L, Langer B, Taylor BR, Falk RE. Examination of patient selection and outcome for hepatic resection for metastatic disease. *Surg Gynecol Obstet* 1987; **165**:239–246.

49. Doci R, Gennari L, Bignami P, Montalto F, Morabito A, Bozzetti F. One hundred patients with hepatic metastases from colorectal cancer treated by resection: analysis of prognostic determinants. *Br J Surg* 1991; **78**:797–801.

50. Egeli RA. Traitement des Métastases Hépatiques, 1991. Thesis, University of Geneva.

51. Ekberg H, Tranberg KG, Andersson R *et al*. Determinants of survival in liver resection for colorectal secondaries. *Br J Surg* 1986; **73**:727–731.

52. Fortner JG, Silva JS, Golbey RB, Cox EB, MacLean J. Multivariate analysis of a personal series of 247 consecutive patients with liver metastases from colorectal cancer treated by hepatic resection. *Ann Surg* 1984; **199**:306–316.

53. Gennari L, Doci R, Bozzetti F, Bignami P. Surgical treatment of hepatic metastases from colorectal cancer. *Ann Surg* 1986; **203**:49–54.

54. Holm A, Bradley E, Aldrete JS. Hepatic resection of metastasis from colorectal carcinoma – Morbidity, mortality, and pattern of recurrence. *Ann Surg* 1990; **209**:428–434.

55. Hughes KS, Simon R, Songhorabodi S. Resection of the liver for colorectal carcinoma metastases: a multi-institutional study of patterns of recurrence. *Surgery* 1986; **100**:278–284.

56. Iwatsuki S, Esquivel CO, Gordon RD, Starzl TE. Liver resection for metastatic colorectal cancer. *Surgery* 1986; **100**:804–810.

57. Lise M, DaPian PP, Nitti D, Pilati PL, Prevaldi C. Colorectal metastases to the liver: present status and management. *Dis Colon Rectum* 1990; **33**:688–694.

58. Sesto ME, Vogt DP, Hermann RE. Hepatic resection in 128 patients: a 24-year experience. *Surgery* 1987; **102**:846–851.

59. Steele G, Ravikumar TS. Resection of hepatic metastases from colorectal cancer. Biologic perspectives. *Ann Surg* 1989; **210**:127–138.

60. Sa Cunha A, Thomas S, Bertoux L, Belghiti J. L'épanchément pleural: causes et conséquences après hépatectomie par voie abdominale. *Gastroenterol Clin Biol* 1996; **20**:A220.

61. Cady B, Monson DO, Swinton NW. Survival of patients after colonic resection for carcinoma having simultaneous liver metastases. *Surg Gynecol Obstet* 1970; **131**:697–700.

62. Goslin R, Steele G, Zamcheck N et al. Factors influencing survival in patients with hepatic metastases from adenocarcinoma of the colon and rectum. *Dis Colon Rectum* 1982; **25**:749–754.

63. Wagner JS, Adson MA, van Heerden JA, Adson MH, Ilstrup DM. The natural history of hepatic metastases from colorectal cancer – a comparison with resective treatment. *Ann Surg* 1984; **199**:502–508.

64. Jaffe BM, Donegan WL, Watson F et al. Factors influencing survival in patients with untreated hepatic metastases. *Surg Gynecol Obstet* 1968; **127**:1–11.

65. Oxley EM, Ellis H. Prognosis of the large bowel in the presence of liver metastases. *Br J Surg* 1969; **56**:149–152.

66. Nordic Gastrointestinal Tumor Adjuvant Therapy Group. Expectancy or primary chemotherapy in patients with advanced asymptomatic colorectal cancer: A randomized trial. *J Clin Oncol* 1992; **10**:904–911.

67. Scheele J, Stangl R, Altendorf-Hofmann A. Hepatic metastases from colorectal carcinoma: impact of surgical resection on the natural history. *Br J Surg* 1990; **77**:1241–1246.

68. Panis Y, Ribeiro J, Chrétien Y, Ballet F, Nordlinger B. Dormant liver metastases: demonstration by experimental study in rats. *Br J Surg* 1992; **79**:221–223.

69. Nordlinger B, Guiguet M, Vaillant JC et al. Surgical resection of colorectal carcinoma metastases to the liver. A prognostic scoring system to improve case selection, based on 1568 patients. *Cancer* 1996; **77**:1254–1262.

70. Soreide O, Berstad T, Bakka A et al. Surgical treatment as a principle in patients with advanced abdominal carcinoid tumors. *Surgery* 1992; **111**:48–54.

71. Carty SE, Jensen RT, Norton JA. Prospective study of aggressive resection of metastatic pancreatic endocrine tumors. *Surgery* 1992; **112**:1024–1032.

72. Diaco DS, Hajarizadeh H, Mueller CR, Fletcher WS, Pommier RF, Woltering EA. Treatment of metastatic carcinoid tumors using multimodality therapy of octreotide acetate, intra-arterial chemotherapy and hepatic arterial chemoembolization. *Am J Surg* 1995; **169**:523–528.

73. Elias D. Treatment of hepatic metastases thought to be confined to the liver. *Lett Cancerol* 1992; **1**:203–209.

74. Dousset B, Saint Marc O, Pitre J, Soubrane O, Houssin D, Chapuis Y. Endocrine hepatic metastases: medical treatment, surgical resection or transplantation. *Gastroenterol Clin Biol* 1996; **20**:A203.

75. Elias D, Rougier P, Lasser P et al. Major surgery and reductional chemotherapy in polymetastatic neuroendocrine tumors. *Ann Chir* 1988; **42**:474–481.

76. Blumgart LH, Allison DJ. Resection and embolization in the management of secondary hepatic tumors. *World J Surg* 1982; **6**:320–345.

77. Hughes KS, Sugarbaker PH. Resection of the liver for metastatic solid liver tumors. In: *Surgical Treatment of Metastatic Cancer*, Rosenberg SA (eds) 1987: 125–164. Philadelphia, JB Lippincott.

78. Maehara Y, Kakeji Y, Takayashi I et al. Non-curative resection for advanced gastric cancer. *J Clin Oncol* 1992; **51**:221–225.

79. Foster JH. Survival after liver resection for secondary tumors. *Am J Surg* 1978; **135**:389–394.

80. Elias D, Lasser P, Desruennes E, Hardy C. Sixty hepatic resections for liver metastases from extra-colorectal cancers [Abstract]. *HPB Surgery* 1990; **2**:111.

81. Goulet RJ, Hadacre JM, Einhorn LH et al. Hepatic resection for disseminated germ cell carcinoma. *Ann Surg* 1990; **212**:290–293.

82. Fernandez-trigo V, Shamsa F, Sugarbaker PH et al. Repeat liver resections from colorectal metastasis. *Surgery* 1995; **117**:296–304.

83. Nordlinger B, Vaillant JC, Guiguet M et al. Survival benefit of repeat liver resections for recurrent colorectal metastases: 143 cases. *J Clin Oncol* 1994; **12**:1491–1496.

Laparoscopic Surgery and Liver Metastasis

Timothy G. John, K.K. Madhavan and O. James Garden

7

Introduction

The evaluation of liver metastases has been a fundamental feature of the history of the development of laparoscopy. In his seminal paper of 1911, Bernheim recognised the utility of 'organoscopy' as a minimal access procedure which might 'reveal general metastases or a secondary nodule in the liver, thus rendering further procedures unnecessary and saving the patient a rather prolonged convalescence'.[1] In the 1930s, Ruddock and Benedict further developed this theme, performing diagnostic 'peritoneoscopy' in the evaluation of liver metastases in association with the investigation of ascites, and gastric, colorectal and gynaecological malignancies.[2,3] Out of 135 patients with clinically suspected hepatic malignancy in whom laparoscopy was performed, Ruddock reported having established the correct diagnosis in 69 out of 79 proven cases (87%), thus establishing the utility of laparoscopy in the diagnosis of liver tumours as early as 1939.[2]

The application of diagnostic laparoscopy in the assessment of suspected liver disease found popularity mostly with hepatologists and medical gastroenterologists who exploited its utility in identifying both focal and diffuse abnormalities affecting the liver, and in facilitating liver biopsy. Conversely, surgical laparoscopists principally championed the staging role of laparoscopy in the detection of intra-abdominal metastases prior to laparotomy in patients with a variety of potentially resectable tumours. The continued development of advanced laparoscopic techniques enabling resection or palliative therapies for a variety of intra-abdominal malignancies has re-emphasized the importance of laparoscopic assessment of liver metastases. The feasibility of treating such metastatic lesions laparoscopically by resection, regional chemotherapy, or by local tumour ablation with laser hyperthermia or cryotherapy further highlights the importance of laparoscopic liver assessment. It seems likely that the advent of laparoscopic ultrasonography (LapUS) will be fundamental to the success of such approaches.

Indications and Current Status

The indications for the laparoscopic evaluation of liver metastases may be considered in the context of the following:

(i) The 'diagnostic dilemma' in patients with clinical or radiological evidence of a focal hepatic lesion. The patient may have presented *de novo*, or be participating in a surveillance programme following resection of a primary malignancy, and it is necessary to confirm or refute the diagnosis of liver metastasis.

(ii) Staging laparoscopy as a prelude to exploratory laparotomy with a view to 'curative' resection of a variety of primary extrahepatic tumours. Laparoscopic methods of liver assessment may also be important in patients undergoing laparoscopic colorectal cancer surgery, and in patients undergoing staging of lymphoma.

(iii) Staging laparoscopy as a prelude to 'curative' hepatic resection in patients with established liver metastases.

The utility of laparoscopy in the former scenario has long been recognized. In the early 1970s, Trujillo performed diagnostic laparoscopy in 37 patients in whom a carcinoma had been resected within the preceding five years and liver metastases were suspected.[4] An elevated serum alkaline phophatase level, hepatomegaly or an abnormal radioisotope scan of the liver, and a normal blind percutaneous liver biopsy had been obtained in each patient. A laparoscopic diagnosis of hepatic metastases was achieved in 29 patients (78%), and no false-negative examinations were identified during follow-up in the remainder. Thus, despite substantial development of hepatic imaging investigations, the continuing relevance of Ruddock's observations of three decades before was underlined.[2]

The advent in the 1980s of non-invasive cross-sectional imaging techniques such as computed tomography (CT), magnetic resonance imaging (MRI) and ultrasonography (US) as the predominant methods of hepatic imaging led to a dramatic decline in the use of diagnostic laparoscopy for suspected liver disease. Nevertheless, despite the universal adoption of these modalities, the fallibility of all imaging techniques in generating false-negative and false-positive results must be remembered. Diagnostic laparoscopy retains an important (and often underrated) role as an adjunct to radiological techniques in the evaluation of suspected liver metastases. This was illustrated by Brady et al. who reported 25 patients with clinically suspected hepatic or peritoneal malignancy in whom the results of abdominal CT had been non diagnostic.[5] Laparoscopy with biopsy established a diagnosis of malignancy in 25 patients (48%), with significant implications for their clinical management.

The high sensitivity (and specificity) of staging laparoscopy in detecting small liver metastases in the staging of a variety of primary malignancies has now been established in a range of studies (Table 7.1). Modern laparoscopic optical and lighting systems enable excellent visualization of >80% of the liver surface, facilitating the identification and biopsy of small metastatic lesions affecting the liver surface (Figure 7.1). Most reports emphasize the laparoscopic detection of unsuspected liver metastases together with minimal volume metastatic deposits on the serosal surfaces of the abdominal

Table 7.1   Laparoscopic detection of intraabdominal metastases (liver and peritoneal) in the staging of patients with abdominal malignancies

Authors	Incidence of metastases at laparoscopy (%)	Sensitivity for metastases (%)	Laparotomy avoided (%)
Pancreatic cancer			
Cuschieri et al.[65, 66]	75	98	30
Ishida[67]	43	–	–
Warshaw et al.[6, 7, 68]	41	96	41
John et al.[69]	35	83	45*
Bemelman et al.[70]	23	76	17*
Fernández-del Castillo et al.[71]	24	93	24
Conlon et al.[72]	29	75**	36
John et al. (unpublished)	30	94	38*
Gastrooesophageal cancer			
Gross et al.[8]	48	100	52
Shandall and Johnson[9]	27**	96	54
Dagnini et al.[10]	10**	97	45
Possik et al.[11]	16**	87**	34
Kriplani and Kapur[12]	40	92	40
Bemelman et al.[13]	9	83	5*
Molloy et al.[14]	38	96	42
Anderson et al.[16]	14	83	16*
Lowy et al.[17]	4**	33**	25
Finch et al.[18]	12	75	19*
Gallbladder cancer			
Kriplani et al.[25]	77	95	75

*   Takes account of the findings of laparoscopic ultrasonography.
** Liver metastases only.

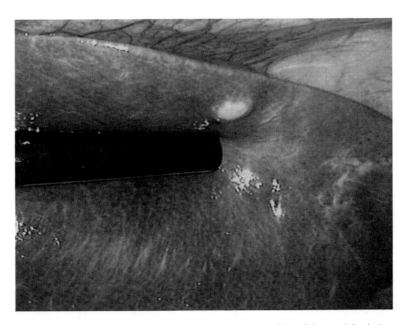

Figure 7.1. Unexpected discovery of a small hepatic metastasis on the undersurface of the left hepatic lobe during staging laparoscopy in a patient with periampullary cancer. Spiral CT scanning had failed to identify this lesion.

cavity, omentum and bowel. The mode of metastatic dissemination is probably transcoelomic rather than blood-borne in the context of peritoneal carcinomatosis, although malignant lesions affecting the mesothelium overlying the hepatic capsule may be difficult to differentiate from superficial liver metastases. However, most clinical reports consider the spectrum of distant intra-abdominal malignant dissemination as an entity, probably because the implications for treatment are similar. Such lesions are frequently beyond the threshold of detection by US, CT and MRI scanning techniques, and it has been established that laparoscopy is unique in its ability to detect such 'occult' intra-abdominal metastases (Table 7.1).

The rationale for the adoption of staging laparoscopy is strongest in circumstances where the discovery of unsuspected intra-abdominal metastases is frequent and would preclude tumour resection. Accordingly, it is now generally accepted that exploratory laparotomy and biopsy is an unacceptable primary method of establishing a diagnosis in patients with suspected pancreatic malignancy. Thus, surgical exploration may be avoided in 20–30% of patients with potentially resectable pancreatic and periampullary cancer because of the availability of non-operative methods for the relief of malignant obstructive jaundice such as endoscopic and percutaneous biliary stent insertion

(Table 7.1). Warshaw and colleagues showed that no single investigation was alone sufficient to evaluate patients with pancreatic cancer, and established the role of laparoscopy in detecting occult intra-abdominal metastases irrespective of preceding normal CT scans.[6,7] The role of staging laparoscopy in patients with malignant obstruction of the distal bile duct may become even more important with the development of laparoscopic methods of palliative biliary and duodenal bypass.

In the staging of gastro-oesophageal cancer, the delayed discovery of disseminated tumour at exploratory laparotomy may preclude radical gastro-oesphageal resections, and avoidance of the implicit morbidity of unnecessary surgery remains an important goal in the management of such patients. Several studies testify to the sensitivity of laparoscopy in the staging of carcinoma of the stomach, gastric cardia and/or oesophagus (Table 7.1).[8-18] Nevertheless, the potential pitfalls of laparoscopy in the detection of liver metastases in such patients were highlighted by Bemelman and colleagues, who reported a low yield in the laparoscopic evaluation of patients with oesophageal carcinoma. However, it should be noted that this low yield for staging laparoscopy was at variance with the results of other studies, and was partly due to a failure to establish a histological diagnosis of metastatic spread in the face of visible abnormalities, thus highlighting the importance of accurate and representative biopsy as part of the laproscopic assessment of liver metastases.

The sensitivity of laparoscopy in detecting liver metastases has been reported in patients with ovarian tumours,[19] bronchogenic carcinoma,[20] carcinoma of the breast,[21] malignant melanoma[22] and lymphoma[23,24] in which the laparoscopic findings directly influenced patient management. In the staging of patients with gallbladder carcinoma, the unique role of staging laparoscopy was highlighted by its superior sensitivity (95% versus 51%) in demonstrating the intra-abdominal metastases which had been present in 41 patients (77%).[25] The combination of transabdominal ultrasonography and laparoscopy resulted in 40 patients avoiding unnecessary laparotomy (75%), while 5 out of 6 patients with resectable disease were correctly identified using this algorithm.

Nevertheless, most studies which have evaluated the role of laparoscopy in the detection of liver metastases in patients with various primary malignancies have either not compared the findings prospectively with alternative imaging modalities, or considered alternative investigations which are now mainly of historical interest (e.g. radioisotope hepatic scintigraphy). In an attempt to address this issue in the context of the staging of pancreatic and periampullary cancers, and also to revisit the work performed by Warshaw and colleagues,[7] prospective 'blind' comparison of laparoscopy with LapUS versus transabdominal ultrasonography (USS), dynamic intravenous contrast-enhanced abdominal CT scanning (CT) and selective visceral angiography (SVA) was performed in the Royal Infirmary Edinburgh (unpublished data). Fifty patients were studied, biopsy-proven distant intraabdominal metastases being demonstrated in 16 patients (32%), and 14 patients proving 'resectable for cure'. Laparoscopic staging was shown to be significantly more sensitive and predictive than USS, CT and SVA in detecting such metastases (94% versus 29%, 33% and 0%, respectively). While prospective comparison with newer techniques such as helical CT scanning is obviously desirable, preliminary data have shown the persistence of false-negative findings, and even this new advanced technology may not be sufficient to challenge the unique role of laparoscopy in the staging of this disease.[26]

The role of staging laparoscopy as a prelude to hepatic resection in patients considered to have potentially resectable liver metastases has long been neglected by liver surgeons. The same has also been largely true for patients with primary liver cancer, although the utility of laparoscopy in the selection of such patients for operative intervention has been reported as a corollary to diagnostic laparoscopy. This reflects the propensity of hepatocellular carcinoma for multifocal or extrahepatic dissemination, and its association with hepatic cirrhosis which may be of sufficient severity to preclude attempts at resection. Similarly, most liver surgeons would consider as unresectable liver metastases associated with extrahepatic tumour dissemination, multifocal or bilobar distribution within the liver, or invasion of the main portal vein, hepatic venous confluence or inferior vena cava. Avoidance of unecessary laparotomy in patients with unresectable disease should be fundamental to their management as there are currently no known advantages for palliative surgery, while laparotomy and closure carries an unacceptable risk of both physical and psychological morbidity.

In this context, the fallibility of existing radiological modalities in the pre-operative detection of extrahepatic tumour dissemination in patients considered on the basis of CT to have resectable colorectal liver metastases was demonstrated by Lefor and colleagues.[27] They reported the unexpected discovery of such findings at laparotomy in 28 out of the 107 patients (26%) studied. The experience in the Royal Infirmary, Edinburgh, between 1988 and 1991, before the adoption of staging laparoscopy, was that of a 58% resectability rate for all patients undergoing exploratory laparotomy with a view to liver resection.[28]

There is now evidence supporting the incorporation of laparoscopy within the staging algorithm for patients being considered for 'curative' resection of hepatic metastases. Babineau and colleagues demonstrated factors contraindicating tumour resection at laparoscopy in 14 out of 29 such patients (48%), despite preceding radiological screening.[29] This experience was reproduced in Edinburgh following the introduction of mandatory staging laparoscopy (with LapUS) as a prelude to exploratory laparotomy for liver resections.[28] Laparoscopic staging was performed in a series of 50 patients with liver tumours (liver metastases, $n = 37$; primary liver tumours, $n = 9$; non-malignant lesions, $n = 6$), having failed to gain access to the peritoneal cavity in another 2 patients due to the presence of adhesions (4% failure rate). Laparoscopy demonstrated previously unsuspected factors contraindicating liver resection in 23 patients (46%), thus reproducing the findings of Babineau et al.[29] Extrahepatic tumour spread was demonstrated in 18 cases and/or bilobar lesions were shown in 11 patients. Consequently, unnecessary laparotomy was averted in these patients, with 13 out of 14 patients (93%) undergoing liver resection following exploratory laparotomy. Comparison with the preceding group of patients in whom staging laparoscopy had not been performed revealed a significant improvement in the resectability rate following the adoption of staging laparoscopy.[28]

Nevertheless, the popularity of current radiological modalities such as CT arterioportography (CTAP) in the pre-operative assessment of patients with liver metastases continues to overshadow the potential benefit of laparoscopy. While the sensitivity of CTAP in detecting small liver metastases undoubtedly represents an improvement over other cross-sectional imaging techniques, the challenge of detecting minimal volume superficial and extrahepatic tumour remains. Furthermore, the dilemma posed by the high incidence of false-positive CTAP results reported in several series is a concern. Preliminary results of a prospective comparison of staging laproscopy (with LapUS) versus CTAP in the pre-operative staging of 37 patients with colorectal liver metastases again supported an ongoing role for laparoscopic assessment.[30] Extrahepatic and/or bilobar metastases below the threshold of detection of CTAP were demonstrated laparoscopically in 10 patients (27%). Furthermore, laparoscopy with LapUS was able to refute false-positive CTAP findings (bilobar lesions and portal vein invasion) in 6 out of 37 patients (16%). These observations support the role of staging laparoscopy at least as an adjunct to existing non-invasive imaging techniques in the pre-operative assessment of such patients.

Laparoscopic Ultrasonography

Despite the aforementioned advantages of laparoscopy in the assessment of liver metastases, there are inherent limitations associated with the technique. Laparoscopic inspection alone is insufficient for the detection of liver tumours in approximately one-third of patients who present with intrahepatic lesions situated away from the visible organ surface, and in those in whom the liver is partially obscured by adhesions. Nor can the laparoscopist determine their exact relationships with the intrahepatic vascular structures since the liver bears few surface anatomical markings. A fundamental component in the planning of hepatic resectional surgery is the ability to document the site, size and number of liver tumours, and their pattern of involvement with respect to the segmental hepatic anatomy. These shortcomings may potentially be addressed by the technique of LapUS which exploits the advantages of intraoperative contact ultrasonography (IOUS) during laparoscopy.

Early studies of B-mode LapUS imaging of the abdominal organs involved prototype laparoscopic probes incorporating the ultrasound transducer within the telescope shaft ('echolaparoscopes'). In the early 1980s, Japanese workers reported their success in using such devices to provide recognizable, high resolution images of intrahepatic lesions during diagnostic laparoscopy, in some cases succeeding where transabdominal ultrasonography had failed.[31,32] Furukawa and colleagues used a 5–7.5 MHz 360° sectoral scanning probe which was introduced through a separate port from the laparoscope, and reported 'diagnostic value' in 36 of 42 cases of liver tumour and 8 of 10 cases of liver cysts.[33]

The development of linear array LapUS probes appears to have improved examination of the liver compared with radial-scanning or sectoral-scanning probes.[34] The potential disadvantages of sectoral-scanning LapUS transducers in the assessment of the liver was reported by Fornari and colleagues who reported their experience with a prototype rigid 180° sector scanning laparosocopic ultrasound probe.[35] 'Blind areas' in the posterolateral sector of the liver resulted in the failure to detect some lesions, adequate sonographic penetration of the hepatic parenchyma was not always achieved and orientation of the image with respect to the intrahepatic vasculature could be difficult with this transducer configuration.[35] Conversely, the stable and more easily manipulated rectilinear image obtained with linear array LapUS probes was found to be better suited for cross-sectional hepatic imaging in the same way as the linear array IOUS probes which had found popularity with liver surgeons.[34] The feasibility of obtaining LapUS-guided needle biopsies of small intrahepatic tumours which were not visible laparoscopically was also demonstrated using this type of instrument.[36,37] In 1984, Okita and colleagues described their success in using LapUS to diagnose tumour invasion of the portal vein, albeit in the context of hepatocellular carcinoma.[38] However, LapUS remained an essentially experimental technique until the revival of interest in minimal access surgery in the early 1990s when a variety of sophisticated LapUS systems became commercially available.

Initially, an improvised LapUS technique was developed in the Royal Infirmary, Edinburgh, whereby a 16-mm diameter 5-MHz linear array ultrasound probe designed for endorectal ultrasonography was introduced into the abdominal cavity via a custom built large port assembly.[39] The improved resolution of this system over preoperative CT, US and SVA was illustrated by the additional diagnostic and staging information obtained in 7 patients with primary and secondary liver tumours under consideration for liver resection. Laparoscopic inspection identified extrahepatic tumour spread and/or bilobar liver tumour in 2 patients. Using LapUS, factors contraindicating surgical intervention were demonstrated in 4 further patients in whom bilobar liver tumour and portal vein invasion were defined.[39]

Having adopted pre-operative laparoscopic evaluation of potential candidates for liver resection (see above), the contribution of LapUS over laparoscopy was assessed.[28] Additional staging information was attributable to LapUS in 18 out of 43 patients examined (42%) (bilobar or multifocal liver tumour, hilar lymphadenopathy and main portal or hepatic venous invasion). In 7 patients, the avoidance of unnecessary laparotomy was attributable to the findings of LapUS alone.[28] However, scrutiny of the contribution of LapUS over staging laparoscopy alone in the pre-operative assessment of patients with colorectal liver metastases has indicated that its impact may be rather more marginal in terms of clinical decision making.[30] Upstaging of tumour status was a direct result of LapUS alone in only 3 out of 37 patients (8%), although this does not take account of its important contribution in refuting the 6 instances of overstaging associated with CTAP (16%).[30]

The insensitivity of pre-operative scanning investigations in detecting occult hepatic metastases in patients undergoing resection of primary colorectal cancers, together with the surgeon's inability to manually palpate the liver during minimal access procedures, inevitably supports a potential role for LapUS in screening the liver during laparoscopic operations for colorectal malignancy. However,

there have been no published studies evaluating LapUS in such a role, although the utility of IOUS in the detection of impalpable synchronous hepatic metastases at open surgery is well established. These observations seem certain to be reproduced in the context of the detection of occult liver metastases during minimal access colorectal cancer operations.

Recent technical innovations in the design of LapUS instruments include the development of flexible LapUS probes which may be used to examine less accessible areas within the abdomen, and scanners incorporating colour flow Doppler technology. In the authors' experience, articulating probes certainly improve the manoeuvrability of the transducer and may facilitate LapUS examination of the posterior reaches of the liver. They may also improve transducer contact in the presence of large intrahepatic tumours causing gross abnormalities in hepatic contour (Figure 7.2). However, the additional expertise required to manipulate the hand-piece control levers may distract the novice laparoscopic ultrasonographer, while such probes have proven to be more vulnerable to breakage. In practice, the simple step of flooding the upper abdomen with warm crystalloid solution usually establishes excellent acoustic contact which permits the rigid LapUS probe to be 'floated' in the sub-phrenic space, providing adequate imaging of the posterolateral hepatic segments (Figure 7.3).

Although colour flow Doppler scanning may highlight vascular intrahepatic lesions, including metastases, its immediate contribution to hepatic laparoscopic ultrasonography may not be sufficient to justify its additional expense. Colour flow imaging usually occurs at the expense of B-mode image quality, and while rapid recognition of ductal, venous and arterial structures may be facilitated by this technique, similar information is readily available using a simple audible Doppler signal which is a feature of most LapUS systems.

Liver Biopsy

Biopsy of a solid liver lesion is indicated in cases of diagnostic doubt, for example when the presence of liver metastasis from a primary malignancy of unknown origin is suspected. Biopsy may also be required during the staging of hepatic malignancy

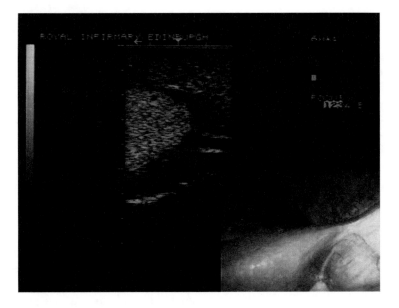

Figure 7.2. Laparoscopic ultrasound demonstration of a laparosopically invisible liver metastasis in hepatic segment IV. Use of a 'flexible' LapUS probe (Aloka, KeyMed Ltd, Southend-on-Sea, UK) ensures optimal apposition of the linear array transducer with the liver surface to demonstrate a hyperechoic liver tumour.

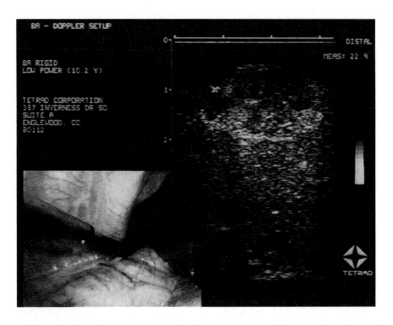

Figure 7.3. The rigid LapUS probe has been 'floated' away from the liver surface in the right subphrenic space to demonstrate a superficially situated haemangioma in hepatic segment VI. Note the hyperechoic appearance associated with posterior acoustic enhancement. Electronic calipers have measured the maximum diameter of this lesion at 22.4 mm (top right of image).

when the resultant information may affect clinical management. It should be emphasized that it is unacceptable to deny a patient potentially curative surgical intervention on the basis of laparoscopic appearances without confirmatory tissue diagnosis. Confirmation of a tissue diagnosis of liver metasta-sis may be important in patients entered into clinical trials where such confirmation is mandatory, while the presence of diffuse parenchymal liver diseases such as steatosis, hepatitis and cirrhosis should be documented through biopsy of the adjacent liver, as the confirmation of such findings may establish a relative contraindication to hepatic resection. However, this is usually more relevant to the management of patients with hepatocellular carcinoma than liver metastases.

Conversely, it is important to exercise restraint when contemplating biopsy of focal liver lesions. Laparoscopic (or percutaneous) biopsy of potentially resectable liver tumour is usually contraindicated because of the risk of malignant seeding into the peritoneal cavity, to the port site or to the needle track. The dissemination of resectable disease in this way is a well-documented complication which should be regarded as an avoidable catastrophe, although most reported cases refer to patients with hepatocellular carcinoma.[40-45] The laparoscopic discovery of liver metastases in an anatomically resectable location and without evidence of extrahepatic dissemination warrants exploratory laparotomy with a view to liver resection. Histological proof of malignancy is rarely required under these circumstances, as the radiological, laparoscopic and biochemical findings and the clinical context of the case are usually sufficient for management decisions. Laparoscopy with biopsy should also be deferred in patients with coagulopathy, and caution should be excercised before attempting biopsy of a superficial liver lesion which might represent a haemangioma with the attendent risk of haemorrhage. Similarly, there should be a high index of suspicion regarding the biopsy of lesions where echinococcal cyst is a possibility (e.g. suspected necrotic metastases with cystic change).

The role of laparoscopically-guided needle biopsy of suspected malignant liver lesions compared with blind percutaneous biopsy or radiologically-guided percutaneous biopsy has long provoked controversy. However, it is recognized that the positive yield of a single random percutaneous liver biopsy is <50% in patients with focal hepatic malignancy, and the benefits of laparoscopic liver biopsy over blind percutaneous biopsy has been emphasized by workers such as Trujillo[4] (see above). Nevertheless, the development of non-invasive radiological imaging technique such as USS, CT and MRI as a means of directing needle biopsy has challenged the role of laparoscopy in the retrieval of targetted-biopsy specimens.[46] In this context there is no evidence supporting a primary role for laparoscopic-guided biopsy over scan-guided biopsy in diagnosis of overt focal liver metastases. A study by Fornari and colleagues underlined this fact, where USS-guided FNAC was compared with laparoscopic biopsy utilising core-cutting needles in 63 patients.[47] There were no significant differences with respect to sensitivity and accuracy (76% versus 74%, and 84% versus 83%, respectively).

Some workers have emphasized the importance of obtaining a wedge biopsy of liver, as opposed to needle biopsy, under certain circumstances such as staging laparoscopy for Hodgkin's lymphoma. Accordingly, Lefor and Flowers have described the technique of laparoscopic wedge biopsy of the liver whereby an Endo-GIA® (Auto-Suture) stapling device is introduced via a 12-mm port.[48] A wedge of liver is excized from the free edge of the left hepatic lobe having created two haemostatic staple lines placed at a 90° angle with overlap of the staple lines at the apex. However, they have urged caution in instances where the liver edge is gauged to be too thick or firm for fear of problems maintaining haemostasis, and it seems unlikely that this techniques will contribute to laparoscopic biopsy in the context of hepatic metastases in other circumstances.

Fukuda et al. first reported LapUS-guided biopsy of focal liver malignancy in 1984,[36] having successfully confirmed the presence of small hepatocellular carcinomas not visible laparoscopically in 4 patients. Bönhof and coworkers later reported being able to exclude focal malignancy and confirm fatty infiltration by LapUS-guided biopsy, thus resolving an instance of diagnostic doubt.[37] It is to be hoped that LapUS sytems incorporating guided-needle biopsy systems will be developed commercially to facilitate accurate and representative sampling of the liver. Until this happens, it will remain necessary to perform laparoscopic and LapUS-guided needle biopsy of the liver by the free-hand technique under direct vision (see below).

Technique of Laparoscopy with Laparoscopic Ultrasonography

While laparoscopic evaluation of the liver is possible using local or general anaesthesia, it is the authors' own practice to perform the procedure under general anaesthesia with endotracheal intubation, mechanical ventilation and muscle relaxation as a separate procedure from any planned exploratory laparotomy. Local anaesthesia may be facilitated by the use of intravenous sedation, and may be performed as a day case, but usually demands the use of small calibre (e.g. 5-mm diameter) laparoscopes, a low-pressure pneumoperitoneum (i.e. <10 mmHg) and nitrous oxide gas for insufflation. Local anaesthetic procedures can be limited by patient discomfort, anxiety and vagal reactions when manipulating the abdominal viscera, especially when LapUS is also performed via a second 10-mm port, and these factors may limit the examination. Bleiberg and coworkers attributed their relatively low success rate in obtaining adequate laproscopic liver biopsies in 66% of 240 patients primarily to the limitations of the local anaesthetic procedure.[49] However, they subsequently observed an improvement in the yield of satisfactory laparoscopic liver biopsies in 90% out of 112 patients examined under general anaesthesia.[50] While it is recognized that many thousands of laparoscopic liver examinations (often with biopsy) are performed as a day case under local anaesthetic every year, it is the authors' belief that the high yield of useful information affecting patient management, plus the absence of additional morbidity, justifies laparoscopy with LapUS as a separate general anaesthetic procedure on clinical as well as health economic grounds.

With the patient placed supine on the operating table, two ports are usually inserted, one at the umbilicus and the other in the right flank (although a left flank port may be preferable in patients with left-sided lesions). This enables the camera and LapUS probe or accessory instrument positions to be alternated. We prefer to employ a direct cutdown technique to achieve access to the peritoneal cavity, avoiding the risk of visceral or vascular injury associated with the blind introduction of a Veress needle. This approach is particularly useful in patients who have undergone previous abdominal surgery, and is also a safer option in the presence of abdominal wall venous collaterals in patients with cirrhosis and portal hypertension. In a series of 52 patients undergoing staging laparoscopy with LapUS in Edinburgh,[28] laparoscopy failed due to adhesions in only 2 cases (4%), despite previous laparotomy having been performed in 78% of patients. Placing the patient in 20° reverse Trendelenberg position facilitating inspection of the liver by the inferior displacement of the upper abdominal viscera.

Systematic laparoscopic inspection of the peritoneal cavity and liver is performed. The use of a 30° oblique viewing laparoscopic telescope facilitates inspection of the undersurfaces of the falciform liga-

ment and anterior abdominal wall, and to view the posterosuperior surfaces of the liver in the subphrenic spaces. It is also important to retract the left hepatic lobe with a probe to inspect its undersurface (Figure 7.1), the lesser omentum and caudate lobe behind. Malignant peritoneal seedlings appear as tiny white plaques and are best biopsied using laparoscopic scissors or biopsy forceps. Small raised plaques discovered on the liver capsule should always be biopsied as it is often impossible to distinguish a variety of benign lesions (hamartomas, von Meyenberg's complex or biliary ectasia) from malignancy, particularly when there is a background of cirrhosis or biliary obstruction. Such superficial liver lesions are amenable to excison biopsy with scissors or toothed biopsy forceps (Figure 7.4). Alternatively, brush cytology with a sheathed nylon brush, similar to that used during fibreoptic endoscopy, has been reported to be accurate in the diagnosis of superficial liver lesions[51] and has the advantage of being non-traumatic.

Laparoscopic ultrasonography is facilitated by the thin film of moisture covering the surfaces of the abdominal organs which provides excellent transducer contact and promotes high resolution contact sonography. As described above, the instillation of up to 500 ml of crystalloid solution into the peritoneal cavity optimizes 'acoustic coupling', minimizing the amount of probe pressure required to achieve satisfactory transducer contact and acting as a 'stand-off' to demonstrate superficially placed lesions in the 'near-field' of the transducer (Figure 7.3). Peritoneal washings may also be retrieved for cytological examination following diagnostic or staging laparoscopy in cases of intra-abdominal malignancy, although is rarely positive in the absence of peritoneal or hepatic carcinomatosis.

The type of LapUS transducer most commonly employed in the examination of the liver consists of a linear array transducer with a flat side-viewing 'footprint' which generates rectilinear shaped sonograms over a distance of approximately 4 cm. Such probes operate with frequencies of 5–10 MHz, thus providing a spatial resolution of <1 mm and tissue penetration of 3–7 cm which is ideal for evaluation of liver lesions. The probe is sterilised by immersion in glutaraldehyde solution (or by exposure to ethylene oxide gas), and is connected by cable to a portable scanning machine which is positioned adjacent to the operating table. While LapUS images may be observed in real-time on the integrated monitor of the scanning machine, the use of an

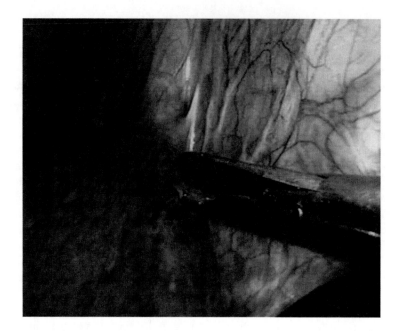

Figure 7.4. Excisional biopsy of a tiny capsular abnormality from the leading edge of hepatic segment IV using straight-bladed laparoscopic scissors confirmed the diagnosis of metastatic adenocarcinoma.

audiovisual mixing device is recommended to permit simultaneous 'picture-in-picture' viewing of both the laparoscopic camera view and the LapUS images on the operating room monitors.

It is convenient to consider LapUS scanning with a rigid linear array probe inserted via the umbilical port as providing images in a predominantly sagittal plane, whereas scanning takes place in a predominantly transverse plane when the probe is operated from a lateral port. In reality, a full range of oblique 'cuts' are produced which enables the laparoscopic ultrasonographer to perceive in real-time the three-dimensional anatomical detail of the liver from the observed sequence of two-dimensional images. It is usually feasible to achieve a complete LapUS examination of the liver using a single 10-mm diameter port inserted at the umbilicus so that evaluation of the liver may be performed during most minimal access therapeutic procedures (Figure 7.5). A second port placed laterally in the right flank affords optimal access for evaluation of the right hemiliver, although the siting of additional ports will be dictated by the presence of adhesions.

Attention is focused on any identified 'reference' lesion, whether by laparoscopic inspection of the liver, or by preceding investigations. Its sonographic appearance is characterized to facilitate comparison with any other abnormalities. A systematic anatomical survey of the liver is then performed to define the precise pattern of liver involvement, ensuring no 'blind areas' of hepatic parenchyma are overlooked. The anatomical survey relies on recognition of intrahepatic vascular landmarks given the paucity of surface markings on the liver capsule. The normal liver parenchyma has a fine homogeneous texture of medium echogenicity. Portal tracts are recognized by their hyperechoic fascial sheaths and divergent course away from the hilum, and visible blood flow may be observed within the larger portal vein branches. The intrahepatic arterial and biliary radicles are usually less obvious. The hepatic veins converge posterosuperiorly towards the inferior vena cava, and are characterized by their relatively attenuated walls and the fluctuating blood flow corresponding with the central venous pulse pressure.

A working knowledge of the hepatic segmental anatomy as described by the French surgical anatomist Couinaud (and later popularised by Bismuth), is fundamental to any hepatic imaging modality (Figure 7.5). Eight hepatic segments are divided into those forming the right hemiliver (V–VIII), the left hemiliver (II–IV) and caudate lobe (segment I). The functional midline of the liver (i.e. the plane of the principal fissure) passes between the gallbladder fossa and the inferior vena cava, has no external markings, but is defined by the course of the middle hepatic vein. This plane may be identified with the probe placed on the diaphrag-

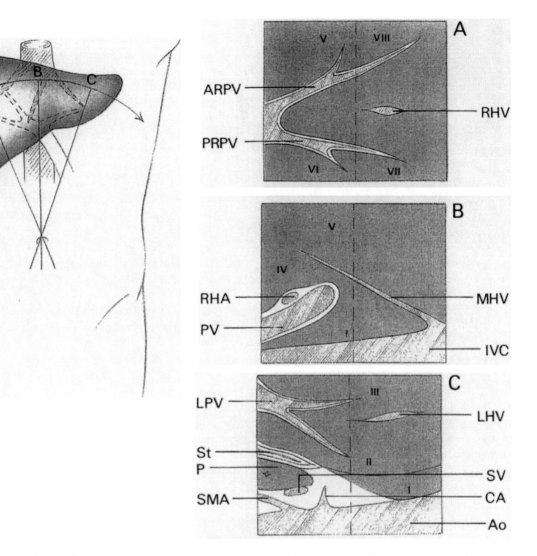

Figure 7.5. Schematic diagram illustrating the orientation of the sonograms obtained using a linear array laparoscopic ultrasound probe via an umbilical port. (A) Oblique scan through the right hemiliver demonstrating the bifurcation of the right portal vein into its anterior (ARPV) and posterior (PRPV) divisions. The right hepatic vein (RHV) is seen passing in the plane between the anterior (V and VIII) and posterior (VI and VII) sectors of the right hemiliver. (B) Parasagittal scan angled slightly to the left through hepatic segment V, the middle hepatic vein (MHV), hepatic segment IV and the caudate lobe (segment I) which separates the hilar structures from the inferior vena cava (IVC). The right hepatic artery (RHA) is depicted passing anterior to the main portal vein (PV). (C) Oblique scan through the left hepatic lobe demonstrating the branches of the left portal vein (LPV) to segments II and III, which are separated from the caudate lobe (I) by the interlobar fissure, and the left hepatic vein. The hepatic parenchyma acts as an acoustic window through which the compressed stomach (St), body of pancreas (P) and paraaortic region may be identified. Ao = aorta; CA = coeliac axis; SMA = superior mesenteric artery; SV = splenic vein; LHV = left hepatic vein.

matic surface of the liver, advancement of the probe serving to trace the course of the middle hepatic vein to its confluence with the inferior vena cava (Figure 7.6). Anteriorly, the structures traversing the liver hilum are identified, and these are separated from the inferior vena cava by the caudate lobe (segment I). From this plane of reference, the anatomical survey is performed with smooth slow sweeps and subtle rotatory movements of the probe over the liver capsule.

The insertion of the falciform ligament and ligamentum teres provides a visual boundary between hepatic segment IV (the quadrate lobe) and the left hepatic lobe (segments II and III) which comprise the left hemiliver. Access to the left subphrenic space for LapUS examination of the left hepatic lobe

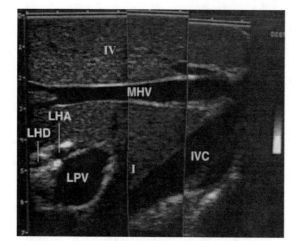

Figure 7.6. Laparoscopic sonograms through the liver in a parasagittal plane slightly to the left of the midline of the liver. The probe was inserted through the umbilical port, and successive cuts obtained as it was gradually withdrawn to show the convergent courses of the middle (MHV) and left hepatic vein (unlabelled) with the inferior vena cava (IVC). The hilar structures (left portal vein, LPV; left hepatic artery, LHA; and left hepatic duct, LHD) surrounded by the hyperechoic Glissonian sheath are shown in cross-section and separate hepatic segments I and IV inferiorly.

well-defined hyperechoic plane demarcating the caudate lobe, the inferior vena cava and the para-aortic region from hepatic segment II (Figure 7.5).

The right hemiliver is divided by the transverse course of the right hepatic vein into anterior (segments V and VIII) and posterior (segments VI and VII) sectors (Figure 7.1). This plane has no surface markings and may be optimally defined with the LapUS probe inserted through a right flank port into the right paracolic gutter and right lateral subphrenic space. The anterior sector comprises segment V inferiorly (readily identified adjacent to the gallbladder fossa), and segment VIII superiorly (forming the 'dome of the liver'). The posterior sector comprises segment VI (adjacent to the right kidney inferiorly), and segment VII (the least accessible segment and concealed with the bare area posterolaterally). The anterior and posterior sectoral divisions of the right portal pedicle are bifurcate perpendicular to the plane of the right hepatic vein, and their respective segmental branches can be defined (Figure 7.5).

Focal hepatic abnormalities may be described as hyperechoic, isoechoic or hypoechoic relative to the background hepatic parenchyma. They may be distinguished from benign lesions such as simple hepatic cysts, focal fatty infiltration and haemangiomas. Simple cysts are anechoic, lack a defined wall and cause posterior acoustic enhancement.

may be achieved by incision of the falciform ligament when exposure is prevented by left upper abdominal adhesions. The fascia of the hepatic insertion of the lesser omentum is identified as a

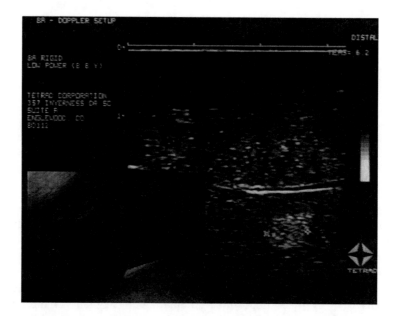

Figure 7.7. Staging laparoscopic ultrasonography for pancreatic cancer with the probe placed upon hepatic segment VI. A hyperechoic metastasis (measuring 6.2 mm in diameter) has been demonstrated lying posterior to the right hepatic vein in hepatic segment VII.

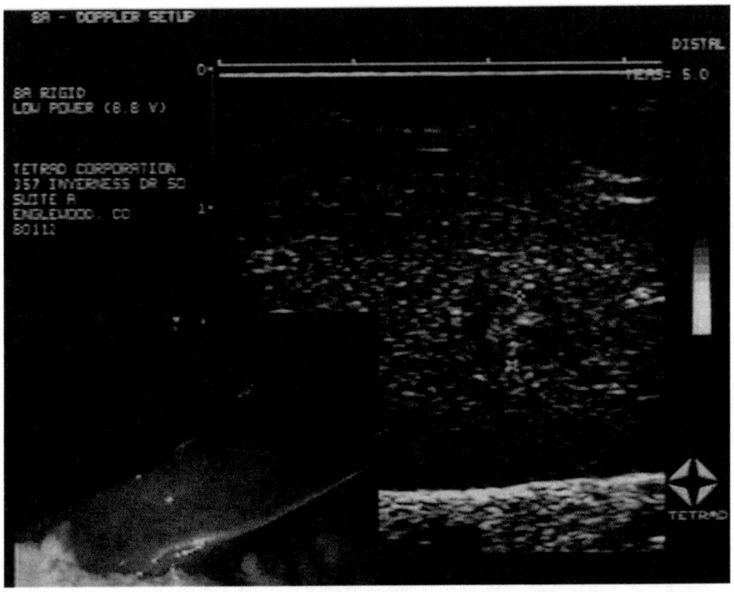

Figure 7.8. Isoechoic intrahepatic metastasis detected by LapUS with the probe placed on the right hepatic lobe. An anechoic halo circumscribes the lesion, and electronic calipers indicate a tumour diameter of 5 mm in diameter (top right).

Fatty infiltration is commonly encountered adjacent to the ligamentum teres insertion and gallbladder fossa, appearing as a well-circumscribed, irregular hyperechoic area. Haemangiomas are hyperechoic lesions which are discovered incidentally in 5–10% of patients and do not cause posterior attenuation of the ultrasound beam ('shadowing'). Rather, they typically cause posterior acoustic enhancement (Figure 7.3). This is an important discriminating feature from hyperechoic metastases of gastrointestinal origin (Figure 7.7) which typically cause posterior acoustic attenuation. Metastatic lesions also vary according to the presence of cystic or necrotic areas, calcification and the presence of satellite nodules. However, it is the presence of an 'anechoic halo' around the lesion which is pathognomonic for liver metastases (i.e. 'bullseye' or 'target' lesions) (Figure 7.8). This feature should be readily recognized by the laparoscopic ultrasonographer. The number, size and site of metastatic lesions and their relationship with important vascular structures is defined so that where appropriate, anatomical liver resections may be planned with adequate tumour clearance to maximize postoperative survival. Occlusion or stenosis of the portal veins, hepatic veins or inferior vena cava should be sought, and the hilar and para-aortic regions should be scrutinized for extrahepatic disease in the form of malignant regional lymphadenopathy.

Focal intrahepatic liver lesions usually require needle biopsy. The needle must be of adequate length to traverse the tissues of the abdominal wall, the cushion of gas formed by the pneumoperitoneum and the intervening liver parenchyma. If necessary, the pneumoperitoneum may be partially deflated to bring the abdominal wall and liver into closer proximity. Temporary cessation of respiration or mechanical ventilation may facilitate placement of the biopsy needle and reduce the risk of liver laceration. A separate needle puncture technique is utilized, whereby the biopsy needle is introduced into camera view from a puncture site distant from the camera port (Figure 7.9). The exact site of needle puncture and the angle of insertion are chosen carefully to avoid abdominal wall blood vessels and to ensure the accessibility of the target lesion.

For LapUS-guided needle biopsy, light abrasion of the needle tip with a scalpel blade produces a well-defined hyperechoic signal which facilitates sonographic identification (Figure 7.10). As with laparoscopic needle biopsy under direct vision, the site of needle puncture must be chosen carefully to facilitate access to the desired area of liver, and to anticipate the angle of the needle within the sonographic field. Large intrahepatic blood vessels, the bile ducts and gallbladder should again be avoided. The needle track appears as a bright point source when the needle enters perpendicular to the sono-

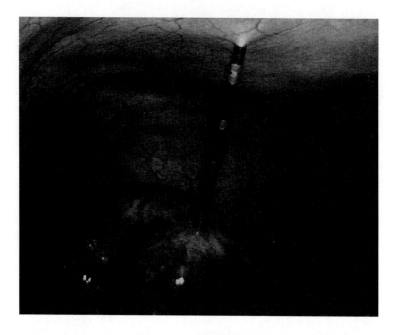

Figure 7.9. Laparoscopic-guided needle biopsy of a large metastasis of colorectal origin arising from the left hepatic lobe.

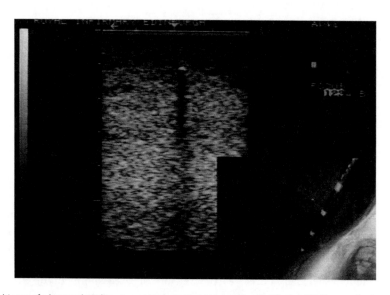

Figure 7.10. Needle biopsy of a hyperechoic liver tumour in hepatic segment IV guided by LapUS. The needle tip generates abright signal casting a posterior acoustic shadow which may be emphasised by abrasion of the needle tip.

graphic 'cut' (Figure 7.10), and as a hyperechoic linear signal when the needle is inserted in the same plane as the ultrasound beam. Slight rotatory or side-to-side movements of the LapUS transducer help to maintain the three-dimensional orientation of the ultrasonographer during the biopsy procedure.

Most needle tracks cease bleeding spontaneously several minutes after withdrawal of the biopsy needle from the liver, but haemostasis must be ensured prior to withdrawal of the ports. Tamponade of the biopsy site using a blunt instrument such as a LapUS probe is usually all that is required. Some workers have reported the utility of laparoscopic thermal probes, the tips of which are placed tangentially over the biopsy site to promote coagulation.[52]

Laparoscopically-Assisted Hepatic Resection

Introduction

Whereas the diagnostic role of laparoscopy and laparoscopic ultrasonography has become increasingly established in the management of hepatobiliary disease, it is not yet clear whether laparoscopic liver surgery will become established in the surgical treatment of hepatic disease. Early experience has shown that a number of simple procedures can be undertaken by laparoscopic means with not inconsiderable benefit to the patient, resulting from the avoidance of laparotomy.[53-56] However, major laparoscopic interventions to the liver are technically demanding and their benefit and safety to the patient have yet to be ascertained. The role of laparoscopy and laparoscopic ultrasonography in facilitating tumour destruction by cryo-ablation and interstitial therapy have been evaluated by some workers, although any advantage over an open surgical or percutaneous approach is not clearly evident.[57]

In the management of benign hepatic pathology, for example, we and others have confirmed the feasibility of undertaking extensive laparoscopic procedures for patients with benign hepatic cysts.[53,55] Decompression and extensive deroofing of cysts is an attractive proposition for the laparoscopic surgeon, since this does not involve the sacrifice of hepatic parenchyma, produces minimal blood loss and does not require the delivery of extensive amounts of tissue from the abdomen. Although some workers have suggested that laparoscopic surgical intervention is ideally suited to the management of benign cysts, we have noted, however, that access to posteriorly-located cysts is difficult and that patients with extensive polycystic involvement do not achieve great benefit from this minimal access procedure.[56] Laparoscopic intervention for more complex cysts, such as those resulting from hydatid disease, is less clear. Early reports have highlighted the possible risk of contamination of the peritoneal cavity by live daughter cysts during the surgery and, as at open surgery, liberal use of scolicidal agents, may give cause for concern.[54] Such laparoscopic procedures raise the question as to whether a potential short-term gain is achieved at the expense of a long-term compromise.

Hepatic Resections

In recent years, postoperative morbidity and mortality rates have been reduced following hepatic resection through the restriction of such procedures to specialist centres.[58] As yet, most attempts at laparoscopic liver surgery have been attempted in non-specialist centres and, whilst this experience has clearly indicated the ability of performing such resections, there are no data which enable assessment of benefit to the patient.[59-62]

A number of techniques which are applicable to open hepatic resectional surgery can be considered for laparoscopic liver surgery. There is no doubt that development of laparoscopic instrumentation will allow mobilization of the liver and dissection of its vascular pedicles. Although water-jet dissection has been proposed as a means of facilitating open hepatic resectional surgery, this technique is unsuitable for laparoscopic use because of the contamination of the operating field and telescope. Furthermore, concerns have been expressed regarding the possibility of disseminating hepatic malignancy as a result of the dislodgement of cells and cellular aggregates by the pressurized jet.[57]

As at open surgery, dissection of the hepatic parenchyma would be greatly facilitated by ultrasonic dissection.[58,63] The cavitational ultrasonic surgical aspirator (CUSA) removes hepatic tissue as a result of the cavitational effect of the oscillating ultrasonic dissector. Irrigation and suction at the tip of this device maintains a clean operating field and enables skeletonization of the intraparenchymal structures. These vessels can be secured before they have the opportunity to retract into the liver tissue. There is, however, still a tendency for mist or spray to result in contamination of the telescope.

Haemostasis can be achieved by multiple application of metal clips and/or diathermy. Bleeding from the transected liver surface can be controlled by use of ion plasma coagulation.[64] A high-frequency current is used to ionize argon, thereby creating an ion plasma within the gas jet which spreads across the tissue surface and produces uniform and shallow coagulation of the tissue. Extensive areas can therefore be spray coagulated without coming into contact or dislodging the coagulum. Where a positive-pressure pneumoperitoneum is employed, however, care must be taken because of the rise in the intra-abdominal pressure due to the inflow of argon gas during coagulation.

Technique

The techniques described have generally required insertion of at least five trocars to enable placement of the telescope, retractors and instrumentation. Mobilization of the liver can be undertaken by division of the falciform and triangular ligaments. The most commonly undertaken resection has involved that of the left lobe (segments II and III). Such a resection would require division of the lesser omentum, taking care to identify any aberrant left hepatic artery.

Gugenheim and his colleagues[61] have described laparoscopic, non-anatomical liver resection in three patients Access was achieved by the insertion of six ports after creation of a pneumoperitoneum of 13 mmHg. Hook diathermy was employed to incise the liver capsule approximately 2 cm from the lesion. The subsegmental pedicles were skeletonized by ultrasonic dissection before being secured by resorbable clips. Haemostasis was achieved by diathermy, argon beam coagulation and the application of fibrin glue. The specimens were retrieved either through an enlarged umbilical incision or via a McBurney incision. No transfusion of blood was required in the patients reported and 2 of the 3 patients were discharged home before the seventh postoperative day.

Azagra and his colleagues[60] have described an anatomical left lobectomy which pursues the same principles as that employed at open surgery. The individual pedicles to segments II and III are identified in the umbilical fissure and secured by a combination of extracorporeal slip-knot, clipping and division by a stapling device. The parenchymatous dissection can be undertaken by means of an ultrasonic laparoscopic hand-piece dissector and the left hepatic vein secured by a tourniquet before division with a stapling device. Delivery of the specimen requires a mini-laparotomy incision of at least 5 cm in length at the umbilicus.

The advantage of such a technique is not entirely apparent from the technique described by Azagra and his colleagues.[60] The operative procedure lasted 6 hours and 30 minutes and was associated with a blood loss of 600 ml. Although there were no postoperative complications, the patient was only discharged from hospital on the eighth postoperative day.

In addition to the conventional risks of open hepatic resectional surgery, concerns have been expressed regarding the risk of gas embolization. This complication was encountered by Cuschieri[57] during an attempted laparoscopic-assisted liver resection and is a major cause for concern. This risk can be minimized if the hepatic resection is undertaken using a gasless technique combined with abdominal wall lift devices. The disadvantage of dispensing with the pneumoperitoneum is that blood loss from the divided hepatic parenchyma may be increased.

In one of the largest series in the literature to date, Kaneko and his colleagues describe 11 consecutive cases of laparoscopic hepatic resection undertaken using a gasless technique.[62] Non-anatomical techniques of resection were employed in most cases and with the assistance of microwave tissue coagulation and ultrasonic surgical aspiration techniques. One of the 10 patients required conversion to an open operation because of haemorrhage and operation times were in the range 1–7 hours. All patients were ambulant by the seventh postoperative day (including the patient converted to an open operation!) but no data were available on duration of convalescence.

Conclusion

The recent development of laparoscopic surgical techniques has caused many surgeons to reconsider the role of diagnostic laparoscopy in the evaluation of hepatic metastases. Peritoneal and overt hepatic dissemination can be detected thereby avoiding unnecessary laparotomy. The limitations of laparoscopy in assessing the depths of the liver substance have been overcome with the development of laparoscopic ultrasound transducers. Detailed information can be obtained on the precise location of the tumour and the presence of further metastases can be excluded. Considerable information is now available to suggest that patients can be better selected for consideration of hepatic resection by including laparoscopic ultrasonography into the investigative algorithm of hepatic metastases.

Whereas laparoscopic surgery has become increasingly established in many areas of gastrointestinal disease, laparoscopic hepatic resection poses a number of challenges which are not easily surmountable. Despite developments in instrumentation, laparoscopic surgeons have tended to be restricted to performing non anatomical liver resections. It remains to be seen whether the potential advantages of earlier discharge from hospital will compromise long term survival.

References

1. Bernheim B. Organoscopy: cystoscopy of the abdominal cavity. *Ann Surg* 1911; **53**:764–767.
2. Ruddock JC. Peritoneoscopy. *Surg Gynecol Obstet* 1937; **65**:623–639.
3. Benedict EB. Peritoneoscopy. *N Engl J Med* 1938; **218**:713–714.
4. Trujillo NP. Peritoneoscopy and guided biopsy in the diagnosis of intraabdominal disease. *Gastroenterology* 1976; **71**:1083–1085.
5. Brady PG, Peebles M, Goldschmid S. Role of laparoscopy in the evaluation of patients with suspected hepatic or peritoneal malignancy. *Gastrointest Endosc* 1991; **37**:27–30.
6. Warshaw AL, Tepper JE, Shipley WU. Laparoscopy in the staging and planning of therapy for pancreatic cancer. *Am J Surg* 1986; **151**:76–80.
7. Warshaw AL, Gu ZY, Wittenberg J, Waltman AC. Preoperative staging and assessment of resectability of pancreatic cancer. *Arch Surg* 1990; **125**:230–233.
8. Gross E, Bancewicz J, Ingram G. Assessment of gastric carcinoma by laparoscopy. *Br Med J* 1984; **288**:1577.
9. Shandall A, Johnson C. Laparoscopy or scanning in oesophageal and gastric carcinoma. *Br J Surg* 1985; **72**:449–451.
10. Dagnini G, Caldironi MW, Marin G, Buzzaccarini O, Tremolada C, Ruol A. Laparoscopy in abdominal staging of esophageal carcinoma: report of 369 cases. *Gastrointest Endosc* 1986; **32**:400–402.
11. Possik RA, Franco EL, Pires DR, Wohnrath DR, Ferreira EB. Sensitivity, specificity, and predictive value of laparoscopy for the staging of gastric cancer and for the detection of liver metastases. *Cancer* 1986; **58**:1–6.
12. Kriplani AK, Kapur ML. Laparoscopy for pre-operative staging and assessment of operability in gastric carcinoma. *Gastrointest Endosc* 1991; **37**:441–443.
13. Bemelman WA, van Delden OM, van Lanschot JJB, de Wit LT, Smits NJ, Fockens P, Gouma DJ, Obertop H. Laparoscopy and laparoscopic ultrasonography in staging of carcinoma of the esophagus and gastric cardia. *J Am Coll Surg* 1995; **181**:421–425.
14. Molloy RG, McCourtney JS, Anderson JR. Laparoscopy in the management of patients with cancer of the gastric cardia and oesophagus. *Br J Surg* 1995; **82**:352–354.
15. Watt I, Stewart I, Anderson D, Bell G, Anderson JR. Laparoscopy, ultrasound and computed tomography in cancer of the oesophagus and gastric cardia: a prospective comparison for detecting intra-abdominal metastases. *Br J Surg* 1989; **76**:1036–1039.
16. Anderson DN, Campbell S, Park KGM. Accuracy of laparoscopic ultrasonography in the staging of upper gastrointestinal malignancy. *Br J Surg* 1996; **83**:1424–1428.
17. Lowy AM, Mansfield PF, Leach SD, Ajani J. Laparoscopic staging for gastric cancer. *Surgery* 1996; **119**:611–614.
18. Finch MD, John TG, Garden OJ, Allan PL, Paterson-Brown S. Laparoscopic ultrasonography for staging of gastroesophageal cancer. *Surgery* 1997; **121**:xxx–xxx. In press.
19. Rosenhoff SH, Young RC, Anderson TC *et al.* Peritoneoscopy: a valuable staging tool in ovarian carcinoma. *Ann Intern Med* 1975; **83**:37–41.
20. Margolis R, Hansen H, Muggia F, Kanhouwa S. Diagnosis of liver metastases in bronchogenic carcinoma. A comparative study of liver scans, function tests, and peritoneoscopy with liver biopsy in 111 patients. *Cancer* 1974; **34**:1825–1829.
21. Van der Spuy S, Levin W, Smit BJ, Graham T, McQuaide JR. Peritoneoscopy in the management of breast cancer. *S Afr Med J* 1978; **54**:402–403.
22. Bleiberg H, La Meir E, Lejeune F. Laparoscopy in the diagnosis of liver metastases in 80 cases of malignant melanoma. *Endoscopy* 1980; **12**:215–218.
23. Huberman M, Bunn P, Matthews M, Ihde D, Gazdar A, Cohen M, Minna J. Hepatic involvement in the cutaneous T-cell lymphomas. Results of percutaneous biopsy and peritoneoscopy. *Cancer* 1980; **45**:1683–1688.
24. Bagley C, Thomas L, Johnson R, Chretien P, DeVita V. Diagnosis of liver involvement by lymphoma: Results in 96 consecutive peritoneoscopies. *Cancer* 1973; **31**:840–847.
25. Kriplani AK, Jayant S, Kapur BM. Laparoscopy in primary carcinoma of the gallbladder. *Gastrointest Endosc* 1992; **38**:326–329.
26. Gmeinwieser J, Feuerbach S, Hohenberger W, Albrich H, Strotzer M, Hofstädter F, Geissler A. Spiral-CT in diagnosis of vascular involvement in pancreatic cancer. *Hepatogastroenterology* 1995; **42**:418–422.
27. Lefor AT, Hughes KS, Shiloni E, Steinberg SM, Vetto JT, Papa MZ, Sugarbaker PH, Chang AE. Intra-abdominal extrahepatic disease in patients with colorectal hepatic metastases. *Dis Colon Rectum* 1988; **31**:100–103.
28. John TG, Greig JD, Crosbie JL, Miles WFA, Garden OJ. Superior staging of liver tumors with laparoscopy and laparoscopic ultrasound. *Ann Surg* 1994; **220**:711–719.
29. Babineau TJ, Lewis WD, Jenkins RL, Bleday R, Steele GD, Forse RA. Role of staging laparoscopy in the treatment of hepatic malignancy. *Am J Surg* 1994; **167**:151–155.
30. John TG, Madhavan KK, Redhead DN, Crosbie JL, Garden OJ. Laparoscopic ultrasonography in the staging of colorectal liver metastases: a prospective comparison with CT arterioportography. *Br J Surg* 1996; **83**:31.
31. Aramaki N, Yoshida K, Yamashiro Y, Namihisa T. Ultrasonic laparoscopy [Abstract]. *Scand J Gastroenterol* 1982; **78**(Suppl 17):185.
32. Ota Y, Sato Y, Takatsui K, Kimura H, Torii M, Yamazaki M, Fujiwara K, Niwa H, Oka H, Oda T. New ultrasonic laparoscope. Improvement in diagnosis of intraabdominal disease [Abstract]. *Scand J Gastroenterol* 1982; **78**(Suppl 17):194.
33. Furukawa Y, Sakamoto F, Kanazawa H, Kohsaka N, Ishida H, Kuroda H, Katsuta N, Tsuneoka K. A new method of B-mode ultrasonography under laparoscopic guidance [Abstract]. *Scand J Gastroenterol* 1982; **78**(Suppl 17):186.
34. John TG, Garden OJ. Clinical experience with sector scan and linear array ultrasound probes in laparoscopic surgery. *Endosc Surg Allied Technol* 1994; **2**:134–142.
35. Fornari F, Civardi G, Cavanna L, Sbolli G, Rossi S, Di Stasi M, Buscarini E, Buscarini L. Laparoscopic ultrasonography in the study of liver diseases: preliminary results. *Surg Endosc* 1989; **3**:33–37.
36. Fukuda M, Mima S, Tanabe T, Suzuki Y, Hirata K, Terada S. Endoscopic sonography of the liver – diagnostic application of the echolaparoscope to localize intrahepatic lesions. *Scand J Gastroenterol* 1984; **19**(suppl 102):24–28.
37. Bönhof JA, Linhart P, Bettendorf U, Holper H. Liver biopsy guided by laparoscopic sonography. A case report demonstrating a new technique. *Endoscopy* 1984; **16**:237–239.
38. Okita K, Kodama T, Oda M, Takemoto T. Laparoscopic ultrasonography. Diagnosis of liver and pancreatic cancer. *Scand J Gastroenterol* 1984; **19**(Suppl 94):91–100.

39. Miles WFA, Paterson-Brown S, Garden OJ. Laparoscopic contact hepatic ultrasonography. *Br J Surg* 1992; **79**:419–420.

40. Keatc RF, Shaffer R. Seeding of hepatocellular carcinoma to peritoneoscopy insertion site. *Gastrointest Endosc* 1992; **38**:203–204.

41. John TG, Garden OJ. Needle track seeding of primary and secondary liver carcinoma after percutaneous liver biopsy. *HPB Surgery* 1993; **6**:199–204.

42. Nduka CC, Monson JRT, Menzies-Gow N, Darzi A. Abdominal wall metastasis following laparoscopy. *Br J Surg* 1994; **81**:648–652.

43. Yamada N, Shinzawa H, Ukai K *et al.* Subcutaneous seeding of small hepatocellular carcinoma after fine needle aspiration biopsy. *J Gastroenterol Hepatol* 1993; **8**:195–198.

44. Russi EG, Pergolizzi S, Mesiti M *et al.* Unusual relapse of hepatocellular carcinoma. *Cancer* 1992; **70**:1483–1487.

45. Ishida H, Dohzono T, Furukawa Y, Kobayashi M, Tsuneoka K. Laparoscopy and biopsy in the diagnosis of malignant intra-abdominal tumors. *Endoscopy* 1984; **16**:140–142.

46. Leuschner M, Leuschner U. Diagnostic laparoscopy in focal parenchymal disease of the liver. *Endoscopy* 1992; **24**:689–692.

47. Fornari F, Rapaccini GL, Cavanna L, Civardi G, Anti M, Fedeli G, Buscarini L. Diagnosis of hepatic lesions: ultra-1sonically guided fine needle biopsy or laparoscopy? *Gastrointest Endosc* 1988; **34**:231–234.

48. Lefor AT, Flowers JL. Laparoscopic wedge biopsy of the liver. *J Am Coll Surg* 1994; **178**:307–308.

49. Bleiberg H, Rozencweig M, Longeval E, Fruhling J, de Maertelaer V. Peritoneoscopy as a diagnostic supplement to liver function tests and liver scan in patients with carcinoma. *Surg Gynecol Obstet* 1977; **145**:821–825.

50. Bleiberg H, Rozencweig M, Mathieu M, Beyens M, Gompel C, Gerard A. The use of peritoneoscopy in the detection of liver metastases. *Cancer* 1978; **41**:863–867.

51. Lightdale CJ, Hajdu SI, Luishi CB. Cytology of the liver, spleen and peritoneum obtained by sheathed brush during laparoscopy. *Am J Gastroenterol* 1980; **74**:21–24.

52. Jeffers LJ, McDonald TJ, Hyder S, Foust R, Reddy KR, Schiff ER. The use of two new coagulation probes for control of haemorrhage in laparoscopic liver biopsy. *Gastrointest Endosc* 1989; **35**:398–402.

53. Paterson-Brown S, Garden OJ. Laser-assisted laparoscopic excision of liver cyst. *Br J Surg* 1991; **78**:1047.

54. Katkhouda N, Fabiani P, Benizri E, Mouiel J. Laser resection of a liver hydatid cyst under videolaparoscopy. *Br J Surg* 1992; **79**:560–561.

55. Morino M, de Giuli M, Festa V, Garrone C. Laparoscopic management of symptomatic nonparasitic cysts of the liver. *Ann Surg* 1994; **219**:157–164.

56. Rasmussen IC, Garden OJ. Benign lesions of the liver. In: *A Comparison to Specialist Surgical Practice – Hepatobiliary and Pancreatic Surgery* Garden OJ (eds), 1996: 49–69. London, WB Saunders.

57. Cuschieri A. Laparoscopic liver surgery. In: *Endosurgery.* Toouli J, Gossot D, Hunter JG (eds), 1996: 473–481. Edinburgh, Churchill Livingstone.

58. Garden OJ, Bismuth H. Hepatic resection. In: *Operative Surgery: Hepatobiliary and Pancreatic Surgery* 5th edn Carter DC, Russell RCG, Pitt HA, Bismuth H (eds), 1996: 30–45. London, Chapman and Hall.

59. Wayland Y, Woisetchlaeger R. Laparoskopische Resektion einer Leber Metastase. *Chirurgie* 1993; **64**:195–197.

60. Azagra JS, Goergen M, Gilbart E, Jacobs D. Laparoscopic anatomical (hepatic) left lateral segmentectomy – technical aspects. *Surg Endosc* 1996; **10**:758–761.

61. Gugenheim J, Mazza D, Katkhouda N, Goubaux B, Mouiel J. Laparoscopic resection of solid liver tumours. *Br J Surg* 1996; **83**:334–335.

62. Kaneko H, Takagi S, Shiba T. Laparoscopic partial hepatectomy and left lateral segmentectomy: Technique and results of a clinical series. *Surgery* 1996; **120**:468–475.

63. Farin G. Ultrasonic dissection in combination with high frequency surgery. *Endosc Surg* 1994; **2**:211–213.

64. Farin G, Grund KE. Technology of argon plasma coagulation with particular regard to endoscopic applications. *Endosc Surg* 1994; **2**:71–77.

65. Cuschieri A, Hall AW, Clark J. Value of laparoscopy in the diagnosis and management of pancreatic carcinoma. *Gut* 1978; **19**:672–677.

66. Cuschieri A. Laparoscopy for pancreatic cancer: does it benefit the patient? *Eur J Surg Oncol* 1988; **14**:41–44.

67. Ishida H. Peritoneoscopy and pancreas biopsy in the diagnosis of pancreatic diseases. *Gastrointest Endosc* 1983; **29**:211–218.

68. Fernández-del Castillo C, Warshaw AL. Laparoscopy for staging in pancreatic carcinoma. *Surg Oncol* 1993; **2**:25–29.

69. John TG, Greig JD, Carter DC, Garden OJ. Carcinoma of the pancreatic head and periampullary region: tumor staging with laparoscopy and laparoscopic ultrasonography. *Ann Surg* 1995; **221**:156–164.

70. Bemelman WA, de Wit LT, van Delden OM, Smits NJ, Obertop H, Rauws EJA, Gouma DJ. Diagnostic laparoscopy combined with laparoscopic ultrasonography in staging cancer of the pancreatic head region. *Br J Surg* 1995; **82**:820–824.

71. Fernández-del Castillo C, Rattner DW, Warshaw AL. Further experience with laparoscopy and peritoneal cytology in the staging of pancreatic cancer. *Br J Surg* 1995; **82**:1127–1129.

72. Conlon KC, Dougherty E, Klimstra DS, Coit DG, Turnbull ADM, Brennan MF. The value of minimal access surgery in the staging of patients with potentially resectable peripancreatic malignancy. *Ann Surg* 1996; **223**:134–140.

Liver Transplantation for Hepatic Metastases

Hauke Lang, Karl Jürgen Oldhafer, Hans Jürgen Schlitt, and Rudolf Pichlmayr†

8

Introduction

The results of hepatic resection for secondary liver tumours have (steadily) improved as a result of advances in surgical technique, perioperative management and diagnostic modalities which enable an earlier and more accurate detection of liver metastasis. Despite the development of extracorporeal liver surgery which enables the possibility of removing centrally located or multilocular intrahepatic tumours, only a small number of patients with secondary hepatic tumours are candidates for radical surgery.[1] Liver transplantation has broadened the limits of potential radicality by removing the diseased liver in total. At the outset in the development of liver transplantation patients with otherwise unresectable hepatobiliary malignancies were thought to be almost ideal candidates for liver grafting due to their superior physical condition compared to patients suffering from end-stage liver disease and portal hypertension.[2-6] Between 1968 and 1988 every fourth liver transplant in Europe was performed for hepatobiliary cancer.[7] However, long-term results of liver transplantation for secondary hepatic tumours were disappointing since the vast majority of patients developed early tumour recurrence.[3,5] With continuing improvements in immunosuppression and operative techniques, it is no longer the technical ability and expertise that determines long-term survival after liver transplantation but careful patient selection. Thus, the indication for liver transplantation in hepatic malignancies, especially of secondary hepatic tumours, has become one of the most controversial issues in liver transplantation. This is reflected by the decreased frequency of liver transplantation for

Table 8.1   Liver transplantation for hepatobiliary malignancies: Comparison between 1968–1988 and 1988–1995 (European Liver Transplant Registry, December 1995)

Transplantation	1968–1987	1988–1995
Liver transplantation (total)	2002	16414
Liver transplantation for cancer	507	1734
hepatocellular	309 (61%)	1094 (63.1%)
cholangiocellular	61 (12%)	172 (9.9%)
biliary tract	38 (7%)	110 (6.3%)
metastasis	60 (12%)	161 (9.3%)
others	39 (8%)	197 (11.3%)

liver malignancies in the last decade. In the European Liver Transplant Registry (ELTR), a total of 16 414 liver transplantations were listed between January 1988 and December 1995 but only 11% (*n* = 1734) were performed for hepatobiliary cancer. Of these patients, only 9% underwent liver grafting for hepatic metastases[7] (Table 8.1).

Although hepatic transplantation for metastases from a variety of primary tumours has been performed up until the present time, there are few conclusive data concerning the role of liver transplantation in the treatment of secondary liver tumours. In one of the first registry reports, Penn summarized data on 40 liver transplantations for various metastatic tumours including adenocarcinoma of the colon (*n* = 10), neuroendocrine tumours (*n* = 14), leiomyosarcoma (*n* = 5), carcinoma of the breast (*n* = 3) and each one of meningioma, neuroblastoma, renal cell carcinoma, cystosarcoma of the pancreas, seminoma and malignant melanoma as well as one haemangiopericytoma and one unknown primary tumour. In this heterogeneous group, eight patients survived for more than 24 months and only two patients survived longer than five years but with recurrent or residual tumour. A life table analysis of these data revealed an overall two-year survival rate of 38% and a five-year survival rate of 21%.[8] The largest single center experience with liver transplantation for metastatic cancer was reported by Iwatsuki and his colleagues from Pittsburgh. Their series of 42 patients comprised 22 cases of neuroendocrine tumours, 12 adenocarcinomas, 7 malignant stromal tumours and 1 malignant melanoma. In 29 patients, the Pittsburgh group performed allografting with liver alone or combined with islet cells and in 13 cases as cluster transplantation (liver, pancreas, duodenum). Mortality at three months was 16.6% for the first group and 38.5% for the latter. Iwatsuki described a high tumour recurrence rate in all tumour groups within the first postoperative year. Most of these patients died within two years after liver grafting. However, they observed an overall tumour-free survival of 45% for neuroendocrine tumours.[9]

These two series show that tumour recurrence is the rule but, on the other hand, it has to be appreciated that long term survival after liver transplantation has been observed in several different tumour types. This emphasizes the problematic nature of the indications for liver transplantation for metastatic disease. In oncologic surgery tumour recurrence and low survival rates are also frequent but there is less discussion regarding the justification of surgery if palliation, prolongation of life or only the hope for cure are possible. The same goals are true for liver transplantation but here the extremely high costs and the limitation of donor organs have to be taken into account. However, all these arguments become somewhat problematic if prolongation of life or at least a good quality of life can be achieved.[10] A detailed analysis of the experience with liver transplantation in transplant centres across the world is presented in an attempt to address these various issues when liver grafting is considered for metastatic disease.

Colorectal Metastases

In the early years of liver transplantation, irresectable colorectal metastases were by far the most frequent indication for secondary liver tumours. The largest single-centre experience was reported in 1987 by Mühlbacher and colleagues who grafted 9 patients with colorectal metastases. The overall one-year survival was 67% with 2 patients alive three years after transplantation and with one of them free of detectable tumour. Up until 1988, a total of 30 transplants for colorectal liver metastases had been performed in seven European centres. Only 6 patients were alive after two years and there was no five-year survivor. The longest reported survival after liver transplantation for colorectal metastases is four years and ten months.[11] In Hannover 4 liver transplantations were performed for colorectal metastases with one of them being undertaken as an urgent transplantation after a failed attempt at extracorporeal liver resection; 2 out of the 4 patients died from septic complications, the other 2 patients died from tumour recurrence at 11 months and 32 months.[12] Although tumour recurrence was noted frequently within the first postoperative year in both the Vienna and Hannover series a few patients remained completely free of symptoms for a considerable period of time. Quality of life was often excellent and even unaffected by recurrence for a period until patients finally had a rapid decline in their physical condition although they succumbed with large tumour loads.[11,12]

Metastases of Mesenchymal Tumours

Data on liver transplantation for metastatic mesenchymal tumours are uncommon. The Pittsburgh group reported 7 transplantations for metastatic malignant stromal tumours with 6 of these patients undergoing cluster transplantation. Despite a relatively high recurrence rate after liver transplantation, the authors suggested a more favourable course compared to metastases of epithelial origin. For the 6 patients undergoing cluster transplantation, the Pittsburgh group noted a recurrence rate of 83%. The incidence and median time of tumour related mortality was 66% (4 of 6 patients) and 938 days, respectively. At the time of reporting, 2 patients were alive at 19 months with recurrence and at 49 months apparently free of tumours. Similarly, Olthoff published a report of a single patient who underwent liver transplantation for irresectable metastases of a leiomyosarcoma of the stomach. This patient was alive 70 months after transplantation without evidence of disease.[9,13,14]

Neuroendocrine Metastases

Neuroendocrine tumours are rare neoplasms which present difficult and complex challenges of diagnosis and treatment. Even when metastatic spread to the liver has occurred, the patient's course is frequently asymptomatic. Initial clinical signs are usually due to large tumourous masses or associated with endocrine activity. Impairment of liver function is uncommon and declares itself late in the course of the disease. All therapeutic options should consider the natural history of the disease, the severity of clinical symptoms as well as the relative contribution of tumour bulk and hormone release to general malaise and discomfort. Current front-line management of metastatic neuroendocrine tumours comprises hepatic resection, embolization, local and systemic chemotherapy and antihormonal medical treatment.

In the vast majority of patients good palliation or even prolonged survival can be achieved by these therapeutic measures.[15-25] In 1989, the first reports of liver transplantation for metastatic neuroendocrine tumours came from Pittsburgh, from King's College Hospital in London as well as from our own unit. Although follow-up was short (seven to 38 months) with several deaths apparently unrelated to the malignant process, these three groups found that liver transplantation for neuroendocrine hepatic metastases appeared more favorable than for any other metastatic group.[5,26,27] In 1993 this initial impression was supported by Iwatsuki and colleagues who noted an overall disease free survival of 45% in 22 patients after liver transplantation for neuroendocrine tumours with some survivors at one year ($n = 3$), two years ($n = 2$), and four years ($n = 3$).[9]

Our own experience is limited to 14 patients (5 male and 9 female) with a median age of 48.5 years

Table 8.2 Patient characteristics and course in liver transplantation for neuroendocrine hepatic metastases (Klinik für Abdominal- und Transplantationschirurgie, Medizinische Hochschule Hannover January 1982 to September 1996)

Case no.	Sex	Age at transplant	Site of primary tumour	Tumour markers (elevated)	Therapy of Liver Metastasis prior to transplant	Extrahepatic tumour at transplant	Transplant potentially curative	Site of recurrence	Survival	Status
77	F	51	Small Bowel	5 HIAA	liver resection	no	yes		11 days	dead
254	F	59	Small Bowel		somatostatin	yes	no	residual intra-abdominal tumour	6.5 months	d.o.d.
325	F	18	Small Bowel	GFRH Prolactin	somatostatin	no	yes		9 years	alive n.e.d.
465	F	47	Pancreas	VIP Neurotensin PTH	liver resection, somatostatin	no	yes	pancreas	84	alive
521	M	49	Pancreas			yes	no	primary tumour, pelvis, bone, liver	68 months	d.o.d.
593	F	18	Stomach			yes	yes	lung	70	alive
682	M	35	Small Bowel	5 HIAA	liver resection, chemoembolization	no	yes		63 months	alive n.e.d.
689	M	50	Pancreas	Gastrin Cortisol	somatostatin	no	yes		62 months	alive n.e.d.
722	F	48	Pancreas	Gastrin		no	yes	bone	58 months	alive
762	M	58	Lung	5 HIAA	liver resection, somatostatin	no	yes	spleen, lymph nodes lung, liver	52 months	alive
787	F	54	Small Bowel			yes	no	primary tumour, pancreas	48 months	alive
1109	F	43	Pancreas			yes	yes		6.5 months	alive n.e.d.
1142	M	61	Pancreas	VIP Calcitonin	Chemotherapy, interferon, somatostatin	yes	?	lung ?	2 months	alive n.e.d.
1148	F	33	Pancreas		chemoembolization, stop-flow perfusion	no	yes		3 weeks	n.e.d.

Abbreviations: 5 HIAA = 5-Hydroxyindoleacetic acid; GRFH = growth factor releasing hormone; PTH = parathyroid hormone; VIP = vasoactive intestinal polypeptide; n.e.d. = no evidence of disease; d.o.d. = died of disease.

(range 18–59 years) who underwent liver transplantation for histologically proven neuroendocrine liver metastases. The primary tumours were located in the small bowel (n = 5), pancreas (n = 7), stomach (n = 1) and the lung (n = 1). In 9 cases the site of the primary tumour had been identified and resected prior to transplantation. Three occult primary tumours were detected and removed during liver transplantation. In 2 other patients, however, the primaries disclosed themselves in the small bowel and pancreas two and four years after liver grafting. Endocrine activity of the tumours with hormone production and associated clinical symptoms was noted in 8 patients (Table 8.2). The median interval between first symptoms of the disease and liver transplantation was 38 months (range from 3 to 90 months) and the median time between detection of liver tumour and liver transplantation was 28 months (3–62 months).

Liver transplantation was considered only when patients were suffering from an otherwise untreatable hormonal release or from massive tumour bulk resulting in disability and general malaise (Figure 8.1). In one patient complications of chemoembolization led to sclerosing cholangitis and secondary biliary cirrhosis with progressive liver insufficiency which required transplantation three years after embolisation. This patient had viable tumour cells demonstrated on histology at the time of transplant and is alive beyond five years. A further case highlights the dilemma faced in the management of such patients.

CASE HISTORY

A 54-year-old man presented with multiple hepatic metastases of neuroendocrine origin and the serum level of the vasoactive intestinal polypeptide (VIP) was elevated. Two years later, computed tomography demonstrated the primary tumour in the tail of the pancreas. Chemotherapy produced an initial complete remission of the primary tumour but after a few months the tumour increased in size. Several courses of chemotherapy plus therapy with interferon and somatostatin were administered without remission or symptomatic relief. In 1996, the patient was suffering from massive diarrhoea (about 20 litres per day) which required treatment in the intensive care unit. A liver transplant and left pancreatectomy was undertaken despite the presence of a probable pulmonary metastasis. After transplantation the patient had complete relief from all tumour symptoms and VIP serum levels returned to normal. The patient was discharged in excellent physical condition without any hormonal symptoms.

Overall, 11 of the 14 patients are currently alive with a median survival of 59 months (range 11 days to 108 months) (Figure 8.2). One patient died 11 days after transplant from cardiopulmonary insufficiency. A second patient died from septic complications 6.5 months after transplant. A third patient died with massive tumour recurrence in the abdomen, chest and bone 5.5 years after transplantation.

After liver grafting, all patients were judged to have excellent symptomatic relief. Similarly,

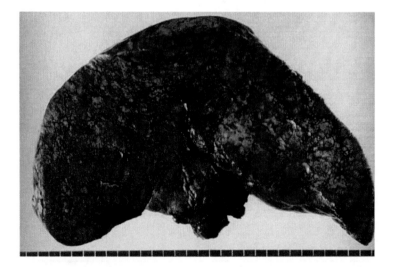

Figure 8.1. Hepatectomy specimen with multiple irresectable neuroendocrine metastases of a gastrin and cortisol producing tumour originating in the pancreas (Case no. 689).

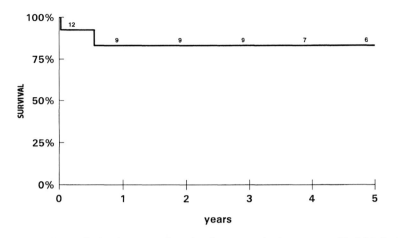

Figure 8.2. Actuarial survival ($n = 14$) after liver transplantation for neuroendocrine tumours (Medizinische Hochschule Hannover 1982–1996; follow-up to 31 August 1996). One patient died due to tumour recurrence 68 months after transplantation.

tumour-associated hormone levels returned to normal ranges in the postoperative period. In 2 patients tumour recurrence was shown to have occurred and was associated with increased gastrin and 5-hydroxyindoleacetic acid levels.

At present, 8 of the surviving 11 patients are in good physical condition without any clinical symptoms despite tumour recurrence in 2 of these patients. The three remaining patients are symptomatic from associated tumour recurrence.

Overall, 7 patients have developed tumour recurrence or had residual tumour at the time of liver transplant. The interval between transplantation and the diagnosis of tumour recurrence ranged between 6 weeks and 48 months. Treatment of recurrence or residual tumour consisted of surgical resection if this was possible and intrahepatic recurrence was treated by chemoembolization. Further therapy included administration of somatostatin, chemotherapy or interferon-alpha. At present, 6 of the surviving 11 patients have no evidence of tumour recurrence 2 to 108 months following transplantation. In 4 of them the primary tumour had been removed prior to transplantation (12, 45, 62 and 62 months before liver transplantation) and in 2 patients a primary tumour in the distal pancreas was resected simultaneously at liver transplantation[28,29] (Table 8.2).

The largest experience of liver transplantation for neuroendocrine hepatic metastases has come from a French multicentric study. Of the 31 transplants from 11 centres, the primary tumour sites were páncreas ($n = 17$), small bowel ($n = 7$), lung ($n = 3$), stomach ($n = 2$), colon and rectum ($n = 1$ each) and lymphatic system ($n = 1$). Tumours were classified as carcinoids

($n = 15$), gastrinomas ($n = 7$), glucagonoma ($n = 1$) and non-functioning tumours ($n = 8$). In only 54% of the cases hormone-related symptoms were present at the time of transplantation and, in 11 patients, the primary tumours were removed during liver transplantation. This included 7 upper abdominal exenterations of which 3 were combined with simultaneous liver and pancreas transplantation.[30]

In the French series, the postoperative mortality was 19%, and 4 of the 7 cluster resections patients died. Four patients died without evidence of recurrence within one year of liver transplantation and another 8 patients died from tumour recurrence 2 to 41 months after transplant. At the time of report only 13 patients were alive with actuarial survival rates of 58% at one year and 36% at five years.

The French group suggested a more favourable outlook for carcinoid tumour patients following liver transplant with survival rates one, three and five years of 80%, 80% and 69% for carcinoids compared to 38%, 15% and 0% for the other neuroendocrine metastases.[30]

Table 8.3 provides a review of the literature of liver transplantation for neuroendocrine hepatic metastases.

Liver Transplantation plus Multimodality Treatment

The desperate prognosis of patients suffering from multiple hepatic metastases and the poor effective-

Table 8.3 Liver transplantation for hepatic metastases of neuroendocrine tumours – review of the literature

Author	Year	Patients (n)	(alive)	Maximal survival (months)
Makowka[26]	1989	5	3	21
Arnold[27]	1989	4	2	38
Alsina[39]	1990	2	2	13
Wenisch[34]	1992	4	2	11
Farmer[40]	1993	2	2	29
Curtiss[42]	1995	3	3	30
Alessiani[14]	1995	14	9	61
Anthuber[41]	1996	4	0	33
Dousset[43]	1996	9	3	62
Le Treut[30]	1996	31	13	>60
Lang[28]	1996	14	11	108

ness of cytotoxic chemotherapy and liver transplantation in these cases encouraged Margreiter and his colleagues to undertake a much more aggressive approach combining radical surgery by means of total hepatectomy and liver replacement with systemic treatment using chemotherapy and radiation. After successful liver transplantation, a protocol of high-dose cyclophosphamide (60 mg/kg for two days) and total body irradiation at 1000 rad was undertaken. This treatment was followed by rescue therapy of autologous bone marrow (harvested prior to transplantation) and reinfusion of buffy-coat cells. Two patients with liver metastases from breast cancer and one with (colorectal) metastases were subjected to this aggressive protocol. The procedure was associated with a surprisingly low mor-

bidity and was tolerated well by the liver graft. However, results were disappointing with 2 of the 3 patients dying within one year due to malignant disease. In the third patient, two skin metastases and breast cancer of the contralateral breast developed and this required repeated surgery with radiotherapy. This patient was alive and free of tumour 45 months after transplantation but Margreiter has abandoned the treatment protocol.[31]

Extended Resection Cluster Transplantation

Long-term results following liver transplantation in most patients with concomitant extrahepatic tumour, whether lymph node metastases or the primary tumour, are poor because of frequent tumour recurrence after supposed curative resection. This observation led to the development of more aggressive surgical strategies. In 1989 Starzl and his colleagues published the first results of abdominal organ cluster transplantation for the treatment of upper abdominal malignancies. By means of a multivisceral upper abdominal resection (cluster resection), they attempted radical excision of most of the tissue embryologically derived from the foregut (Figure 8.3). This excenteration may entail removal of the liver, stomach, spleen, pancreaticoduodenal complex and part of

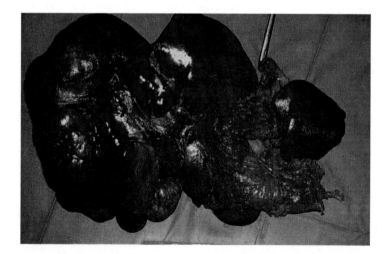

Figure 8.3. Resection specimen after cluster resection (liver, stomach, pancreas, duodenum, spleen) for adenocarcinoma of the pancreas with multiple liver metastases.

the colon. Transplantation can be performed as an isolated liver transplant, as a cluster transplant or as liver transplantation combined with islet cell transplantation.[32]

The largest experience with this approach for hepatic metastases was reported by Alessiani and colleagues in 1995. Of 57 cluster transplantations, they performed 24 for hepatic metastases from primary endocrine tumours ($n = 14$), sarcomas ($n = 6$) and adenocarcinoma of the pancreas ($n = 2$) or the colon ($n = 2$). The actuarial survival rates at one and three years were 64% and 64% for the endocrine tumours, 100% and 44% for sarcomas but only 25% and 25% for the adenocarcinomas, respectively.[14] In the French multicentric study on liver transplantation for neuroendocrine hepatic metastases, 7 cluster resections were reported. In their series four of the patients died from procedure-related complications.[30] Similarly, Knechtle and coworkers reported 3 patients who underwent abdominal cluster transplantation for neuroendocrine malignancies. They described 2 deaths due to tumour recurrence (13 and 19 months after liver transplantation) and only 1 disease-free survival (28 months posttransplant).[33] Comparable data came from Wenisch's group who performed 4 upper abdominal exenterations combined with liver transplantation for metastatic endocrine pancreas tumours. They described 2 deaths within the first year and 2 disease-free survivors about seven and eight months after liver grafting.[34]

Discussion and Future Aspects

The most obvious reason for witholding liver transplantation for hepatic metastases derives from the fact that metastatic spread of an extrahepatic tumour to the liver has to be regarded as a systemic disease. In addition, the influence of immunosuppression on tumour growth has not yet been clarified in detail. Changes in ploidy from diploidy to aneuploidy have been observed after chemotherapy: similarly, the assumption that growth of residual tumour could be accelerated as a consequence of immunosuppression can neither be denied nor confirmed.[35] Even the late recurrence four years after liver transplantation in one of our patients

with neuroendocrine tumours does not argue against possible acceleration of tumour growth.

The major concern in considering liver transplantation for cancer is still the reluctance to use limited donor organs to transplant patients who have significantly lower survival rates compared to those candidates who undergo liver grafting for benign diseases (European Liver Transplant Registry) (Figure 8.4).

The use of right liver lobes for tumour patients when a split liver transplant has been undertaken might be an attractive alternative. However the cancer patient would also have to take on the increased risk of transplanting a reduced-size-liver with higher morbidity and mortality risk. On the assumption that tumour patients are usually in a better general physical condition compared with patients suffering from end-stage liver disease, this approach might be ethically justified. Similarly transplantation of tumour patients with low quality donor livers might by considered. These donor organs can usually not be accepted for critically ill recipients (i.e. in fulminant hepatic failure) in our experience but might be tolerated by a patient in good physical condition. The ethics of providing these patients with a suboptimal liver has to be balanced with whether it is justified to exclude patients from a procedure which offers the only possibility of cure. Looking at the long-term results for liver grafting in hepatobiliary malignancies it does appear that liver metastases have a similar prognosis to other malignancies (Figure 8.5).

Patients with neuroendocrine tumours should be looked upon as a special group with regard to liver grafting. Not only possible cure but also dramatic relief of associated symptoms can be obtained with liver transplantation. However, a critical evaluation of the results of liver grafting for neuroendocrine metastases has to consider the biologically less aggressive characteristics and comparatively slower growth rates of neuroendocrine tumours. In contrast to most other neoplasms, an aggressive treatment of neuroendocrine liver metastases is often unnecessary because of the commonly asymptomatic and indolent course with long survival even of untreated patients.[17] Treatment is usually not indicated until hormonal syndromes or abdominal discomfort and pain occur,[22,24] and medical therapy with long-acting somatostatin analogues often controls hormonal syndromes.[16,18,20] In cases of solitary or well-localized liver metastases, conventional hepatic resection is the treatment of choice.[15,21,36]

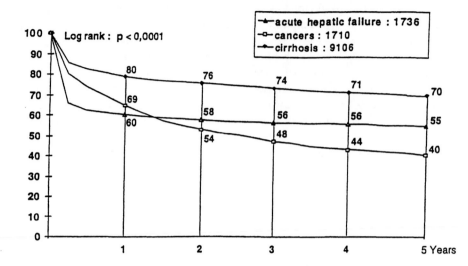

Figure 8.4. Patient survival after liver transplantation for acute hepatic failure, liver cirrhosis and hepatic cancer (January 1988–December 1995) (European Liver Transplant Registry, December 1995).

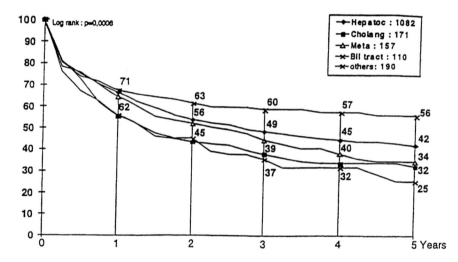

Figure 8.5. Patient survival after liver transplantation for hepatobiliary malignancies (January 1988–December 1995) (European Liver Transplant Registry, December 1995).

The largest series with liver resection in 74 patients was reported by Que who found an overall symptomatic response rate of 90% with an operative mortality rate of 2.7% and a mean four-year survival of 73%. In their analysis, survival among patients with assumed curative resection did not differ significantly from those with palliative approaches.[37] Good symptomatic relief can be achieved by cyto-reductive hepatic resection when not all of the tumourous mass is removed. However, the value of surgery is often compromised by multilocular intrahepatic metastatic spread of tumour and only few patients are candidates for liver resection.[22,37] A variety of chemotherapeutical treatment regimens have been introduced with response rates for islet cell tumours up to 69% and a duration of response up to 20 months. This treatment has been shown to be less effective in carcinoid tumours.[19,25] Better results have been claimed by a combination of hepatic artery occlusion and subsequent alternating chemotherapy with doxorubicin plus decarbazine and streptozocin plus fluouracil. With this approach Moertel and his colleagues reported a median survival time of 49 months for patients with advanced carcinoid tumours compared to only 27 months for hepatic artery occlusion alone. The response rate was 80% for devascularization plus chemotherapy and 60% for artery occlusion alone with a duration of response of 18 months and 4 months, respectively.[24] Recently Perry and coworkers published data on 30 patients with either carcinoid or islet cell tumour metastases treated with intra-arterial doxorubicin followed by embolization with gelatin powder or pledgets. They described a 50% reduction of tumour size and/or hormone markers in 79% of patients with a median survival of 24 months. A minor response rate of even 92% could be obtained and no procedure-related death was observed.[38]

In this context, the median survival of 59 months after liver transplantation in our series compares favourably with all other reported management protocols. Only 3 patients have died but in 2, death was entirely related to the transplant procedure itself or septic complications. Only one patient has died due to the underlying disease, but in this patient, quality of life remained good for a long period of time despite extensive tumour recurrence. In advanced carcinoid tumours with liver metastases death most often results from hepatic or cardiac failure and yet our own experience demonstrates that removal of the diseased liver may result in significant symptomatic relief and perhaps prolonged survival.[26] This is also reflected by the good results of cytoreductive hepatic surgery and by the asymptomatic clinical course of some of our patients with extrahepatic tumour recurrence after liver transplantation.[22]

The follow-up of the reported series of liver transplantation for neuroendocrine hepatic metastases is still too short for useful evaluation although the early results indicate that patients without extrahepatic tumour at the time of transplantation should be considered as candidates for liver grafting. In addition, the symptomatic relief seen after transplant raises the issue as to whether those cases with extrahepatic tumour and poorly controlled symptoms should also be considered.

It remains a matter of considerable debate as to whether liver transplantation is justified as palliation when almost comparable effectiveness can be obtained by chemoembolization and without the risks of surgery and immunosuppression. However, in certain conditions when all other therapeutic options are no longer effective total hepatectomy and liver transplantation broadens the therapeutic options in the management of neuroendocrine tumours. Further experience and studies are required to determine whether a subgroup of neuroendocrine tumours (e.g. carcinoid) presents a more favourable indication for liver transplantation as suggested by the French multicentre study.

With regards to other metastatic tumours of either epithelial or mesenchymal origin, the role of liver transplantation is viewed with extreme caution by many. Results in general are poor but the transplant may be considered in selected cases of colorectal carcinoma or metastases of leiomyosarcoma since effective palliation and rehabilitation may be possible. Further study is certainly warranted and liver transplantation should only be entertained within trial protocols.

Similar concerns exist for multivisceral resection when combined with liver transplantation alone or with cluster transplantation. Experience with this approach is limited and survival rates are still hampered by procedure-related complications which have not allowed assessment of the risk of tumour recurrence following this aggressive surgical treatment strategy. Similarly, combined treatment protocols with liver transplantation as part of the management programme need to be worked out satisfactorily. There is hope for more effective chemotherapeutic drugs and for progress in immunotherapy of tumours. Perhaps future efforts will be directed at the molecular biological analysis of tumour cell DNA prior to liver transplantation[35] and thus may be a helpful selection criteria.

In conclusion, hepatic transplantation for selected patients with hepatic metastases seems justified in a limited number of patients since not only cure but also symptomatic relief and rehabilitation can be achieved. Further efforts will be directed to the crucial question of proper patient selection. The potential value of liver transplantation has to be justified in every individual case because of the extent of the procedure, the associated complications and risks, the false expectations which might be raised for the individual patient and, because of the costs and the limited availability of donor organs.

References

1. Pichlmayr R, Grosse H, Hauss J, Gubernatis G, Lamesch P, Bretschneider HJ. Technique and preliminary results of extracorporeal liver surgery (bench procedure) and of surgery on the *in situ* perfused liver. *Br J Surg* 1990; 77:21–26.

2. Bechstein WO, Neuhaus P. Liver transplantation for hepatic metastases of neuroendocrine tumors. *Ann New York Acad Sci* 1994; **733**:507–514.

3. O'Grady JG, Polson RJ, Rolles K, Calne RY, Williams R. Liver transplantation for malignant disease. Results in 93 consecutive patients. *Ann Surg* 1989; **207**:373–379.

4. Pichlmayr R, Weimann A, Oldhafer KJ et al. Role of liver transplantation in the treatment of unresectable liver cancer. *World J Surg* 1995; **19**:807–813.

5. Ringe B, Wittekind C, Bechstein WO, Bunzendahl H, Pichlmayr R. The role of liver transplantation in hepatobiliary malignancy. A retrospective analysis of 95 patients with particular regard to tumor stage and recurrence. *Ann Surg* 1989; **209**:88–98.

6. Pichlmayr R, Weimann A, Ringe B. Indications for liver transplantation in hepatobiliary malignancy. *Hepatology* 1994; **20**:33.

7. European Liver Transplant Registry December 1995.

8. Penn I. Hepatic transplantation for primary and metastatic cancers of the liver. *Surgery* 1991; **110**:726–735.

9. Iwatsuki S, Tzakis A, Todo S, Selby R, Starzl TE. Liver transplantation for metastatic hepatic malignancies. *Hepatology* 1993; **18**:723.

10. Pichlmayr R. Is there a place for liver grafting for malignancy? *Transplant Proc* 1988; **20**:478–482.

11. Mühlbacher F, Piza F. Orthotopic liver transplantation for secondary malignancies of the liver. *Transplant Proc* 1987; **19**(1):2396–2398.

12. Lang H, Oldhafer KJ, Duebener L, Ringe B, Pichlmayr R. The role of liver transplantation in the treatment of metastatic hepatic tumors. *Br J Surg* 1994; **81**(Suppl 1):87.

13. Olthoff KM, Millis M, Rosove MH, Goldstein LI, Ramming KP, Busuttil RW. Is liver transplantation justified for the treatment of hepatic malignancies? *Arch Surg* 1990; **125**:1261–1268.

14. Alessiani M, Tsakis A, Todo, Demetris AJ, Fung JJ, Starzl TE. Assessment of five-year experience with abdominal organ cluster transplantation. *J Am Coll Surg* 1995; **180**:1.

15. Ahlman H, Westberg G, Wängberg B, Nilsson O, Tylen U, Schersten T. Treatment of liver metastases of carcinoid tumors. *World J Surg* 1996; **20**:196–202.

16. Arnold R. Medical treatment of metastasizing carcinoid tumors. *World J Surg* 1996; **20**:203–207.

17. Delcore R, Friesen SR. Gastrointestinal neuroendocrine tumors. *J Am Coll Surg* 1994; **178**:187–211.

18. Hajarizadeh H, Ivancev K, Mueller CR, Fletscher WS, Woltering EA. Effective palliative treatment of metastatic carcinoid tumors with intra-arterial chemotherapy/chemoembolization combined with octreotide acetate. *Am J Surg* 1992; **163**:479–482.

19. Kvols LK, Buck M. Chemotherapy of metastatic carcinoid and islet cell tumors. *Am J Med* 1987; **82**(Suppl 5B):77–83.

20. Kvols LK, Moertel CG, O'Connell MJ, Schutt AJ, Rubin J, Hahn RG. Treatment of the malignant carcinoid syndrome. Evaluation of a long-acting somatostatin analogue. *N Engl J Med* 1986; **315**:663–666.

21. Martin K Jr, Moertel CG, Adson MA, Schutt AJ. Surgical treatment of functioning metastatic carcinoid tumors. *Arch Surg* 1993; **118**:537–542.

22. McEntee GP, Nagorney DM, Kvols LK, Moertel CG, Grant CS. Cytoreductive hepatic surgery for neuroendocrine tumors. *Surgery* 1990; **108**:1091–1096.

23. Moertel CG. Karnofsky Memorial Lecture: an odyssey in the land of small tumors. *J Clin Oncol* 1987; **5**:1503–1522.

24. Moertel CG, Johnson CM, McKusick MA et al. The management of patients with advanced carcinoid tumors and islet cell carcinomas. *Ann Intern Med* 1994; **120**:302–309.

25. Moertel CG, Lefkopoulo M, Lipsitz S, Hahn RG, Klaassen D. Streptozocin–doxorubicin, streptozocin–fluorouracil, or chlorozotocin in the treatment of advanced islet-cell carcinoma. *N Engl J Med* 1992; **326**:519–523.

26. Makowka L, Tzakis AG, Mazzaferro V et al. Transplantation of the liver for metastatic endocrine tumors of the intestine and pancreas. *Surg Gynecol Obstet* 1989; **168**:107–111.

27. Arnold JC, O'Grady JG, Bird GL, Calne RY, Williams R. Liver transplantation for primary and secondary hepatic apudomas. *Br J Surg* 1989; **76**:248–249.

28. Lang H, Oldhafer KJ, Weimann A et al. Liver transplantation for metastatic neuroendocrine tumors. *Ann Surg* 1997; **225**:347–354.

29. Lang H, Oldhafer KJ, Schlitt HJ, Scheumann GFW, Ringe B, Pichlmayr R. Ist die Lebertransplantation als chirurgisches Therapiekonzept bei Metastasen neuroendokriner Tumoren gerechtfertigt? *Langenbecks Arch Chir* 1996; Suppl II. 416–418.

30. Le Treut YP, Delpero JP, Houssin D et al. Is liver transplantation (OLT) a rational approach for neuroendocrine metastases (NEM)? Report of a French multicentric study of 31 cases. *HPB Surgery* 1996; **9**(Suppl 2):19.

31. Margreiter R, Niederwieser D, Frommhold H, Schönitzer A, Huber C. Tumor recurrence after liver transplantation followed by high-dose cyclophosphamide, total body irradiation, and autologous bone marrow transplantation for treatment of metastatic liver disease. *Transplant Proc* 1987; **19**(1):2403–2404.

32. Starzl TE, Todo S, Tzakis A et al. Abdominal organ cluster transplantation for the treatment of upper abdominal malignancies. *Ann Surg* **210**:374–386.

33. Knechtle SJ, Kalayoglu M, D'Alessandro AM et al. Should abdominal cluster transplantation be abandoned? *Transplant Proc* 1993; **25**:1361–1363.

34. Wenisch HJC, Markus BH, Herrmann GH, Usadel KH, Encke A. Multiviscerale Oberbauchresektion und orthotope Lebertransplantation – ein chirurgisches Behandlungskonzept für regionär metastasierende Tumoren des endocrinen Pancreas. *Zentbl Chir* 1992; **117**:334–342.

35. Gulanikar AC, Kotylak G, Bitter-Suermann H. Does immunosuppression alter the growth of metastatic liver carcinoid after orthotopic liver transplantation? *Transplant Proc* 1991; **23**:2197–2198.

36. Soreide O, Berstad T, Bakka A. Surgical treatment as a principle in patients with advanced abdominal carcinoid tumors. *Surgery* 1992; **111**:48–54.

37. Que FG, Nagorney DM, Batts KP, Linz LJ, Kvols LK. Hepatic resection for metastatic neuroendocrine carcinomas. *Am J Surg* 1995; **169**:36–43.

38. Perry LJ, Stuart K, Stokes KR, Clouse ME. Hepatic arterial chemoembolization for metastatic neuroendocrine tumors. *Surgery* 1994; **166**:1111–1117.

39. Alsina AE, Bartus S, Hall D. Liver transplantation for metastatic neuroendocrine tumors. *J Clin Gastroenterol* 1990; **12**:533–537.

40. Farmer DG, Shaked A, Colonna JO. Radical resection combined with liver transplantation for foregut tumors. *Am J Surg* 1993; **59**:806–812.

41. Anthuber M, Jauch KW, Briegel J et al. Results of liver transplantation for gastroenteropancreatic tumor metastases. *World J Surg* 1996; **20**:73–76.

42. Curtiss SI, Mor E, Schwartz ME et al. A rational approach to the use of hepatic transplantation in the treatment of metastatic neuroendocrine tumors. *J Am Coll Surg* 1995; **180**:184–187.

43. Dousset B, Saint-Marc O, Pitre J, Soubrane O, Houssin D, Chapuis Y. Metastatic endocrine tumors: medical treatment, surgical resection, or liver transplantation. *World J Surg* 1996; **20**:908–915.

Cryotherapy and Other Ablative Procedures

Howard M. Karpoff, Yuman Fong and Leslie H. Blumgart

9

Introduction

Hepatic malignancies represent a substantial medical problem. Not only is the liver a common site for primary cancers, it is also a common site for growth of a variety of metastatic cancers. Because of its vascularity, and its position at the delta of the portal circulation, growth of metastatic gastrointestinal cancers in the liver is particularly common. For example, 25% of patients presenting with colorectal cancer will be found to have metastases to the liver at the time of diagnosis,[1,2] and 50% of patients treated with colonic/rectal resection will have tumour recurrence in the liver within five years.[3] One series of patients with advanced colorectal cancer showed a 77% incidence of liver metastases.[4] It is well established that surgical resection of metastatic disease isolated to the liver represents potentially curative therapy, and even short of cure can improve long-term survival from colorectal cancers.[5-7] However, other local treatments are being investigated for patients with metastatic colorectal cancer isolated to the liver for whom resection is not feasible, or who have recurred after resection. Furthermore, techniques are being investigated to determine if a less invasive alternative to resection can be found to provide cure for metastatic lesions.

Many ablative procedures are being proposed for destruction of liver tumours. These include methods of freezing, heating, or chemically ablating tumours (Table 9.1). It is important to preface this chapter on ablative therapies with a warning against using such techniques as alternatives to liver resection. There is little doubt that these physical methods can kill tumour. Such tumour killing can usually be per-

Table 9.1   Types of ablative therapy

Cryotherapy
Hyperthermia
Electrocautery
Laser
Microwave
Radiofrequency
Tissue-destroying agents
Percutaneous ethanol injection
Percutaneous hot saline injection
Others
Focused ultrasound
Piezoelectric crystals

formed with less destruction of non-neoplastic liver parenchyma than formal liver resections. So in the clinical setting of treatment of hepatocellular carcinoma, where the majority of patients also suffer from cirrhosis of the liver and have poor hepatic reserve, it is advantageous to preserve non-neoplastic parenchyma. For treatment of metastatic cancers, which usually occur in patients with no cirrhosis, the advantages are less clear. Established data for resection of hepatic colorectal metastases demonstrate that resection of ≤80% of liver tissue is associated with an operative mortality <5%, hospital stay of less than two weeks, and a potential for cure.[5-8] It would be difficult to accept ablative therapy as an alternative to resection without direct comparative data from random assignment trials. No such trials have been performed and currently in metastatic colorectal cancer, there is no role for ablative therapy when tumours are completely resectable. These ablative procedures should be considered for non-resectable disease *and using them in treatment of resectable disease should be restricted to formal clinical trials.* The surgeon interested in treating a patient with ablative therapies not only must be versed in the different ablative techniques, but also must be experienced in standard surgical resections, so that no patient is deprived of an opportunity at potential cure.

The majority of patients with metastatic disease arising from primary colorectal cancers are not candidates for surgical resection however, due to anatomic considerations or due to extrahepatic disease. In fact, only 5–10% of these patients will have surgically resectable disease.[9] In addition, in those patients undergoing resection with curative intent, recurrence will occur in upwards of 60% of patients and the liver will be the first site of recurrence in the majority.[7,10,11] Thus a major cause of death for patients with unresectable metastatic colorectal cancer is the liver disease. This is the reason that local ablative techniques have been developed. In other cancers such as neuroendocrine tumours[12] or hepatocellular carcinoma[13] ablative therapy has been show to provide good palliation. Whether such benefit will be found for metastatic colorectal cancer has been speculated and not yet proven, and is the topic of much ongoing investigations.

In this chapter, we discuss the various ablative techniques, including cryotherapy, laser therapy hyperthermia and other methods of hyperthermia, and percutaneous ethanol injection. We will not discuss the use of brachytherapy for tumour ablation.[10,14]

Cryotherapy

Cryotherapy is the use of the freeze–thaw process to produce tissue destruction. Although topical freezing has been used as an ablative modality for over a century, it was not until recent development and marketing of vacuum-insulated, liquid nitrogen-cooled cryoprobes[15,16] that cryotherapy of liver lesions became widely popularized. The application of this technology was further facilitated by the recent improvements in intra-operative ultrasound. Current ultrasound techniques allow localization of tumours, identification of smaller lesions and more accurate delivery of cryoprobes. In addition, intra-operative ultrasound is a superb tool for monitoring the progress of freezing, ensuring both complete freezing of tumours as well as preventing unnecessary damage

to neighbouring vasculature and biliary structures. These developments have made cryoablation a widely accessible tool for ablation of liver tumours.

A major advantage of cryoablation is the limited amount of 'normal' liver tissue that is destroyed. This makes it particularly attractive for patients with poor liver reserve. This has resulted in much enthusiasm for using this technique as a surgical alternative to resection for patients with hepatocellular carcinoma, in whom cirrhosis is a frequent comorbid condition. Since cirrhosis is an uncommon comorbid condition for patients with metastatic colorectal cancer, and non-cirrhotic livers have great functional reserve and rapid regenerative capacity, the advantages of cryoablation over resection are less clear. Resection of ≤80% of the liver parenchyma is associated with rapid recovery from surgery and rapid recovery of liver function. Further, cryoablation is not without side-effects and mortality. At present, cryoablation cannot be considered an alternative to resection, though formal trials comparing the two would undoubtedly be an important contribution to the care of patients with metastatic colorectal cancer. Comparative trials to other ablative modalities or chemotherapy are also needed to define the role for cryoablation in the care of patients with unresectable metastases.

Patient Selection

Since most cryoablation is performed under general anaesthesia and through a formal laparotomy incision, patients chosen for cryoablation must be deemed an acceptable risk for major surgery. Patients should not have extrahepatic metastatic disease. Excepting for patients enrolled in formal clinical trials designed to compare resection with cryoablation, the liver tumour should be deemed unresectable. Finally, tumours must be encompassable by cryoablation (Table 9.2).

In evaluation of the general health of patients in preparation for cryoablation, pulmonary status is particularly important because most hepatic cryoablative procedures are performed through a large subcostal incisions that may limit respiratory excursion postoperatively, and also because almost all patients will develop a sympathetic pleural effusion postoperatively. Renal status must be thoroughly investigated, as renal failure from a tumorolysis syndrome after cryoablation is a well-documented potential complication (see below).

Table 9.2 Selection and monitoring of patients

Pre-operative evaluation
Patient selection
  Good general health: particularly pulmonary and renal function
  Tumours isolated to liver
  Tumours unresectable due to location or number
  Tumours encompassable by therapy
  Able to tolerate general anaesthesia
Workup
  Chest, abdominal and pelvic CT
  Complete blood counts, prothrombin time, liver function tests
  CEA

Post-operative care
Hydration ± alkalinization of urine
Antibiotics
Respiratory therapy
Monitor liver/renal/pulmonary functions
Evaluate tumour response with CEA/CT scan with intravenous contrast

Chest X-ray, abdominal and pelvic computed tomographic (CT) scans, and a recent colonoscopy should be performed to rule out extrahepatic disease, as well as to define the liver lesions for treatment planning. Baseline liver function tests are essential. A complete blood count as well as prothrombin time should be obtained because thrombocytopenia, coagulopathy and haemorrhage are possible consequences of cryoablation. Levels of tumour marker carcinoembryonic antigen (CEA) should be ascertained to provide a parameter for evaluation of treatment response. The CT scan of the liver used to define lesions to be treated by cryoablation should be performed with intravenous contrast so as to demonstrate the relative locations of the major portal and hepatic veins to tumour. Patients with severe contrast allergy should have a magnetic resonance imaging (MRI) study performed to define these vessels, since knowledge of the locations of major vasculature relative to tumour is essential in the planning of the safe placement of cryoprobes for ablation.

Number and size of lesions, as well as proximity to major vasculature, are important criteria for selecting patients for cryoablation. Most surgeons will not freeze more than five lesions. Although tumours as large as 10 cm can be ablated by using multiple cryoprobes, lesions ≤5 cm in size can be treated with much more confidence. The limitations in number and size of tumours are due to the technical limits of freezing by currently available cryoprobes and since 20–40 min is required for freezing of each lesion, cryoablation is also limited by the length of time that is reasonable for the pro-

cedure. Finally, the risk, including the risk of vascular or biliary injury, as well as the severity of the tumorolysis syndrome increases with the amount of tumour ablated. If a major hepatic vein or portal pedicle is closely adjacent to the tumour, complete freezing is unlikely since the flow of warm blood though these vessels will protect adjacent regions of the tumour from freezing. Temporary occlusion of the vascular inflow to the liver will increase the effectiveness of freezing but also increases the risk of vascular or biliary injury. Lesions that involve a significant length of a major vascular structure should be considered with caution. Furthermore, the authors consider involvement of the hilus of the liver by tumour a complete contraindication to cryotherapy since the risk of biliary injury and fistula is too high to be acceptable for a non-curative procedure.

Technique

Exposure is generally through a bilateral subcostal incision. Complete mobilization of the liver as for liver resections is performed since this not only facilitates probe placement but allows for control of haemorrhage should this occur. The peritoneal cavity is searched for extrahepatic disease. The liver is examined carefully using a combination of direct visualization, palpation, and intraoperative ultrasound with transducers (3.5–7.5 MHz) allowing different depths of penetration.[17] The number and location of metastases are determined, and the relation of the metastatic deposits to major vascular and biliary structures are scrutinized. The edges of the abdominal incision, as well as other abdominal viscera are then covered with warm saline-soaked pads to protect them from inadvertent injury.

The cryoprobes to be used are then chosen according to the size of lesion to be frozen. A 5-mm probe will generally produce an ice ball of approximately 3 cm in size, while a 10-mm probe will produce an iceball of approximately 6 cm in size. Multiple 10-mm probes can be placed in a parallel fashion, 2–3 cm apart to produce confluent ice balls of up to approximately 10 cm in size. The trajectory of the cryoprobes is chosen so as *not* to direct the probe at any major hepatic vein or portal pedicle even if this means traversing more hepatic parenchyma. For most tumours, the probe can be directly introduced under ultrasound guidance. For deeply placed lesions, a variation of the Seldinger technique may be helpful. Under ultrasound monitoring, a peel-away sheath from either a commercially available cryoprobe-introducer kit or a standard vascular access introducer kit may be placed into the tumour. The cryoprobe is then introduced into the tract of this sheath as it is withdrawn. The final position of the probe is confirmed by ultrasound.

Liquid nitrogen is then circulated through the cryoprobe while freezing is monitored by ultrasound. The area that is frozen will appear hypoechoic on intraoperative ultrasound. Freezing is continued until this hypoechoic rim reaches an area approximately 1–2 cm beyond the edge of the tumour. A temperature of –160°C to –180°C is generally achieved. For large lesions, portal inflow occlusion by clamping the gastrohepatic ligament (Pringle manoeuvre) may be used to increase the rapidity of freezing. Control of the gastrohepatic ligament also allows rapid control of haemorrhage should this arise from hepatic, arterial or portal venous branches; however, the risk of vascular and biliary injury increases with a Pringle manoeuvre since the portal pedicle is deprived of the warm blood that protects it against the effects of freezing. After freezing, the lesion is thawed until the rim of freezing recedes 1–2 cm before a second freeze cycle is initiated. At least two freeze–thaw cycles are used since multiple cycles are more effective.[18,19] Between freeze–thaw cycles, thawing a rim of only 1–2 cm is adequate since the vascular necrosis that occurs in this rim of tissue deprives the central portion of tumours of nutrient blood and results in necrosis of the entire tumour. During freezing, the cryoprobe must be held as steadily as possible, since twisting the probe with resultant cracking of the frozen liver surface is a major cause of haemorrhage after thawing. After freezing, the probe is warmed, withdrawn from the liver, and haemostatic agents packed into the probe tract. A drain is left near the port of entry to monitor and control bile leaks.

Perioperative Care

Renal failure from tumorolysis is a dreaded complication of cryoablation. Perioperative fluid management is therefore of utmost importance. The patient should receive intravenous fluids adequate to maintain a urine output of >50 cc hour. Alkalinization of the urine by sodium bicarbonate administration should also be considered for patients for whom

large volumes of tumour have been ablated.[17] Some investigators have also advocated pre-operative endoscopic biliary stent placement to prevent biliary fistulae after cryoablation. The authors have not found this necessary when lesions involving the hilus are avoided and the path of the cryoprobe chosen to avoid impalement of the major portal pedicles.

Postoperatively, radiological studies and serum tumour markers are used to evaluate the efficacy of treatment.[16,20–24] Contrast-enhanced CT scans are the most common method for evaluating lesions after cryoablation. After treatment, the ablated region evolves to become a fibrous scar which does not enhance after contrast injection.[16,20] Other imaging modalities such as whole body positron emission tomography (PET) after ^{18}F-FDG (fluorodeoxyglucose) injection, or functional MRI may yet provide even more sensitive methods for evaluating treatment results. The tumour marker CEA is still the most commonly used test for evaluation of effectiveness of cryoablation.

Complications

Mortality associated with cryoablation has been reported from 0 to 5% (Table 9.3), and seems to correlate with the aggressiveness of the cryoablation. Most of the early studies had few or no deaths.[18,25–27] It is only as a more aggressive approach has developed that mortality and complication rates have significantly increased. Deaths are due mainly to liver failure,[17] or infection. Intra-operative complications due to cryoablation include haemorrhage, most often due to cracking of the frozen liver.[28] Biliary injury may occur leading to postoperative biliary fistula.[29,30] Inadvertent cryo-injury to adjacent organs, including the diaphragm, stomach and colon have all been reported.[31] Hypothermia has also been reported,[29] though the authors have never found this to be significant even when freezing large volumes of tumour, and certainly have never found it necessary to use special warming devices as advocated by other investigators.[32]

Postoperatively, nearly all patients develop a right pleural effusion, which may contribute to atelectasis and other pulmonary complications (Table 9.3).[29] Patients may also develop a tumorolysis syndrome, characterized by fever, thrombocytopenia,[29,33] and 'myoglobinuria'.[17] The severity of this tumorolysis syndrome also appears to correlate with the volume

Table 9.3 Complications associated with cryoablation

Author	n	Mortality (%)	Hospital stay (days)	Complications
Ravikumar[18]	32	0	6	Fever, leukocytosis, abscess, wound dehiscence, transient elevation of liver enzymes
Onik[30]	18	0	–	Pleural effusion, haemorrhage, biliary fistula, hepatic abscess, renal failure
Onik[17]	57	5	–	Pleural effusion, haemorrhage, biliary fistula, renal failure, hepatic failure, myocardial infarction
Cozzi[12]	6	0	9	Coagulopathy/bleeding
Shafir[31]	39	0	–	Coagulopathy and haemorrhage, renal failure, cyro-injury of other organs
Morris and Ross[36]	162	1	7	Sepsis, thrombocytopenia, elevation of liver enzymes, renal failure, bleeding, myocardial infarction, liver abscess

of tumour ablated. Severe cases may result in acute tubular necrosis and renal failure. Infections, including liver abscesses or subphrenic abscesses are known complications associated with cryoablation. Finally, experimental animal models have shown cardiac arrhythmias due to transient hyperkalaemia,[34] but this has not been borne out in humans.

Long-term Results

Three groups have been major contributors to the growing, published experience in the use of cryotherapy for metastatic colorectal carcinoma (Table 9.4). Morris and his colleagues have certainly contributed most extensively.[26,27,35] Since their first report of 7 patients in 1989,[26] they have accumulated an experience of over 162 patients.[36] They have documented a median survival exceeding 1000 days in a group of 92 patients with colorectal metastases treated by cryotherapy.[36] However, this is not a disease-free survival since 75% of patients undergoing cryosurgery alone had relapse of their preoperative CEA levels by six months.[27] The authors advocate adjuvant intra-arterial chemotherapy as a potential solution to this problem.

Ravikumar and his colleagues have also demonstrated cryoablation to be a safe palliative technique.[18,25] In 25 patients treated for metastatic colorectal cancer to the liver, with a median follow-up of two years, 28% of the patients (7) have remained in remission.[25] Onik et al. treated 57 patients with metastatic colorectal disease and had a disease-free survival of 27% at 21 months.[17]

Discussion

It is clear that cryoablation can be performed safely in well-selected populations, though it is rarely curative. Cryoablation of limited numbers of lesions that are not centrally placed can be accomplished with safety. Patients with small numbers of periph-

Table 9.4 Hepatic cryosurgery for colorectal cancer

Author	Year	n	Follow-up (months)	Median survival (days)	Survival at follow-up (%)
Ravikumar[18]	1991	24	24 (5–60)	not reached	28%
Onik[30]	1991	18	29	–	–
Onik[17]	1993	57	21	–	27%
Preketes[35]	1995	38	–	570	–
Shafir[31]	1995	25	14 (1–34)	not reached	–
Morris[36]	1996	92	36	800	–

eral lesions, however, are also the prime candidates for surgical resection. Data also demonstrate that as aggressiveness of cryotherapy has increased the complication rates and mortality rates have significantly increased. The closer a tumour is to major vasculature and biliary radicals, the greater the chance for incomplete freezing and for complications. Therefore, the large central lesions that are difficult to resect are also difficult to freeze. No clinical trial has yet directly compared cryoablation with resection. Median length of hospital stay for patients undergoing cryoablation has been reported to be between six and nine days (Table 9.3),[12,18] while median hospital stays after even the most major liver resections has been reduced to approximately nine days.[37] Since resection has been shown to be potentially curative,[5,7] until data from direct comparative trials with resection prove otherwise, cryoablation must be regarded as a no substitute for resection. Furthermore, it is important that decisions to ablate or to resect be undertaken by surgeons experienced in liver surgery. Patients should not be relegated to palliative therapy who may otherwise be offered potentially curative treatment.

The major advantage of cryoablation over other ablative techniques is clear. Cryoablation can produce larger areas of tissue destruction than can be accomplished by ethanol injection, laser ablation or microwave ablation (see below). In the treatment of metastatic colorectal cancers, cryoablation is therefore more applicable for unresectable tumours. The major disadvantages of cryotherapy compared to other ablative techniques is that it necessitates a laparotomy. That is why investigations of the feasibility of laparoscopic cryotherapy[38,39] or percutaneous cryotherapy[40] are underway.

The biggest limitation to any ablative method is the possibility of leaving behind viable tumour. Even with the large tumours that may be ablated by cryoablation, incomplete tumour destruction, particularly for larger lesions, remains a common occurrence.[38] Furthermore, as with conventional hepatic resection, the treatment of obvious metastases may not eliminate micrometastases. The role for systemic or regional chemotherapy in conjunction with cryoablation demands thorough investigation. There is already data that the combination of cryotherapy or regional chemotherapy with ablation may be more effective than either alone.[41] Whether these findings will be sustained by random assignment trials is an important question whose answer will greatly effect future treatment of unresectable colorectal metastases to the liver.

Hyperthermia

The use of heat or other forms of energy to raise the temperature of tumour cells may be exploited to produce tumour ablation. A wide variety of techniques have been developed to deliver energy to heat tissues including microwave, lasers, ultrasound and radiofrequency. The most important feature is not the mechanism by which energy is delivered but the ability to deliver the energy focally to destroy tumour tissue while sparing normal tissue. Attempts at hyperthermia have been carried out for cancers of different organ systems with varied effects.[42] Such hyperthermic ablation of tumours must be distinguished from another variety of hyperthermic treatment of tumours consisting of raising the temperature of the tissue only a few degrees above normal. This form of mild hyperthermia has been shown to enhance the local effects of chemotherapy.[43] This 'mild' hypothermia treatment modality will not be discussed in this chapter.

Clinical investigation of hyperthermia has been directed at the same clinical population deemed most suitable for cryotherapy, namely patients with unresectable liver tumours either due to anatomical considerations or due to poor liver reserve. Since some forms of hyperthermic ablation may be delivered without general anaesthesia and laparotomy, these treatment modalities are also being investigated for patients who are poor surgical risks, or those who refuse surgery. Unlike cryoablation, however, where warm blood circulating through the major vessels often protects major vasculature against freezing, hyperthermia is less discriminant, and injury to major vascular or biliary structures theoretically more likely. Thus, unresectability of tumour due to proximity to major vasculature may also be a contraindication to hyperthermic ablation. It is safe to say that the role of hyperthermic ablation for metastatic colorectal cancer has not been defined.

Microwave

Microwave ablation is usually accomplished percutaneously, but certainly can also be delivered in an operative setting. The patient is sedated and locally anesthaetized. Then, a microwave electrode is placed within the tumour under ultrasound guidance, and microwaves of 2450 MHz in frequency are produced for a fixed length of time, usually 60 s. The high-frequency energy induces tissue coagulation by local heat production. The microwave electrodes may be repositioned to administer ablation to other parts of the tumour. Seki *et al.* also apply microwave radiation to the puncture site to prevent bleeding when the probe is removed.[44] Only a limited amount of tissue around the microwave electrode is destroyed, and multiple treatment sessions may be necessary for tumours >2 cm in diameter.[44] Sessions may be carried out twice weekly. To monitor tissue destruction, various imaging modalities may be used. Necrosis may be noted by echogenic change on ultrasound, loss of contrast enhancement on CT or decrease in intensity in T2-weighted images in MRI.[44] As with other techniques, serum tumour markers can be used as a reflection of effectiveness of microwave treatments.[45]

Side-effects of microwave therapy include a transient fever, mild discomfort during the procedure seen in 50% of cases, and transient increase in liver function tests, which return to normal within a week.[44]

Most of the experience with microwave therapy of liver tumours has been with hepatocellular carcinoma[44,46,47] and have mainly been feasibility studies showing microwaves to be an effective source of ablative energy. Pathologically, coagulation necrosis is seen with a fibrous capsule around the necrosed tissue. Needle biopsies post-treatment have confirmed necrosis.[45] Data on ablating metastatic tumours with microwaves are sparse.[48] Shibata used microwave therapy in 22 patients with metastatic disease via a percutaneous approach and showed ablation of tumour.[48] These same authors also attempted microwave ablation during laparotomy in 67 metastatic lesions in 10 patients and found a 60% rate of tumour ablation.[48] Ogawa showed long-term survival in 2 patients with multiple metastases treated by microwave coagulation.[49] These data are hardly sufficient to advocate this form of ablation as standard therapy for metastatic colorectal cancer in any clinical setting, but certainly encourage future comparative studies to other methods of tumour ablation.

The main advantage of microwave ablation is that is can be performed percutaneously. However, when used percutaneously only small tumours can be ablated. Tumours >2 cm in diameter cannot be destroyed in a single session and require multiple sessions.[44] When applied during laparotomy, multiple microwave electrodes can be placed into the same tumour to allow ablation of larger tumour volumes. However, when used during laparotomy, microwave ablation is no less invasive than cryoablation, and certainly, the risks of injuring major vasculature is theoretically greater. Trials are clearly needed to compare percutaneous microwave ablation with chemical ablative methods such as ethanol injection (see below) for small tumours. Additional comparative trials are needed to determine the relative safety and efficacy of surgical microwave ablation and cryoablation for large tumours.

Radiofrequency

Radiofrequency ablation is mentioned only for completeness. Little clinical data exist to support its use. A recent study analysed the effects of radiofrequency hyperthermia in 67 tumours, 20 of whom had metastatic cancers. A 33% complete response and 89% partial response was found.[50] Much more data is needed to support a role for this technique in the treatment of metastatic colorectal cancer.

Laser

The use of lasers to ablate tumours was described in 1983[50] and first performed in 1985.[51] A comprehensive discussion of the effects of lasers on tissue is given by Jacques[52] and a review of interstitial laser therapy (ILP) is given by Masters[53] and Schneider.[54] The most common laser in use today is the neodymium–yttrium–aluminium garnet (Nd:YAG, 1064 nm) laser, although diode lasers (805 nm) may also be used.[55] Energy is delivered via fibreoptics placed interstitially under ultrasound guidance. Each fibre produces a spherical area of necrosis of approximately 1.5 cm in diameter.[24] Additional fibres can be added to increase the size of the area of necrosis. The procedure may be monitored with ultrasound or MRI[56] and the area of necrosis can be seen on ultrasound, contrast CT[57,58] or MR.[56]

Side-effects of laser therapy include air embolism when high flow co-axial gas is used to cool the probe.[59,60] Reducing the flow rate may eliminate this problem. As with any ablative procedure that leaves the necrotic tumour *in situ*, infection of the necrotic tumour is possible. Pain, asymptomatic subcapsular haematoma and pleural effusion have also been described as complications of ILP.[57]

A study by Nolsoe *et al.* in 11 patients showed ablation of 12 out of 16 colorectal metastases with ILP.[58] An early pilot study of ILP by Masters in 1992 had a 44% overall objective response in 18 lesions.[61] Another study of ILP in 21 patients with 55 liver metastases showed at >50% necrosis in 82% of lesions.[57] However, ILP appears to be less effective in lesions >2 cm in diameter.[56,62] In metastatic colorectal cancer, there are few 2-cm lesions, residing away from major vessels that are not resectable. Even though this technique is capable of ablating tumour, a clinical role for ILP has yet to be found.

Discussion

Microwave, radiofrequency and laser ablation are all effective in destroying tumour tissue. The main advantage of these techniques over cryotherapy is the potential for ablation of tumour without laparotomy. However, percutaneous application of these hyperthermic ablative procedures is greatly limited by the small size of lesions that can be ablated. This is the reason that laparoscopic placement of microwave probes is under investigation.[63,64] Whether any of these techniques will find a role in the treatment of metastatic colorectal cancer is uncertain. Furthermore, the cost of the required equipment, particularly the laser apparatus is not inconsiderable.[44]

Tissue-Destroying Agents

Techniques other than heat and cold have been used to destroy tumorous tissues, such as alcohol injection and hot saline injection. Alcohol injection has a long history of medical use in ganglion blocks. The safety and efficacy of percutaneous ethanol injection (PEI) has now also been established in the treatment of primary liver cancer in cirrhotic patients.[65,66] There have been several large series establishing the low cost and efficacy of PEI in the treatment of hepatocellular carcinoma, one with over 700 patients.[67,68] Recently, there have been reports of success of PEI in the destruction of metastatic disease as well.[69,70] In a report that strongly advocates PEI, Giovannini showed complete necrosis in 31 of 55 cases of metastatic disease and a three-year actuarial survival of 39%.[71] Others have had less encouraging results. In a report by Amin et al., with 22 metastatic colorectal cancers treated by PEI, none

had complete necrosis.[70] The reason that results with percutaneous injection of any ablative agent for metastatic colorectal cancer may be more disappointing than such treatments for hepatocellular carcinoma is that hepatocellular carcinoma are generally soft tumours. Metastatic colorectal cancer on the other hand are generally very hard tumours, making placement of ablative agents by thin relatively-flexible needles technically difficult. At present these percutaneous ablative procedures are still investigational. The authors reserve use of these to patients with metastatic colorectal cancers who have had multiple resection and who have small unresectable recurrences.

Ethanol Injection Techniques

Technical factors limit the tumours that may be injected percutaneously. Most interventional radiologists would only inject lesions that are <4 cm in diameter and fewer in numbers than four. Tumours that are high in the liver are difficult to treat with any percutaneous injections because of the risk of injuring the lung.

Percutaneous ethanol injections may be directed by either ultrasound guidance or CT guidance to deliver absolute ethanol to the tumour tissue. Lee et al. provide a more detailed description of the procedure.[72] Briefly, the patient is lightly sedated with midazolam, and the lesion is visualized using real-time ultrasonography or CT. The volume of ethanol needed is calculated prior to injection by noting the dimensions of the tumour. Enough should be delivered to ensure an adequate margin. After placement of a gauge 19 needle within the tumour, absolute ethanol is injected. However, the alcohol may diffuse away from the tumorous tissue rendering the true area of necrosis unpredictable, particularly for larger lesions. The distribution of ethanol also is not uniform, with ethanol tending to move away from more fibrotic areas. It must be reiterated that because of the dense nature of metastatic colorectal cancers, it is particularly difficult to evenly distribute the alcohol. This may be overcome by repeating the injections within a week of the first injection and after initial softening of the tumour. This is why multiple treatments are usually more effective.[73] Distribution of ethanol can be seen with ultrasound as echodense droplets, or on CT as hypodense areas.[74]

Although some investigators will perform follow-up of the patient with a CT approximately two weeks later,[74] the authors generally will not check tumour necrosis until approximately eight weeks later. A contrast enhanced CT scan will demonstrate necrotic tumours to be hypodense areas. Patients with elevated CEA levels before treatment should also be followed using this tumour marker.

Complications

Pain with injection has been noted and is often associated with reflux of alcohol into the peritoneum but this side-effect may be limited by slow injection of ethanol and slow withdrawal of the needle.[69] Bile collections have also been described after treatment for hepatocellular carcinoma[75] as well as abscess formation,[76,77] though infections are rare. Both may be treated with percutaneous drainage. The risk of needle tract tumour seeding exists for all percutaneous treatments and has been documented after PEI.[78-81] Because of the small volume of tumour that is treatable by PEI, generally there is little of the tumorolysis syndrome that is seen with cryoablation. Pneumothorax is a possible consequence of these treatments if the tumour is high in the liver.

Results

Use of PEI has been effective in treating small hepatocellular carcinoma.[82-84] Livraghi suggested a 52.3% complete necrosis rate in 21 lesions in 14 patients with hepatocellular carcinoma.[82] Data for the treatment for metastatic colorectal cancer are still sparse. Giovannini used PEI in 40 patients with hepatic metastases and found a three-year actuarial survival of 39% and reports a 54% complete necrosis rate and a 32% partial necrosis rate.[69] Amin et al. have been less than enchanted, finding no case of complete necrosis with PEI.[70] Certainly, no comparison of PEI with hepatic resection has been performed in a formal random assignment trial. It must be emphasized that PEI is generally used only for smaller lesions. Therefore, indirect comparisons of results of such treatment to most published resectional series must be avoided. The authors recommend that except for the setting of formal clinical trials, or until further definitive results from trials,

PEI should be reserved for advanced recurrent disease isolated to the liver that has failed conventional chemotherapy.

Hot Saline Injection

Hot saline has been used[85,86] in an attempt to overcome some of the difficulties in the toxicity seen with ethanol. The technique is similar. However, pain during injection ceases upon infusion interruption. Since the injected liquid is non-toxic, larger volumes of liquid can be delivered to ablate larger volumes of tumour, possibly reducing the number of treatments necessary.[85] Honda et al. examined percutaneous saline in the treatment of 20 patients with 23 nodules of hepatocellular carcinoma and found it to be effective and without significant side effects.[86,87] No data using this modality in treatment of metastatic colorectal cancer have been published to date. Other difficulties in using PEI, such as difficulties in treating large tumours, dense tumours and tumours high in the liver must be anticipated for ablation using hot saline.

Discussion

Percutaneous chemical ablation, such as PEI, may be administered at low cost with reasonably low toxicity and side-effects. Advantages of PEI are ease of performance using minimal equipment with low mortality, ability to treat multiple lesions in different locations and low expense. Normal parenchyma is also spared. Disadvantages include irritation and sclerosis of bile ducts and vessels, pain due to leakage of ethanol into the peritoneum, limited size of the lesions that may be treated and difficulty in controlling the area of treatment. In addition, multiple treatment sessions are usually necessary. Therapy may be limited by the size of the lesion, with most investigators recommending PEI only for lesions <4 cm.[69,83]

Since both ethanol and saline injections come with relatively minimal morbidity and can potentially provide curative treatment, investigation aiming to extend indications for treatment using this modality will continue, particularly as palliation for small lesions <4 cm.

Other Techniques

The use of electrocautery for tumour ablation uses techniques similar to other ablative techniques such as ILP or microwave and are also performed under ultrasonic guidance and monitoring.[88] The size of the ablated tissue is proportional to the energy delivered through the tip. This technique is very inexpensive but has yet to be fully evaluated. Another new technique employs high-energy shock waves generated by piezoelectric crystals to destroy tumour.[89] Focused ultrasound can destroy tissue totally non-invasively and has been examined experimentally but to date, it has been difficult to accurately focus the area of destruction.[90,91]

Conclusions

Patients with cancer of the liver generally have a poor prognosis; surgical resection represents the only established effective cure. For patients who are not candidates for surgical resection, current chemotherapeutic regimens are inadequate, and ablative *in situ* therapies may offer alternative strategies. Ablative treatments offer two main advantages: firstly, tumours can be treated focally and, secondly, liver tissue can be conserved. These two advantages may increase the number of patients who are candidates for treatment.

The role of each ablative modality has yet to be defined and a comparison of the ablative modalities under investigation are listed in Table 9.5. Cryotherapy has been shown to be safe treatment for colorectal metastases. The addition of laparoscopy and percutaneous techniques will likely

further expand its use. Other ablative methods, including hyperthermia via microwave or interstitial laser phototherapy, and percutaneous ethanol injections are also efficacious in the treatment of small and medium-sized lesions. Percutaneous ethanol injection in particular holds promise for treatment of primary hepatocellular carcinoma and small non-resectable recurrences in the liver after prior liver resection. Advantages include its simplicity, its minimal invasiveness, low expense and ease of administration. Investigations into use of these ablative methods should be directed at three main areas.

Firstly and most obviously, efficacy studies comparing various modalities in random assignment trials are sorely needed. The number of ablative techniques and their use have increased dramatically in the past decade. Which techniques are more suitable for certain types of tumours or locations awaits these prospective multicentre studies. Secondly, the need for and the optimum drugs for adjuvant therapy should be investigated. Thirdly, continued studies of imaging modalities for guiding and monitoring ablative therapy require study. Further improvements in CT, sonography or magnetic imaging will further extend our ability to use ablative techniques. Developments in PET and functional MRI are also likely to revolutionize our ability to assess the effects of therapy. Finally, increasing awareness of need for cost-containment assumes that minimally invasive techniques will become popular. We need to be sure that use of these modalities is based on data demonstrating efficacy, and that patients not be refused potentially curative resection based solely on cost considerations. Which techniques or combinations of techniques are most effective will require definition in future prospective controlled studies of both efficacy and cost.

Table 9.5 Comparisons of various ablative therapies

Parameter	Cryotherapy	Laser	Microwave	PEI	Saline
Anaesthesia	General	General/local	Local/general	Local	Local
Cost of equipment	Moderate	High	Moderate	Low	Low
Discomfort	High	Moderate	Moderate	Moderate	Low
Ease of performance	Moderate	Moderate	Moderate	Easy	Easy
Amount of equipment	Moderate	Moderate	Moderate	Minimal	Minimal
Ease of repeat treatment	Poor	Poor	Moderate	Easy	Easy
Personnel	Surgeon	Surgeon/radiologist	Surgeon/radiologist	Radiologist	Radiologist
Precision of treatment	High	Moderate	Moderate	Low	Low
Size of lesion treatable	Large	Moderate	Moderate	Small	Small

References

1. Lise M, Da Pian PP, Nitti D, Pilati PL. Colorectal metastases to the liver: present results and future strategies. *J Surg Oncol* (Suppl) 1991; **2**:69–73.

2. Fong Y, Blumgart LH, Cohen AE. Surgical resection of colorectal metastases. *Ca: Cancer J Clin* 1995; **45**:50–62.

3. Kavolius J, Fong Y, Blumgart LH. Surgical resection of metastatic liver tumors. *Surg Oncol Clin N Am* 1996; **5**:337–351.

4. Bengtsson G, Carlsson G, Hafstrom L *et al*. Natural history of patients with untreated liver metastases from colorectal cancer. *Am J Surg* 1981; **141**:586–589.

5. Scheele J. Liver resection for colorectal metastases. *World J Surg* 1995; **19**:59–71.

6. Nordlinger B, Jaeck D, Guiget M *et al*. (eds) *Surgical Resection of Hepatic Metastases: Multicentric Retrospective Study by the French Association of Surgery* 1992: 129–146. Paris, Springer.

7. Fong Y, Cohen AM, Fortner JG *et al*. Liver Resection for colorectal metastases *J Clin Oncol* 1997; **15**(3): 938–946.

8. Fong Y, Blumgart LH, Fortner JG, Brennan MF. Pancreatic or liver resection for malignancy is safe and effective for the elderly. *Ann Surg* 1995; **222**:426–437.

9. Holm A, Bradley E, Aldrete S. Hepatic resection of metastasis from colorectal carcinoma. *Ann Surg* 1989; **209**:428–434.

10. Armstrong JG, Anderson LL, Harrison LB. Treatment of liver metastases from colorectal cancer with radioactive implants. *Cancer* 1994; **73**:1800–1804.

11. Pederson IK, Burcharth F, Roikjaer O, Baden H. Resection of liver metastases from colorectal cancer: indication and results. *Dis Colon Rectum* 1994; **37**:1078–1082.

12. Cozzi PJ, Englund R, Morris DL. Cryotherapy treatment of patients with hepatic metastases from neuroendocrine tumors. *Cancer* 1995; **76**:501–509.

13. Lau WY, Leung TW, Leung KL, Ho S, Leung N, Chan M, Lin J, Li AK. Cryoreductive surgery for hepatocellular carcinoma. *Surg Oncol* 1994; **3**:161–166.

14. Nauta RJ, Heres EK, Thomas DS, Harter KW, Rodgers JE, Holt RW, Lee TC, Walsh DB, Dritschilo A. Intraoperative single-dose radiotherapy. Observations and staging. *Arch Surg* 1987; **122**:1392–1395.

15. Copper IS. Cryogenic surgery: a new method of destruction or extirpation of benign or malignant tissues. *New Engl J Med* 1963; **268**:743–749.

16. Dutta MM, Gage AA. Large volume freezing in experimental hepatic cryosurgery. *Cryobiology* 1979; **16**:50–55.

17. Onik GM, Atkinson D, Zemel R, Weaver ML. Cryosurgery of liver cancer. *Semin Surg Oncol* 1993; **9**:309–317.

18. Ravikumar TS, Kane R, Cady B, Jenkins R, Clouse M, Steele G, Jr. A 5-year study of cryosurgery in the treatment of liver tumors. *Arch Surg* 1991; **126**:1520–1523.

19. Stewart GJ, Preketes A, Horton M, Ross WB, Morris DL. Hepatic cryotherapy: double-freeze cycles achieve greater hepatocellular injury in man. *Cryobiology* 1995; **32**:215–219.

20. McLoughlin RF, Saliken JF, McKinnon G, Wiseman D, Temple W. CT of the liver after cryotherapy of hepatic metastases: imaging findings. *Am J Roentgen* 1995; **165**:329–332.

21. Charnley RM, Thomas M, Morris DL. Effects of hepatic cryotherapy on serum CEA concentration in patients with multiple inoperable hepatic metastases from colorectal cancer. *Aust NZ J Surg* 1991; **61**:55–58.

22. Preketes AP, King J, Caplehorn JRM, Clingan PR, Ross WB, Morris DL. CEA reduction after cryotherapy for liver metastases from colon cancer. *Aust NZ J Surg* 1994; **64**:612–614.

23. Ravikumar TS, Kane R, Cady B. Hepatic cryosurgery with intraoperative ultrasound monitoring for patients with metastatic colon carcinoma. *Arch Surg* 1987; **122**:403–409.

24. Masters A, Steger AC, Bown SG. Role of interstitial therapy in the treatment of liver cancer. *Br J Surg* 1991; **78**:518–523.

25. Ravikumar TS, Steele G, Jr., Kane R, King V. Experimental and clinical observations on hepatic cryosurgery for colorectal metastases. *Cancer Res* 1991; **51**:6323–6327.

26. Charnley RM, Doran J, Morris DL. Cryotherapy for liver metastases: a new approach [see comments]. *Br J Surg* 1989; **76**:1040–1041.

27. Sako S, Seitzinger GL, Garside E. Carcinoma of the extrahepatic ducts. Review of the literature and report of six cases. *Surgery* 1957; **41**:416–417.

28. Ross WB, Horton M, Bertolino P, Morris DL. Cryotherapy of liver tumours – a practical guide. *HPB* 1995; **8**:167–173.

29. Goodie DB, Horton MD, Morris RW, Nagy LS, Morris DL. Anaesthetic experience with cryotherapy for treatment of hepatic malignancy. *Anaesthesia Intensive Care* 1992; **20**:491–496.

30. Onik G, Rubinsky B, Zemel R, Weaver L, Diamond D, Cobb C, Porterfield B. Ultrasound-guided hepatic cryosurgery in the treatment of metastatic colon carcinoma. Preliminary results. *Cancer* 1991; **67**:901–907.

31. Shafir M, Shapiro R, Sung M, Warmer R, Sicular A, Klipfel A. Cryoablation of unresectable malignant liver tumors. *Am J Surg* 1996; **171**:27–31.

32. Onik GM, Chambers N, Chernus SA, Zemel R, Atkinson D, Weaver ML. Hepatic cryosurgery with and without the Bair Hugger. *J Surg Oncol* 1993; **52**:185–187.

33. Cozzi PJ, Stewart GJ, Morris DL. Thrombocytopenia after hepatic cryotherapy for colorectal metastases: correlates with hepatocellular injury. *World J Surg* 1994; **18**:774–776.

34. Ross WB, Morris DL, Morris R, Warlters A. Cardiac rhythm disturbances due to caval occlusion during hepatic cryosurgery. *Cryobiology* 1994; **31**:501–505.

35. Preketes AP, Caplehorn JRM, King J, Clingan PR, Ross WB, Morris DL. Effect of hepatic artery chemotherapy on survival of patients with hepatic metastases from colorectal carcinoma treated with cryotherapy. *World J Surg* 1995; **19**:768–771.

36. Morris DL, Ross WB. Australian experience of cryoablation of liver tumors. *Surg Oncol Clin N Am* 1996; **5**:391–397.

37. Blumgart LH, Fong Y. Surgical management of colorectal metastases to the liver. *Curr Probl Surg* 1995; **5**:333–428.

38. Cuschieri A, Crosthwaite G, Shimi S, Pietrabissa A, Joypaul V, Tair I, Naziri W. Hepatic cryotherapy for liver tumors. Development and clinical evaluation of a high efficiency insulated multineedle probe system for open and laparoscopic use. *Surg Endosc* 1995; **9**:483–489.

39. Cuschieri A. Laparoscopic management of cancer patients. *J Roy Coll Surg (Edin)* 1995; **40**:1–9.

40. Maeda T, Hasebe Y, Hanawa S, Watanabe M, Nakazaki H, Kuramoto S, Yoshio T. Trial of percutaneous hepatic cryotherapy: preliminary report [in Japanese]. *Nippon Geka Gakkai Zasshi [J Jap Surg Soc]* 1992; **93**:666.

41. Morris DL, Horton MD, Dilley AV, Warlters A, Clingan PR. Treatment of hepatic metastases by cryotherapy and regional cytotoxic perfusion. *Gut* 1993; **34**:1158–1161.

42. Kakehi M, Ueda K, Mukojima T, Hiraoka M, Seto O, Akanuma A, Nakatsugawa S. Multi-institutional clinical studies on hyperthermia combined with radiotherapy or chemotherapy in advanced cancer of deep-seated organs. *Int J Hyperthermia* 1990; **6**:719–740.

43. Kondo M, Itani K, Yoshikawa T, Tanaka Y, Watanabe N, Hiraoka M, Noguchi M, Miura K. [A prospective randomized clinical trial comparing intra-arterial chemotherapy alone and when combined with hyperthermia for metastatic liver cancer.] *Gan to Kagaku Ryoho [Jap J Cancer Chem]* 1995; **22**:12, 1807–11.

44. Seki T, Wakabayashi M, Nakagawa T, Itho T, Shiro T, Kunieda K, Sato M, Uchiyama S, Inoue K. Ultrasonically guided percutaneous microwave coagulation therapy for small hepatocellular carcinoma. *Cancer* 1994; 74:817–825.

45. Hamazoe R, Hirooka Y, Ohtani S, Katoh T, Kaibara N. Intraoperative microwave tissue coagulation as treatment for patients with nonresectable hepatocellular carcinoma. *Cancer* 1995; 75:794–800.

46. Zhou XD, Tang ZY, Yu YQ, Ma ZC, Xu DB, Zheng YX, Zhang BH. Microwave surgery in the treatment of hepatocellular carcinoma. *Semin Surg Oncol* 1993; 9:318–322.

47. Saitsu H, Mada Y, Taniwaki S, Okuda K, Nakayama T, Oishi K, Yoshida K. [Investigation of microwave coagulo-necrotic therapy for 21 patients with small hepatocellular carcinoma less than 5 cm in diameter.] *Nippon Geka Gakkai Zasshi* [*J Jap Surg Soc*] 1993; 94:4, 359–65.

48. Shibata T, Takami M, Fujimoto T, Takada T, Kitada M, Tsukahara Y, Okumura Y, Saito M, Murotani M, Sugimoto K. [Microwave tumor coagulation (MTC) in liver tumor: indication and percutaneous approach.] *Gan to Kagaku Ryoho* [*Jap J Cancer Chem*] 1994; 21:13, 2128–31.

49. Ogawa M, Shibata T, Takami M, Tsujinaka T, Takada T, Kitada M, Tsukahara Y, Murotani M, Niinobu T, Iihara K. [Long-term survival in two cases of multiple liver metastasis successfully treated with intraoperative ultrasound-guided microwave tumor coagulation (MTC)] *Gan to Kagaku Ryoho* [*Jap J Cancer Chem*] 1995; 22:11, 1679–83.

50. Cheung AY. Microwaves and radiofrequency techniques in hyperthermia. *Br J Cancer* 1982; 45:16–24.

51. Hashimoto D, Takami M, Idezuki Y. In depth radiation therapy by Nd:YAG laser for malignant tumors of the liver under ultrasonic imaging. *Gastroenterology* 1985; A1663:88.

52. Jacques SL. Laser–tissue interactions: photochemical, photothermal and photomechanical. *Surg Clin N Am* 1992; 8:242–249.

53. Masters A, Bown SG. Interstitial laser hyperthermia. [Review.] *Semin Surg Oncol* 1992; 8:242–249.

54. Schneider PD. Liver resection and laser hyperthermia. [Review.] *Surg Clin N Am* 1992; 72:623–639.

55. Perring S, Hind R, Fleming J, Birch S, Batty V, Taylor I. Dosimetric assessment of radiolabelled lipiodol. *Nucl Med Commun* 1994; 15:34–38.

56. Vogl TJ, Muller PK, Hammerstingl R, Weinhold N, Mack MG, Philipp C, Deimling M, Beuthan J, Pegios W, Riess H. Malignant liver tumors treated with MR imaging-guided laser-induced thermotherapy: technique and prospective results. *Radiology* 1995; 196:257–265.

57. Amin Z, Donald JJ, Masters A, Kant R, Steger AC, Bown SG, Lees WR. Hepatic metastases: interstitial laser photocoagulation with real-time US monitoring and dynamic CT evaluation of treatment. *Radiology* 1993; 187:339–347.

58. Nolsoe CP, Torp-Pedersen S, Burcharth F, Horn T, Pedersen S, Christensen NE, Olldag ES, Andersen PH, Karstrup S, Lorentzen T. Interstitial hyperthermia of colorectal liver metastases with a US-guide Nd-YAG laser with a diffuser tip: a pilot clinical study. *Radiology* 1993; 187:333–337.

59. Malone DE, Lesiuk L, Brady AP, Wyman DR, Wilson BC. Hepatic interstitial laser photocoagulation: demonstration and possible importance of intravascular gas. *Radiology* 1994; 193:233–237.

60. Hahl J, Haapianen R, Ovaska J, Puolakkainen P, Schroder T. Laser-induced hyperthermia in the treatment of liver tumors. *Lasers Surg Med* 1990; 10:319–321.

61. Masters A, Steger AC, Lees WR, Walmsley KM, Bown SG. Interstitial laser hyperthermia: a new approach for treating liver metastases. *Br J Cancer* 1992; 66:518–22.

62. Vogl TJ, Muller P, Hirsch H, Philipp C, Hammerstingl R, Bottcher H, Riess H, Beuthan J, Felix R. Laser-induced thermotherapy of liver metastases with MRI control. Prospective

63. Saitsu H, Nakayama T. Microwave coagulo-necrotic therapy for hepatocellular carcinoma. *Jap J Clin Med* 1993; 51:4, 1002–7.

64. Watanabe Y, Sato M, Abe Y, Horiuchi S, Kito K, Kimura S. Laparoscopic microwave coagulo-necrotic therapy for hepatocellular carcinoma: a feasibility study of an alternative option for poor-risk patients. *J Laparoendosc Surg* 1995; 5:169–175.

65. Shiina S, Tagawa K, Niwa Y, Unuma T, Komatsu Y, Yoshiura K, Hamada E, Takahashi M, Shiratori Y, Terano A. Percutaneous ethanol injection therapy for hepatocellular carcinoma. *Am J Roentgen* 1993; 160:1023–1028.

66. Ebara M, Ohto M, Sugiura N *et al.* Percutaneous ethanol injection for the treatment of small hepatocellular carcinoma. Study of 95 patients. *J Gastroenterol Hepatol* 1990; 5:616–620.

67. Livraghi T, Giorgio A, Marin G, Salmi A, de Sio I, Bolondi L, Pompili M, Brunello F, Lazzaroni S, Torzilli G. Hepatocellular carcinoma and cirrhosis in 746 patients. *Radiology* 1995; 197:101–108.

68. Livraghi T, Bolondi L, Buscarini L, Cottone M, Mazziotti A, Morabito A, Torzilli G. No treatment, resection and ethanol injection in hepatocellular carcinoma: a retrospective analysis of survival in 391 patients with cirrhosis. *J Hepatol* 1995; 22:522–526.

69. Giovannini M, Seitz JF. Ultrasound-guided percutaneous injection of small liver metastases. *Cancer* 1994; 73:294–297.

70. Amin Z, Bown SG, Lees WR. Local treatment of colorectal liver metastases: a comparison of interstitial laser photocoagulation (ILP) and percutaneous alcohol injection (PAI). *Clin Radiol* 1993; 48:166–171.

71. Giovannini M, Seitz JF, Rosello R, Gauthier A. Treatment of minor hepatic tumors with ultrasonically-guided percutaneous ethanol injection. *Clinique et Biologique* 1989; 13:974–977.

72. Lee MJ, Mueller PR, Dawson SL, Gazelle SG, Hahn PF, Goldberg MA, Boland GW. Percutaneous ethanol injection for the treatment of hepatic tumors: indications, mechanism of action, technique and efficacy. *Am J Roentgen* 1995; 164:215–220.

73. Livraghi T, Lazzaroni S, Pellicano S, Ravasi S, Torzilli G, Vettori C. Percutaneous ethanol injection of hepatic tumors: single-session. *Am J Roentgen* 1993; 161:1065–1069.

74. Ebara M, Kita K, Sugiura N, Yoshikawa M, Fukuda H, Ohto M, Kondo F, Kondo Y. Therapeutic effect of percutaneous ethanol injection on small hepatocellular carcinoma: evaluation with CT. *Radiology* 1995; 195:371–377.

75. Kohno E, Chen S, Numata K, Nakamura S, Tanaka K, Endo O, Inoue S, Takamura Y. A case of biloma: complication of percutaneous ethanol injection therapy for hepatocellular carcinoma. *Jap J Gastroenterol* 1992; 89(11), 2719–2724.

76. Solinas A, Erbella GS, Distrutti E, Malaspina C, Fiorucci S, Clerici C, Bassotti G, Morelli A. Abscess formation in hepatocellular carcinoma: complications of percutaneous ultrasound-guided ethanol injection. *J Clin Ultrasound* 1993; 21:531–533.

77. Okada S, Aoki K, Okazaki N, Nose H, Yoshimori M, Shimada K, Yamamoto J, Takayama T, Kosuge T, Yamasaki S. Liver abscess after percutaneous ethanol injection (PEI) therapy for hepatocellular carcinoma. A case report. *Hepato-gastroenterology* 1993; 40:496–498.

78. Shimada M, Maeda T, Saitoh A, Morotomi I, Kano T. Needle track seeding after percutaneous ethanol injection therapy for small hepatocellular carcinoma. *J Surg Oncol* 1995; 58:278–281.

79. Borghetti M, Reduzzi L, Bonardi R, Parziale M. The dynamic computed tomography of small hepatocarcinomas treated by US-guided percutaneous ethanol injections. The short- and long-term follow-up aspects. *Radiol Med* 1992; 83:361–365.

80. Cedrone A, Rapaccini GL, Pompili M, Grattagliano A, Aliotta A, Trombino C. Neoplastic seeding complicating percuta-

results of an optimized therapy procedure. *Radiologie* 1995; 35:188–199.

neous ethanol injection for treatment of hepatocellular carcinoma. *Radiology* 1992; **183**:787–788.

81. Goletti O, De Negri F, Pucciarelli M, Sidoti F, Bertolucci A, Chiarugi M, Seccia M. Subcutaneous seeding after percutaneous ethanol injection of liver metastasis. *Radiology* 1992; **183**:785–786.

82. Livraghi T, Vettori C, Lazzaroni S. Liver metastases: Results of percutaneous ethanol injection in 14 patients. *Radiology* 1991; **179**:709–712.

83. Livraghi T, Festi D, Monti F, Salmi A, Vettori C. US-guided percutaneous alcohol injection of small hepatic and abdominal tumours. *Radiology* 1986; **161**:309–312.

84. Kotoh K, Sakai H, Sakamoto S, Nakayama S, Satoh M, Morotomi I, Nawata H. The effect of percutaneous ethanol injection therapy on small solitary hepatocellular carcinoma is comparable to that of hepatectomy. *Am J Roentgen* 1994; **89**:194–198.

85. Veltri A, Martina C, Bonenti G, Dore D, Cirillo S, Grosso M, Fava C. Therapy of malignant hepatic tumors using percutaneous hot saline injections. Feasibility study and preliminary results. *Radiol Med* 1995; **90**:463–469.

86. Honda A, Martina C, Bonenti G, Dore D, Cirillo S, Grosso M, Fava C. Percutaneous hot saline injection therapy for hepatic tumors: an alternative to percutaneous ethanol injection therapy [see comments]. *Radiology* 1994; **190**:53–57.

87. Honda A, Guo Q, Uchida H, Nishida H, Hirai T, Ohishi H, Hiasa Y. Percutaneous hot water injection therapy (PHoT) for hepatic tumors: a clinical study. *Nippon Igaku Hoshasen Gakkai Zasshi* [*Nippon Acta Radiologica*] 1993; 53(7), 781–789.

88. McGahan JP, Browning JP, Brock JM *et al.* Hepatic ablation using radiofrequency electrocautery. *Invest Radiol* 1990; **25**:267–270.

89. Darzi A, Goldin R, Guillou PJ, Monson JR. High-energy shock waves pyrotherapy. A new concept in extracorporeal tumor therapy. *Surg Oncol* 1993; **2**:197–203.

90. Chapelon JY, Prat F, Sibille A, Abou El Fadil F, Henry L, Theillere Y, Cathignol D. Extracorporeal, selective focused destruction of hepatic tumours by high intensity ultrasound in rabbits bearing VX-2 carcinoma. *Minimally Invasive Therapy* 1992; **1**:287–293.

91. Vallencien G, Harouni M, Veillon B, Mombet A, Prapotnich D, Brisset JM, Bougaran J. Focused extracorporeal pyrotherapy: feasibility study in man. *J Endourol* 1992; **6**:173–181.

Systemic Therapy

Roberto Labianca, Giuseppe Dallavalle, M. Adelaide Pessi and Giuseppina Zamparelli

10

Introduction

Most neoplastic diseases will develop liver metastases along their progression. Liver metastases represent a major problem among cancer patients, their high incidence only being exceeded by that of nodal involvement. The proportion of patients with metastatic liver disease has increased in the latest years, as a consequence of technical improvements in diagnostic instruments (e.g. Computed tomography scans, ultrasonography, MRI, markers, nuclear medicine).

One of the neoplasms most frequently metastasizing to the liver is colorectal cancer, due to its portal supply as well as to preferential organ colonization. For this reason, much clinical experience has accumulated with regard to the medical treatment of liver metastases from primary colorectal cancer. Most of this chapter will focus on this condition.

Liver Metastases from Colorectal Cancer

5-Fluorouracil (5FU)

Since 5-fluorouracil (5-FU) was discovered in 1957 by Heidelberg,[1,2] following the observation that hepatoma cells of rat use uracil more efficiently that normal intestinal cells, it continues to represent the standard treatment of gastrointestinal tract cancer. Although 5-FU and its deoxynucleoside 5-fluorodeoxiuridine (FUdR) have been known as antitumoural agents for 30–35 years, preclinical and clinical research concerning these drugs are ongoing and recently have progressed due to a new understanding of intracellular pharmacology and its therapeutic relevance. Interesting new areas include intracellular activation steps, pharmacological interactions and cellular mechanisms of resistance.

Because of the large choice of modalities and route of administration, the study of 5-FU pharmacokinetics is particularly important. 5-FU is converted to FUdR by thymidine phosphorylase and the phosphorylation of FUdR by thymidine kinase results in development of the active 5-FU metabolite, FdUMP, which inhibits thymidylate synthase in the presence of the reduced folate 5,10-methylenetetrahydrofolate. Therefore 5-FU may be converted to fluorouridine monophosphate (FUMP) through the sequential action of uridine phosphorylase and uridine kinase or through direct conversion by orotic acid phosphoribosyltransferase in the presence of 5'-phosphoribosyl-1-pyrophosphate (PRPP). FUMP may be further metabolized to fluorouridine triphosphate (FUTP) which may be incorporated into RNA or converted to FdUMP.[3] Finally, FdUMP may be subsequently phosphorylated to the triphosphate form which may be incorporated into DNA.[4]

The cytotoxic effects of 5-FU are due to three main mechanisms: (1) thymidylate synthase inhibition by 5-fluorodeoxiuridine-monophosphate (5-FdMP) in presence of 5,10-methylenetetrahydrofolate (CH2FH4) through the formation of a ternary stable complex which causes cellular death by thymine deprivation; (2) direct assimilation of 5-FU into RNA and consequent interference in its maturation and function; (3) recently demonstrated direct assimilation of 5-FU into DNA which leads to chain fragmentation and to cellular death.[4]

Oral bioavailability of 5-FU is erratic, as <75% of an oral dose reaches the systemic circulation and it is now widely accepted that 5-FU should not be given by oral route. Usually 5-FU is administered intravenously. After conventional single doses of 400–600 mg/m^2 peak plasma concentration reaches 0.2–1 mM, but rapid metabolic breakdown to dihydrofluorouracil in the liver and other tissues leads to an abrupt fall in plasma concentration. More than 80% of administered 5-FU by the intravenous or intraarterial route is eliminated by its metabolic conversion to dihydrofluorouracil (DHFU) and 20% is excreted intact in the urine. The liver, kidney, white blood cells and gastrointestinal mucosa are the primary sites of 5-FU metabolism. Because a large part of metabolism occurs in extrahepatic tissues, the doses should not be necessarily modified in the presence of hepatic dysfunction.

Elimination of 5-FU obeys non-linear pharmacokinetics characteristics resulting in recycling of the drug consequent persistantly elevated doses. For these considerations, much research now is devoted to evaluate new modalities of administration (with more efficacious and less toxic schedules): the so-called 'biochemical modulation'. The following section reviews this subject area.

Modalities of Administration

5-FU can be given by bolus injection, short infusion or long-term infusion. In 1989, the Mid Atlantic Oncology Program[5] reported the results of a prospective randomized comparison of continuous infusion 5-FU with administration of the drug by intravenous bolus injection.

The tumour response rate was 7% for the bolus arm and 30% for the infusion arm ($P < 0.001$). Toxicity was different for the two arms with major leukopenia observed only in the bolus arm.

Hand–foot syndrome was observed only in the infusional arm, although this had little impact on quality of life. In spite of the major different in objective response rate, overall survival for the two groups was comparable. Subsequently other trials, comparing 5-FU i.v. bolus to 5-FU continuous infusion, were conducted by the NCIC,[6] France,[7] ECOG[8] and SWOG.[9] In these two last trials, other random arms were included.

Table 10.1 summarizes the results from these trials; in general, it was possible to observe an advantage of 5-FU continuous infusion over bolus administration in terms of objective tumour response. The 30% response rate observed for infusional 5-FU is comparable to that found with the use of several biochemical modulation strategies, raising the possibility that the efficacy of 5-FU might be enhanced further by the addition of leukovorin or other agents.

In 1991 Ardalan et al.,[10] using high-dose 5-FU (2600 mg/m^2) by 24-hour infusion with leukovorin (500 mg/m^2), reported a 30% objective response. Prompted by these results, other multicentric studies started in order to evaluate the benefit and tolerability of this kind of treatment. The results of five studies are summarized in Table 10.2.[11-14] In all of these studies toxicity consisted mainly of mucositis, diarrhoea, nausea and hand–foot syndrome. Leukopenia and thrombocytopenia were moderate. In some patients, cardiotoxicity was observed. In comparison to protracted continuous infusion of 5-FU, the toxicity seems to be somewhat higher.

Pretreated patients with metastatic colorectal cancer can probably benefit from weekly high-dose 5-FU + leukovorin particularly when they have had documented progression of disease on 5-FU bolus-containing regimens.

Table 10.1 Randomized clinical trials comparing 5-FU continuous infusion to 5-FU bolus in patients with advanced colorectal cancer

Institution	5-FU continous infusion	5-FU bolus	patients (n)
France (Rougier, 1992)[7]	5-FU 750 mg/m^2/day 1–day 7, q 21 d	5-FU 500 mg/m^2 day 1–day 5, q 28 d	155
NCIC (Weinerman, 1992)[6]	5-FU 350 mg/m^2, day 1–day 15, q 28 d	5-FU 400–450 mg/m^2 day 1–day 5, q 28 d	185
MAOP (Lokich, 1989)[5]	5-FU 300 mg/m^2 without interruption	5-FU 500 mg/m^2 day 1–day 5, q 35 d	179
ECOG (Hansen, 1992)[8]	5-FU 300 mg/m^2 without interruption	5-FU 500 mg/m^2 day 1–day 5, then 5-FU 600 mg/m^2 day, q 7 d	± 320
SWOG (Leichman, 1993)[9]	5-FU 300 mg/m^2 day 1–day 28, q 35 d	5-FU 500 mg/m^2 day 1–day 5, q 35 d 5-FU 2600 mg/m^2 day 1, q 7 d	± 400
	5-FU 200 mg/m^2 day 1–day 28, q 35 d, plus folinic acid 20 mg/m^2 i.v. q 7 d	5-FU 425 mg/m^2 plus folinic acid 20 mg/m^2 i.v. day 1–day 5, q 28 d ×2, then q 35 d	

Table 10.2   5-FU 24-h infusion plus folinic acid weekly in refractory colorectal cancer

Authors	Patients (n)	CR (%)	PR (%)	PR + MR + NC	Median duration (months)	Survival (months)
Ardalan et al. 1991[10]	10	–	30%	n.a.	n.a.	10
Weh et al. 1994[11]	57	–	9%	65%	3	8
Jaeger et al. 1995[12]	69	–	25%	86%	7	9
Loef er et al 1995[13]	55	–	35%	81%	n.a.	n.a.
Lorenz et al. 1996[14]	38	–	32%	77%	n.a.	n.a.

CR = complete response; PR = partial response; MR = minor response; NC = no change

Biochemical Modulation

Folinic Acid or Leukovorin

The limited number of objective responses obtained with 5-FU in monochemotherapy (about 20%) led to development of clinical studies whose aim was to increase the activity of this drug. Modulation of 5-FU by leukovorin has been analysed in phase I and II studies, and subsequently in confirmatory phase III trials. The results of ten phase III studies results are now available. They have been conducted by the following (see Table 10.3): GITSG;[15] NCOG,[16] GOIRC;[17] GISCAD;[18] Genova;[19] Toronto;[20] City of Hope;[21] RPCI;[22] Bologna;[23] NCCTG/Mayo Clinic.[24] All trials randomised groups into 5-FU in mono-

chemotherapy compared to 5-FU plus leukovorin. In two studies (NCOG, NCCTG) the authors also compared these groups with methotrexate (MTX) ± leukovorin rescue. In one trial (NCCTG), one arm of randomization incorporated the use of cisplation. Other differences among the trials concerned included: the dose of leukovorin (in the studies of GITSG and NCCTG it was used both in low and high doses) and (ii) the schedule, which in some trials consisted of weekly administration, in others monthly (five times daily) dosing.

The characteristics of each study according to these points are listed in Table 10.3. From these trials it is possible to observe that haematological toxicities were mild or moderate either when 5-FU was

Table 10.3   Randomized trials of leukovorin + 5-FU versus 5-FU

Group	Patients (n)	Schedule	% CR + PR	Survival
Nobile (1988)[19]	82	5-FU 600 mg/m² + leukovorin 500 mg/m² week vs. 5-FU 600 mg/m² weekly	16% vs. 5% (p = 0.05)	No significant difference
Petrelli (1987)[15]	318	5-FU 600 mg/m² + leukovorin 500 or 25 mg/m² 6 out 8 weeks vs. 5-FU 500 mg/m² × 5 every 4 weeks	30.3% vs. 18.8% vs. 12.1% (p < 0.01)	55–45 and 46 weeks (p = 0.08)
Petrelli (1989)[22]	44	5-FU 600 mg/m² + leukovorin 500 mg/m² 6 out 8 weeks vs. 5-FU 450 mg/m² × 5	48% vs. 11% (p = 0.0009)	No significant difference (p = 0.6)
Valone (1989)[16]	153*	5-FU 400 mg/m² × 5 + leukovorin 200 mg/m² × 5 every 4 weeks vs. 5-FU 480 mg/m² followed by 600 mg/m²/week	18.8% vs. 17.3% (p = 0.4)	24 vs. 20 weeks (p = 0.4)
Di Costanzo (1989)[17]	181	5-FU 400 mg/m² × 5 + leukovorin 200 mg/m² × 5 every 4 weeks vs. 5-FU 540 mg/m² × 5	15% vs. 16%	25 vs. 21 weeks
Labianca (1991)[18]	182	5-FU 400 mg/m² × 5 + leukovorin 200 mg/m² × 5 every 4 weeks vs. 5-FU 400 mg/m² × 5 every 4 weeks	20.6% vs. 10% (p = 0.046)	46 vs. 44 weeks
Poon (1989)[24]	208	5-FU 370 mg/m² × 5 + leukovorin 20 or 200 mg/m² × 5 vs. 5-FU 500 mg/m² × 5	43% vs. 26% (p = 0.001)	53 vs. 52 vs. 34 weeks (p = 0.05)
Doroshow (1990)[21]	74	5-FU 370 mg/m² × 5 + leukovorin 500 mg/m² × 5 every 4 weeks vs. 5-FU 370 mg/m² × 5	44% vs. 13% (p = 0.0019)	62 vs. 55 weeks (p = 0.25)
Erlichman (1988)[20]	124	5-FU 370 mg/m² × 5 + leukovorin 200 mg/m² × 5 vs. 5-FU 370 mg/m² × 5	33% vs. 7% (P < 0.0005)	54 vs. 41 weeks (P = 0.05)
Cricca (1988)[23]	64	5-FU 600 mg/m² + leukovorin 200 mg/m² weekly vs. 5-FU 600 mg/m² weekly	26.4% vs. 3.3%	No significant difference

* Randomization 2 : 1.

Table 10.4 Randomized clinical trials comparing low-dose with high dose leukovorin as modulator of 5-FU in advanced colorectal cancer

Group (patients), n	Low-dose leukovorin + 5-FU		High-dose leukovorin + 5-FU		Response rate	
					Low	High
GTTSG[22] (230)	Leukovorin 25 mg/m² (10 min infusion) 5-FU 600 mg/m² i.v.	weekly (6/8)	Leukovorin 500 mg/m² (2 h infusion) 5-FU 600 mg/m² i.v.	weekly (6/8)	18.8%	30.3% (P = 0.046)
PALL I Study Group[27] (298 evaluable)	Leukovorin 20 mg/m² (2 h infusion) 5-FU 500 mg/m² i.v.	weekly	Leukovorin 500 mg/m² (2 h infusion) 5-FU 500 mg/m² i.v.	weekly		
NCCTG[24] (142:73 measurable)	Leukovorin 20 mg/m² i.v. 5-FU 370–425 mg/m² i.v.	× 5 days every 4–5 weeks	Leukovorin 200 mg/m² i.v. 5-FU 370 mg/m² i.v 4–5 weeks	× 5 days every	43%	26% (P = 0.001)
GISCAD[29] (422)	L-Leukovorin 10 mg/m² i.v. 5-FU 370 mg/m² (15 min infusion)	× 5 days every 4 weeks	L-Leukovorin 100 mg/m² i.v. 5-FU 370 mg/m² (15 min infusion)	× 5 days every 4 weeks	10.7%	9.3% (P = 0.78)
NCCTG[28] (372: 201 measurable)	Leukovorin 20 mg/m² i.v. 5-FU 425 mg/m² i.v.	× 5 days every 4–5 weeks	Leukovorin 500 mg/m² (2 h infusion 5-FU 600 mg/m² i.v.	weekly (6/8)	95%	31% (P = 0.51)
FFCD/GERCOD/SFNMI[30] (437)	Leukovorin 20 mg/m² i.v. 5-FU 425 mg/m² i.v.	× 5 days every 4 weeks	Leukovorin 200 mg/m² (2 h infusion) 5-FU 400 mg/m² i.v. + 600 mg/m² (22 h infusion)	days 1–2 every 2 weeks	17%	34% (P = 0.51)
SWOG[9] (240)	Leukovorin 20 mg/m² i.v. 5-FU 425 mg/m² i.v. Leukovorin 20 mg/m² i.v. every week 5-FU 200 mg/m² continuous infusion days 1 to 28, every 5 weeks	× 3 days every 4–5 weeks	Leukovorin 500 mg/m² (2 h infusion) 5-FU 600 mg/m² i.v.	weekly (6/8)	27%	21%

administered alone or with leukovorin. However, episodes of grade 3–4 toxicity were observed in a certain number of patients. The dose-limiting toxicity was oral mucositis and gastrointestinal side-effects where diarrhoea was predominant. In 1992 a meta-analysis[25] of these trials was conducted to evaluate the tumour response and overall survival. It confirmed the advantage of 5-FU plus leukovorin over 5-FU alone in terms of objective tumour response; the overall response rate of 5-FU plus leukovorin was more than twice that of 5-FU alone (23% vs. 11%; $P < 0.001$).

The benefit of 5-FU plus leukovorin was observed both in trials using the weekly and in those using the monthly administration schedule. Because of the limited number of patients, in these trials, it is not possible to evaluate the influence of leukovorin dose on outcome. A proper comparison of low-dose leukovorin versus high-dose leukovorin was further performed in a randomized trial conducted by NCCTG/Mayo Clinic and published in 1994.[26] This trial showed that low-dose leukovorin has a better therapeutic index than the high-dose regimen. Other trials[27-30] summarized in Table 10.4 confirm these results; in particular it seems that the weekly schedule requires high doses, whereas in the five times daily regimen low doses appear to be at least equally effective in terms of response rate, symptomatic relief and overall survival.

In summary, these studies demonstrate that the combination of 5-FU + leukovorin may give higher tumour response rate than 5-FU alone in patients with advanced colorectal cancer, but that the possible benefit of this combination in overall survival was still doubtful. There is no consensus from these trials about the best dose or schedule of administration for 5-FU and leukovorin.

Despite this rather modest advantage over 5-FU alone, the general opinion among medical oncologists is that leukovorin +5-FU represents a step forward in the treatment of advanced colorectal cancer.

Methotrexate (MTX)

Methotrexate exerts its cytotoxic effects through inhibition of the enzyme dihydrofolate reductase resulting in an imbalance of all the reactions that need folinic coenzymes. Transfer reactions of monocarboniose unity, essential for the *ex novo* synthesis of purine nucleotides and thymidylate, are arrested with subsequent block of DNA and RNA synthesis. Additionally an accumulation of oxidized folates occurs which are able to directly inhibit different enzymes of synthesis of purine and pyrimidine bases. Except in the maintenance regimens, the drug is usually administered intravenously. At the used dose elimination occurs, in a three-dimensional curve with a terminal half-life of

8–10 hours. MTX is excreted via the kidneys without significant metabolism in the liver.

Many studies have examined the modulation of MXT with 5-FU, including dosages, intervals and schedules treatment. The sequence and interval of administration of these two antimetabolites seem to be important in achieving optimal therapeutic efficacy. Marsh and colleagues[31] in their randomized study have confirmed the importance of a 24-hour interval between administration of MTX and 5-FU: 168 untreated patients with advanced measurable colorectal cancer received MTX 200 mg/m^2 followed by 5-FU 600 mg/m^2 either 24 hours or 1 hour after MTX. Leukovorin at the dose of 10 mg/m^2 was administered orally every 6 hours for six doses beginning 24 hours after MTX administration. Compared with the 1-hour interval, the 24-hour scheduling interval resulted in a significantly better objective response rate (29% vs. 14,5%), median time to progression (9.9 vs. 5.9 months) and median survival (15.3 vs. 11.4 months).

The combination of MTX and 5-FU, generally with LV rescue, has been evaluated in phase II studies showing good activity with response rates of approximately 35%. Since 1983 several randomized trials comparing 5-FU alone with 5-FU and MTX have been performed. The principal characteristics are summarized in Table 10.5.[16,24,32–34]

A meta-analysis[35] was performed in 1994 to assess the benefit of 5-FU and MTX on tumour response rate and overall survival. The meta-analysis, based on individual data of 1178 patients included in eight randomized clinical trials, concluded that the modulation of 5-FU by MTX doubles the response rate obtained with 5-FU and achieves a small improvement in survival.

This modulation can be utilized in the treatment of advanced colorectal cancer as an alternative to 5-FU and leukovorin, or as second-line therapy in controlled clinical trials.

Interferon (IFN)

The IFNs are a group of proteins with antiviral, antiproliferative, immunomodulating and differentiating properties. Synergistic action between 5-FU and gamma-IFN or alpha-IFN has been shown against different cancer cell lines. This action depends on the administration route, and seems higher when 5-FU is administered after IFN. Pretreatment with alpha-IFN, in fact, results in a reduction in the activity of thymidylate synthase, and increases the levels of fluorodeoxyuridylate.

Clinical trials have investigated the efficacy of 5-FU and IFN in the treatment of advanced colorectal cancer. The first clinical study was reported in 1989 by Wadler[36] as a phase II trial. Seventeen previously untreated patients received a loading course of 5-FU (750 mg/sm^2 by continuous i.v. infusion daily for 5 days) followed by a 1-week interval, then weekly bolus therapy at 750 mg/sm^2. Alpha-2a-IFN was administered subcutaneously at the dose of 9×10^6 IU three times weekly, starting on day 1. This clinical trial demonstrated a response rate of 76%.

These results were confirmed in a subsequent update by the same authors but an important toxicity was observed with two toxic deaths and a high percentage of mucositis, diarrhoea, fever and neurotoxicity. Although the side-effects were severe, these results were considered very interesting and several confirmatory trials were started to evaluate the efficacy of the association of 5-FU with IFN.

Table 10.5 Randomized trials comparing 5-FU alone with 5-FU/MTX in patients with advanced colorectal cancer

Group	5-FU alone	Patients (n)	5-FU/MTX	Patients (n)	CR + PR (%)
NGTATG[34]	5-FU 600 mg/m^2 days 1 and 2 every 14 days × 8, then every 21–28 days	127	MTX 250 mg/m^2 over 2 h; 5-FU 500 mg/m^2 at 3 h and 23 h; Leukovorin at 24 h; every 14 days × 8, then every 21–28 days	122	2 vs. 17 (P = 0.001)
NCCTG Mayo Clinic[24]	5-FU 500 mg/m^2 days 1–5, every 35 days	70	MTX 40 mg/m^2; 5-FU 700 mg/m^2 at 24 h, days 1 and 8 every 28 days	71	10 vs. 26 vs. 12 (P = 0.04)
			MTX 200 mg/m^2 over 4 h; 5-FU 900 mg/m^2 at 7 h; leukovorin at 24 h, every 21 days × 2, then every 28 days	71	
AIO[32]	5-FU 450 mg/m^2 days 1–5, every 21 days	82	MTX 300 mg/m^2 over 4 h; 5-FU 900 mg/m^2 at 7 h; leukovorin at 24 h, every 14 days × 3, then every 21 days	82 88	15 vs. 28 (P = 0.08)
NCOG[16]	5-FU 12 mg/kg/day days 1–5, then 15 mg/kg/day day 1, every 7 days	55	MTX 50 mg/m^2 orally every 6 h × 5; 5-FU 500 mg/m^2 at 24 h; leukovorin at 30 h, every 14 days	55	17.3 vs. 19.8 (n.s.)
GOCS[33]	5-FU 1200 mg/m^2 over 2 h, every 14 days		MTX 200 mg/m^2; 1200 mg/m^2 over 2 h at 20 h; leukovorin at 24 h, every 14 days	61 64	18 vs. 28 (P <0,.05)
RPCI[22]	5-FU 450 mg/m^2 days 1–5 + 5-FU 200 mg/m^2 every other day × 6 doses, every 46 days	23	MTX 50 mg/m^2 over 4 h, then 5-FU 600 mg/m^2, every 7 days × 4, then every 14 days	23	11 vs. 5 (n.s.)

CR = complete response; PR = partial response.

Table 10.6 Main studies with 5-FU + IFN (Wadler-like regimen)

Author	Patients (n) (evaluable)	Pretreated	Complete response	Partial response	Percentage complete + partial responses
Fornasiero[37]	21 (21)	no	4	5	43%
Kemeny[38]	38 (34)	no	–	9	26%
Pazdur[39]	52 (46)	no	1	15	35%
Wadler[40]	27 (27)	yes (9)	1	5	22%
Wadler[41]	32 (32)	no	1	20	63%
ECOG[42]	36 (36)	no	1	14	42%
Ajani[43]	46 (45)	no	–	6	13%
Huberman[44]	42 (33)	no	–	13	39%
Donillard[45]	22 (16)	no	1	4	31%
John[46]	18 (15)	no	1	5	40%
Dufour[47]	21 (21)	no	1	4	24%
Totals	355 (326)		10	101	34

Later clinical trials using this schedule, reported in Table 10.6,[37-47] have not duplicated this initially high response rate and have documented greater toxicity. The final reports of two large phase III trials, conduced by York[48] and Hill,[49] did not show any advantage for 5-FU + IFN versus 5-FU alone.

In other phase II and III trials, the double modulation of 5-FU with IFN and leukovorin was studied.[50-68] Using 5-FU at the dose of 370–425 mg/m^2 (from days 2 to 6) and IFN at the dose of 5×10^6 IU from days 1 to 7, recycled every 28 days Grem[50] obtained a 44.4% response rate in 18 patients with advanced colorectal cancer.

Later, in a phase II trial Grem studied 44 patients with advanced colorectal cancer in order to appraise this combination. The overall response rate was 54%, median survival was 16.3 months and median disease-free survival was 9.3 months. The grade 3 and 4 toxicity included diarrhoea, rash, asthenia, mucositis and neutropenia.

In 1995 the Corfu[68] study was conducted comparing 5-FU plus alpha-IFN with 5-FU plus leukovorin in 496 patients. The observed response rates were 21 and 19% respectively. In the 5-FU plus alpha-IFN arm, significantly more haematological toxicity was observed. In conclusion, the benefits of therapy with IFN + 5-FU ± leukovorin are not clearly defined and for now one should not encourage these combinations in current clinic practice outside the context of controlled clinical trials.

Uracil/Ftorafur (UFT)

UFT, commercially available in Japan and several other countries, is composed of 1-(2-tetrahydro-furyl)-5-fluorouracil (Ftorafur, FT or Tegafur) and uracil in a molar ratio 1:4. FT is converted to 5-FU *in vivo*. It was found that the co-administration of uracil enhanced the concentration of 5-FU in tumours and the resulting antitumor activity of FT. In *in vitro* studies, uracil strongly inhibited the degradation of 5-FU to 2-fluoro-β-aniline (F-β-analine). From *in vivo* studies conducted in Japan, UFT and FT gave a comparable distribution of 5-FU in blood and other normal tissues, but UFT resulted in a 5–10 times greater distribution of 5-FU in tumours.

In 3–9-month toxicity studies, UFT was not found to possess greater toxicity than 5-FU. UFT was more effective than FT in Lewis lung carcinoma, B-16 melanoma and human mammary, gastric and pancreatic carcinoma transplanted in nude mice.[69-72]

Effect of Uracil on 5FU metabolism

Using rat liver homogenates, metabolites of FT using ^{3}H-labelled FT were measured. Although FT is activated to 5-FU by liver enzymes and further degraded to F-β-alanine, the addition of uracil inhibited the formation of fluorouridine propionic acid (FUPA) and F-β alanine in a dose-dependent manner suggesting that uracil inhibits the degradation of 5-FU.

Pharmacology

Following oral administration of UFT, uracil and ftorafur are rapidly and completely absorbed from the gut into the systemic circulation.[73] FT is subsequently metabolized to 5-FU by one of two different pathways and enzyme systems, thereby behaving as a prodrug to 5-FU.[74-76] FT either undergoes hepatic microsomal oxidation at the C5′ position to release 5-FU and succinaldehyde, or cytosolic cleavage of the C2′–N1′ bond forming 5-FU and 4-hydroxybutanal. The succinaldehyde and 4-hydroxybutanal moieties are subsequently converted to succinic acid or butyrolactone and hydroxybutyric acid, respectively. Cytosolic conversion of FT to 5-FU may occur in any tissue and thus may be an important source of intratumoral 5-FU. Other stable metabolic products of FT include 3′OH-ftorafur and 4′OH-ftorafur, both of which are eliminated in the urine and are not converted to 5-FU.

Animal Tumor Data

UFT, FT and 5-FU were administered orally for seven consecutive days in subcutaneously transplanted Walker carcinoma 256, Yoshida sarcoma, AH 130, AH 44 and AH 13. The antitumour effects of the drugs were evaluated by the percentage inhibition of tumour weight. UFT exerted approximately the same degree of tumour inhibitory effect as 5-FU and was about fivefold as potent as that of FT. Tumour inhibitory effects of the drugs on subcutaneously transplanted tumours in mice were studied with Sarcoma 180 and Ehrlich ascites carcinoma. UFT exerted approximately the same degree of tumour inhibitory effect as 5-FU. The effect was about fivefold as potent as that of FT. The effects of the drugs on human mammary, pancreatic and gastric tumour xenografts transplanted in nude mice were studied by determining their tumour inhibitory effects: UFT at one-fifth the dose of FT had a marked inhibitory effect on all of the tumour xenograft. The action of the drugs on syngeneic tumours was studied in YM-12, Lewis lung carcinoma and B-16 melanoma, which proliferate relatively slowly, and mouse leukaemia, which proliferates rapidly.

In the case of YM-12, Lewis lung carcinoma and B-16 melanoma, the drugs were administered orally once daily for 21 consecutive days beginning the day on which the transplanted tumour had grown to about 5 mm in diameter. Compared to 5-FU, UFT exhibited considerable antitumour activity as evidenced by an increased life span in the L1210 and P388 leukaemia models. The antitumour effect of UFT against L1210 was greater than that of FT and 5-FU. The effects of the drugs in the P388 model were unremarkable.

Results of Phase I/II Studies of UFT

'High-Dose' Leukovorin

Phase I studies were conducted at MD Anderson Cancer Center and Roswell Park Cancer Institute utilizing the same treatment regimen of escalating doses of UFT with a fixed dose of 150 mg Leukovorin per day for 28 days followed by a 7-day rest period. At 450 mg m²/day, dose-limiting toxicities of UFT were diarrhoea, abdominal pain and reversible small bowel damage (partial obstruction). These toxicities required hospitalization in 3 of 6 patients entered at this dose level. At 450 mg m²/day, other toxicities included the following: grade II granulocytopenia, grade II nausea, grade III stomatitis (1 patient) and grade I fatigue. The recommended phase II dose of single-agent UFT in combination with leukovorin was 350 mg/mq daily when given for 28 days (three divided doses per day).

In the phase II portion of the trial the UFT starting dose at MD Anderson Cancer Center was 350 mg/m²/day in the first 7 patients while the subsequent 38 patients were treated at 300 mg/m²/d.[77] The dose of leukovorin was 50 mg t.i.d. Grade III toxicities at the 350 mg/m²/day dose of UFT were diarrhoea, anorexia, fatigue, nausea and vomiting. Essentially the same grade III toxicities were seen at 300 mg/m²/day dose of UFT but in a smaller percentage of patients. In this study, 18 of 45 evaluable patients attained a partial response while 1 had a complete response. At Roswell Park Cancer Institute, the UFT was administered at 350 mg/m²/day with high-dose leukovorin. Grade III toxicities included diarrhoea and fatigue, which were considered to be definitely related to protocol therapy. Hyperbilirubinaemia was considered possibly related to protocol therapy; 2 of 8 evaluable patients at Roswell Park Cancer Institute attained a partial response.

'Low Dose' Leukovorin

Phase I trials were conducted at Memorial Sloan-Kettering Cancer Center and the University of Southern California using low-dose leukovorin (15 mg/day) and varying doses of UFT administered for 28 days followed by 7 days of rest. Twenty-one patients were enrolled at the Memorial Sloan-Kettering Cancer Center. At the 200 mg/m²/day and 300 mg/m²/day UFT dose levels, there were no grade III or IV events related to protocol therapy. At the 250 mg/m²/day dose of UFT, grade III headache was reported. At the 350 mg/m²/day dose of UFT, grade III diarrhoea was observed. These events were all strongly related to therapy.

Fifteen patients were enrolled in the phase I trial at the University of Southern California. At the 250 mg/m²/day dose level, one patient reported grade III diarrhoea. At this institution, the following grade III toxicities were observed at the UFT dose of 300 mg/m²/day: asthenia, diarrhoea, convulsions and apnoea. Grade IV events at the same dose level included sepsis, stomatitis, leukopenia, hypotension and neutropenia. The following grade III toxicities were reported at 350 mg/m²/day of UFT: anaemia, asthenia, diarrhoea, nausea and paraesthesia. Grade IV anaemia was also observed at this dose level. All of the above events were possibly, probably or definitely related to study medications.

Twenty-one patients were treated, with 20 evaluable, in a phase II study conducted at the Memorial Sloan-Kettering and Kenneth Norris Jr. Cancer Centers. UFT at 350 mg/m²/day for 28 days followed by 7 days of rest was given with 15 mg of leukovorin. One complete and 4 partial responses were seen (overall response rate: 25%). Grade III/IV diarrhoea was seen in 4 patients. Hand–foot syndrome was not seen and there were only 2 episodes of mucositis.[78]

Conclusion

Data are emerging which suggest that infusional 5-FU is more efficacious than bolus administration. UFT also allows prolonged exposure to the drug without the need for a central catheter or infusion pump. Leukovorin is given with the UFT to further increase its efficacy. Although the optimal timing of leukovorin dosing remains controversial, the 8-hour dosing scheme used allows prolonged exposure to leukovorin and has been well tolerated. The effectiveness and favourable toxicity profile of this approach in metastatic colorectal cancer has been well demonstrated in phase II studies. Confirmation is now required in randomized phase III trials designed to compare the combination of UFT and oral leukovorin with an established regimen of 5-FU + LV given as short intravenous injections over five consecutive days.

Doxifluridine (dFUR)

Doxifluridine (5′-deoxy-5-fluorouridine, dFUR) is a synthetic 5-deoxynucleoside derivative that has been shown to have a therapeutic index that is 10–15 times greater than that of 5-FU or other fluoropyrimidines when tested against several experimental rodent tumours.[79] Consisting of an 5-FU molecule linked to a pseudo-pentose, the drug cannot be phosphorylated and therefore cannot be taken up into nucleic acid without its metabolic conversion to FU.

The biotransformation to 5-FU occurs enzymatically be means of the action of pyrimidine phosphorylases, which, in animal models, have been shown to be present in higher concentrations in tumoral tissues and therefore lead to higher 5-FU concentrations within tumoral cells. Experimental data related to the cytotoxicity of dFUR on human bone-marrow stem cells and human tumour cell lines conform its cytotoxic selectivity for human tumoral cells. Although this selectivity of action has been shown to lead to a lower incidence of side-effects in clinical trials, the data provided by a randomized phase III study that compared dFUR and 5-FU support the better therapeutic index of dFUR.[80]

Experimental data in tumour-bearing rats treated with dFUR and 5-FU show a significant difference in therapeutic activity after the oral administration of these two agents.[81] Unlike 5-FU, dFUR has been shown to be an effective agent when administered orally, with 50–80% of the dose reaching the systemic circulation in unchanged form. Previous studies using the intermittent oral administration of dFUR indicate that doses of between 1000 and 1400 mg/m² have antitumoral activity and an acceptable rate of side-effects.[82,83]

It has recently been shown that the combination of leukovorin and fluoropyrimidine has greater clinical activity in advanced colorectal cancer. Pharmacokinetic data indicate optimal gastrointestinal absorption with the oral administration of low-dose leukovorin, the systemic levels of which are sufficient to enhance the cytotoxicity of 5-FU.

A study[84] was designed to test the activity and feasibility of an all-oral regimen of laevo-leukovorin and dFUR in the treatment of advanced colorectal cancer and to establish whether the pharmacokinetics of dFUR and 5-FU are affected by a demographic and/or biological parameters. One hundred and eight patients with histologically proven colorectal cancer received orally administered levo-leukovorin 25 mg followed 2 hours later by dFUR 1200 mg/m² on days 1–5, with the cycle being repeated every 10 days.

Among 62 previously untreated patients, two complete responses (CR) and 18 partial responses

(PR) were observed (overall response rate, 32%; 95% confidence interval, 21–45%). The median response duration was 4 months (range 2–13 months) and the median survival time 14 months. Among 46 pretreated patients, there were three CR and three PR (response rate, 13%; 95% confidence interval, 5–26%). In this group of patients, the median response duration was 4 months (range 1–12 months) and the median survival time, 12 months. No toxic deaths were observed. The only grade 3–4 side-effect was diarrhoea (32 patients).

Raltitrexed or Tomudex®

Tomudex® (ZD1694) is a new antifolate agent which acts as a pure and specific inhibitor of thymidylate synthase. This enzyme is considered an important target for the development of new anticancer drugs: the folate binding site in thymidylate synthase is believed to offer better opportunities for the design of highly specific inhibitors than the pyrimidine (dUMP) binding site. This belief led to the design of a quinazoline-based drug ICI155387 (CB3717), which has antitumour activity against a variety of solid tumours.[85] Occasional but life-threatening nephrotoxicity prevented the development of this compound. More water-soluble and non-nephrotoxic analogues became available;[86,87] these agents also presented an interesting diversity in biochemical profile, particularly with respect to interactions with folate transport proteins, the reduced folate cell membrane carrier (REC), and the folate-metabolizing enzyme, folypolyglutamate synthase (EPGS). The first new drug to emerge from this program was Tomudex.

Mechanism of Action

Tomudex is 500-fold more cytotoxic than CB3717 against a variety of cell lines, although as an inhibitor of isolated thymidylate synthase it is not among the most potent that have been reported.[88] Cytotoxic potency has been shown in two proteins, the cell membrane transporter and FPGS.[89] Experiments *in vitro* suggest that Tomudex is taken up into L1210 cells by the RFC.

Acquired resistance to Tomudex and reduced ability to take up the drug have been developed in the human ovarian line 41M:R which is cross-resistant to compounds that utilize the RFC, such as MTX.[90] These data support the fact that Tomudex activity is highly dependent on cellular uptake via the RFC.

Polyglutamation plays a further important role in the potency activity of Tomudex. Once the drug has entered cells, it is highly polyglutamated by FPGS; the specifity of Tomudex for the inhibition of thymidylate synthase within the cells was assessed by examining its activity against drug-resistant cell lines and by measuring directly intracellular enzyme inhibition. The polyglutamated forms (tri-tetra- and pentaglumtamates) of Tomudex are retained within the cells for long periods of time and are to 100 times more potent than the parent compound. A further evidence for the importance of polyglutamation carriers comes again from the L1210 cell line with acquired resistance to Tomudex. This line is able to take up Tomudex, but not to metabolize it to polyglutamate analogues to any significant extent.

The antitumour activity of Tomudex was prevented by co-administration of thymidine, indicating that thymidylate synthase is the sole locus of action *in vivo*. Thymidine also prevented leukopenia and weight-loss suggesting that these toxicities are related to the enzyme inhibitory properties of the drug.[91]

It can be concluded that Tomudex is a potent antitumour agent whose mechanism of action is inhibition of thymidylate synthase. This potency is related to rapid cellular uptake and intracellular metabolism to polyglutamate analogues that are both retained by the cells and are substantially more potent as inhibitors of thymidylate synthase.

Clinical Trials

Tomudex entered clinical development in 1991. Clinical phase I, II and III studies were conducted in Europe, the United States, South Africa and Australia.

Phase I Studies

Two Phase I studies were initiated, one in Europe and the other in the United States. The European study was conducted from February 1991 to January 1993, at the Institute for Cancer Research in the UK and the Rotterdam Institute in The Netherlands; this study reported a maximum tolerated dose (MTD) of 3.5 mg/m² i.v. every 3 weeks, with dose limiting toxicity at the gastrointestinal (diarrhoea) and haematological (leukopenia, neutropenia and thrombocytopenia) level as well as asthenia and/or malaise. Other side-effects included asymptomatic reversible rises in liver transaminases and skin rash. Objective responses were seen in patients who had failed to respond to previously cytotoxic regimens.[92] Accordingly, phase II studies were initiated using a dose of 3.0 mg/m^2.

A second phase I study was conducted in the United States at the National Cancer Institute, from August 1991 to December 1993. This study included mainly patients with advanced colorectal cancer, most of whom had received 5-FU and leukovorin regimens beforehand. Dose limiting toxicity was similar to that found in the European study, but the MTD was 4.5 mg/m^2.[93] A dose of 4.0 mg/m^2 was investigated in later trials, but was subsequently discontinued due to greater toxicity.

Phase II Studies

A large phase II clinical programme started in October 1992 in Europe, Australia and the United States. Tomudex was tested at the dose of 3.0 mg/m^2 in several solid tumours, including colorectal, breast, ovarian, pancreatic and non-small lung cancer, producing reproducible objective responses.

In the phase II trial conducted by Zalcberg and colleagues[94] from October 1992 to September 1993, a good response was seen with Tomudex at a dose of 3.0 mg/m^2 every 3 weeks in 176 patients affected with advanced or metastatic colorectal cancer. Over 80% of patients had liver involvement at entry, but many also had extrahepatic metastases. Only 5% of the patients had previously been treated with a 5-FU-based regimen. The total objective response rate was 25.5%, with a further 49% of patients showing stable disease. The time to progression was 4.2 months; the median survival was estimated to be 9.6 months. Toxicity appeared acceptable.

Tomudex therefore appears to have substantial activity in colorectal cancer.

Phase III Studies

Encouraging results reported from phase II studies led to the planning of a large international programme in order to compare Tomudex with 5-FU + leukovorin regimen in terms of survival, time to disease progression, quality of life, tolerance and response rate.

The first study was that described by investigators at the Mayo Clinic consisting of 5-FU 425 mg/m^2 plus leukovorin 20 mg/m^2 by i.v. infusion daily for 5 days cycled 4–5 weekly. In the first trial[95] conducted in Europe, South Africa and Australia, 439 patients

Table 10.7 Tomudex vs. 5-FU + leukovorin: the first Phase III trial

Response	Tomudex (222 patients)	5-FU + leukovorin (212 patients)
Complete response	2.3%	1.9%
Partial response	17.6%	10.8%
Overall response	19.9%	12.7%
Stable disease	35%	32.4%
Median survival	4.8 months	3.6 months
Survival	10.3 months	10.3 months

Table 10.8 Tomudex vs. 5-FU + leukovorin: comparison of toxicity for grades 3 and 4

Event	Tomudex[*]	5-FU + leukovorin[**]
Leukopenia	10%	26%
Anaemia	5%	1%
Thrombocytopenia	3%	1%
ALT and/or AST increased	10%	0%
Mucositis	2%	22%
Diarrhoea	13%	12%
Nausea and vomiting	12%	9%
Fever	3%	2%
Infection	5%	5%
Constipation	3%	3%
Pain	4%	7%
Asthenia	5%	2%
Drug-related deaths	3.2%	2.4%

[*] 222 patients
[**] 212 patients

were randomized to receive either Tomudex at a dose of 3.0 mg/m^2 as a single agent i.v. every 3 weeks or 5-FU + leukovorin by rapid i.v. injection. The data from this study for each treatment arm are reported in Table 10.7.

Tomudex treatment was associated with a statistically significantly lower incidence of side effects such as grade 3 or 4 leukopenia and severe mucositis. Increase in transaminases (grade 3 or 4) was reported in 10% of patients receiving Tomudex and 0% in patients receiving 5-FU + leukovorin. This difference is statistically significant. However these elevations were usually reversible, asymptomatic and were of limited clinical significance. The grade 3 or 4 adverse events are reported in Table 10.8. In both groups, the few drug-related deaths appeared to be related to combinations of gastrointestinal toxicity (diarrhoea in patients who received Tomudex and mucositis in patients who received 5-FU + leukovorin) and myelosuppression.

A further trial is being conducted in North America. A preliminary communication suggests it that objective response rates were similar to either Tomudex or 5-FU + leukovorin. Median survival in patients randomized to Tomudex was 8.8 months compared to a median of 11.1 months in patients receiving 5-FU + leukovorin. This difference may be related to the shorter time on treatment with Tomudex. The tolerability profiles of Tomudex and 5-FU + leukovorin were similar to those seen in the international study. Final results have been not yet published. A third trial, comparing Tomudex to 5-FU + leukovorin (Machover regimen) has been recently concluded in Europe and results are pending.

Irinotecan Hydrochloride Trihydrate (CPT-11)

Mechanism of Action

Irinotecan hydrochloride trihydrate (irinotecan, CPT-11), a water-soluble analogue of comptothecin (CPT), is an antitumour drug extracted from the Chinese tree Camptotheca acuminata.[96] 7-Ethyl-10-hydroxycamptothecin (SN-38) is the active metabolite of CPT-11.[97] CPT-11 and SN-38 are selective inhibitors of the DNA enzyme topoisomerase I. This enzyme is ubiquitous and plays a pivotal role in DNA transcription, replication and repair: its inhibition leads ultimately to cell death.[98]

Preclinical Studies

The preclinical studies of CPT-11 and its active metabolite have demonstrated consistent activity in a variety of cancer cell lines in vitro and of tumour models in vivo (including cell lines of colorectal, ovarian, non small-cell lung, breast cancer, soft tissue sarcoma and mesothelioma,[99] including those that express multidrug resistance (in particular those resistant to doxorubicin, vincristine and vinblastine). CPT-11 has also shown synergistic or additive activity in combination with 5-FU and cisplatin in vitro.[100] With CPT-11, In animal studies, no irreversible or unusual toxicity was observed.

Clinical Studies

Phase I Studies

Phase I studies of CPT-11 were conducted in Europe, Japan and the United States to determine the MTD and the most appropriate intravenous administration schedule for further investigation in phase II studies.[101] Diarrhoea and/or neutropenia were the major dose-limiting toxicities in all phase I studies.

Two very distinct types of diarrhoea were identified. The first occurs during or within 30 minutes of CPT-11 infusion. This is part of a cholinergic syndrome and is very easy to control with anticholinergic therapy. The second one may appear 6–10 days after drug administration. The mechanism appears to be linked to abnormal intestinal ion transport.[102]

Neutrophil nadir appears to occur earlier (median time to nadir: 5 days), and the incidence of grade 4 neutropenia is approximately 6%. The duration of neutropenia is short (<5 days) and usually asymptomatic.[101] Other toxicities include nausea and vomiting, asthenia, early cholinergic-like syndrome (consisting of diaphoresis, early diarrhoea and abdominal cramps) and alopecia.

In Japanese and American studies, the CPT-11 MTD was defined as 240–250 mg/m^2 using a once every 3 weeks schedule and 100–150 mg/m^2 using a weekly schedule. In European studies the MTD was 90–100 mg/m^2 day i.v. infusion over three consecutive days every 3 weeks and 100–115 mg/m^2 with a weekly infusion over 3 weeks at 4 weekly internals. The European experience with a single infusion every 3 weeks showed diarrhoea to be dose limiting at 350 mg/m^2, but concomitant administration of high-dose loperamide allowed administration of CPT-11 at doses of up to 600 mg/m^2.[101,102] This schedule was selected because it appeared to be associated with the least toxicity (in terms of haematological and gastrointestinal adverse events at a higher dose intensity in phase I investigations (compared with those of the once weekly and 3 consecutive days schedules). It was also considered to be the most convenient for outpatient use, requiring less frequent administration.

European phase II studies were therefore commenced using a CPT-11 schedule consisting of a single intravenous infusion every 3 weeks at a dose of 350 mg/m^2.[101]

Phase II Studies

The results of preclinical studies has been confirmed in clinical trials conducted in Japan, Europe and the United States. The response rates reported with CPT-11 in patients with non-small cell range from 32–34%, and are better in combination with cisplatin (43–54%). CPT-11 is also active in small cell lung cancer, with a single agent response rate of 47% in patients previously treated with cisplatin.

Clinical experience with CPT-11 in the treatment of other solid tumours has demonstrated variable activity. This has been seen in phase II trials in patients with squamous cell carcinoma of the uterine cervix or skin, and in those with cancer of the ovary, breast, stomach, pancreas including patients with lymphoma.

Treatment of Colorectal Cancer

The efficacy of CPT-11 given as a monotherapy has been evaluated both as first- and second-line treatment of advanced colorectal cancer in over 300 patients. Five phase II studies have been conducted to date in Europe, the Unites States and Japan using different dosing schedules.[103–107] In the US and Japanese studies, response rates with CPT-11 are 15–32% in patients with newly diagnosed disease and 22–25% in patients with 5-FU refractory disease.[103–105] One of these studies also reported a median duration of response of approximately 7 months and a median survival of approximately 9.4 months for pretreated patients.

The largest phase II study of CPT-11 has been conducted in Europe. In this trial, response rates to CPT-11 given at the dose of 350 mg/m^2 every 3 weeks were similar in chemotherapy-naive (18.8%; $n = 48$) and pretreated (17.7%; $n = 130$) patients.[108] In a subgroup of refractory patients to a previous 5-FU-based chemotherapy, the similar response rate of 16.1% suggests a lack of cross-resistance between the two drugs. In both pretreated and chemotherapy-naive patients, the median duration of response was 9.1 months and the median survival was 10.6 months; 34% of all patients and 32% of pretreated patients had no evidence of disease progression at 6 months (Table 10.9). The above study confirmed the major adverse effects of CPT-11 to be neutropenia and delayed diarrhoea.

The incidence of these effects was not cumulative, and the incidence of delayed severe diarrhoea could be reduced with early high-dose loperamide. Other adverse effects of CPT-11 include the early cholinergic-like syndrome (manageable with atropine), nausea and vomiting, fatigue and alopecia needed (Table 10.10).[108]

The efficacy of CPT-11 in combination with 5-FU has still to be fully assessed (three studies are ongoing with 5-FU in Japan and the USA).[109]

Table 10.9   CPT-11: Phase II European trial

	Eligible patients (n)	Response rate (%)
Overall population	178	18%
Chemotherapy-naive patients	48	18.8%
Patients pretreated with one 5-FU regimen	130	17.7%
Patients progressing while on 5-FU	62	16.1%
Patients progressing after 5-FU termination	68	19.1%

Table 10.10   Incidence of adverse events associated with CPT-11

Adverse event	All grades (%)	Grade 3 or 4 (%)
Leukopenia	81%	36%
Neutropenia	80%	47%
Anaemia	61%	10%
Thrombocytopenia	6%	2%
Nausea and vomiting	78%	20%
Delayed diarrhoea	87%	39%
Fatigue	81%	35%
Alopecia	81%	53%
Infection	13%	4%
Stomatitis	10%	0%
Dermal toxicity	7%	0%

Conclusion

CPT-11 is a novel antitumour agent that has demonstrated activity in both first- and second-line treatment in patients with advanced colorectal cancer, including those refractory to 5-FU-based regimen. CPT-11 appears to have activity similar to that of 5-FU in first-line treatment, and further clinical studies are required to evaluate its role in combination therapy with 5-FU.

Oxaliplatin

Mechanism of Action

Trans-l-diaminocyclohexane oxaliplatinum (Oxaliplatin, L-OHP) is a new platinum complex and an alkylating agent.[110] The mechanism of action of oxaliplatin appears to be almost identical to that of other platinum derivatives: after cellular penetration and hydrolysis, the platinum binds to the guanine bases of DNA, leading to the formation of intra- and intercatenary links, which prevent the replication of DNA and lead to cell death. Whereas total binding is slow in the case of cisplatin (12 hours) and that of carboplatin (18 hours), it is very fast in the case of oxaliplatin (approximately 15 minutes).[111]

Preclinical Studies

Oxaliplatin, in preclinical studies, has shown consistent activity in a variety of cancer cell lines *in vitro* (cell lines sensitive to cisplatin, cell lines naturally resistant to cisplatin, specifically colon cell lines, cell lines secondarily resistant to cisplatin)[112] and of tumour models *in vivo*.[113] Oxaliplatin has also shown synergistic activity with cyclophosphamide, 5-FU, mitomycin C, cisplatin and carboplatin. In animal studies, no irreversible or unusual toxicity was observed: only mild haematological, mild renal and significant digestive side-effects were reported.

Clinical Studies

Phase I Studies

Six phase I studies of oxaliplatin were conducted. The dose administered varied from 0.45 to 200 mg/m^2: the dose recommended for the phase II studies was 130–135 mg/m^2 as a 2-hour infusion.

Peripheral sensitive neuropathy was the major dose-limiting side-effect in all the phase I studies; in addition digestive toxicity (nausea/vomiting) was observed, with no renal or ototoxicity.

Phase II Studies in Advanced Colorectal Cancer

Oxaliplatin in monotherapy showed a response rate of 10% (both in patients pretreated and resistant to fluoropyrimidines and in chemonaive patients).[114,115,116] Combination studies have been conducted using an association of oxaliplatin, leukovorin and 5-FU, mostly by continuous infusion. Response rates between 28% and 53% have been reported with this combination.[117,118] An equivalent response rate was obtained in both first- and second-line treatments. This compares well with response rates of approximately 40% achieved with continuous infusion of 5-FU alone. Progression free survival ranging from 8 to 15 months and overall survival ranging from 15 to 19 months were observed in these studies.

The above studies showed that the major adverse effects of oxaliplatin were nausea and vomiting, and neurological toxicity characterized by peripheral and/or pharyngolaryngeal dysaesthesia and distal paraesthesias (observed in the majority of cases). These side-effects are dose-dependent in terms of duration and intensity and may, in some cases, cause functional impairment (the clinical symptoms are reversible upon treatment cessation or dose reduction). Other adverse effects include minimal haematological toxicity and infrequent diarrhoea or stomatitis.

A large international phase III trial is ongoing in order to evaluate if the association of the three drugs is superior to leukovorin + 5-FU alone, given according to the above reported regimen.

Liver Metastases from Non-colorectal Cancer

Metastatic malignant tumours of the liver are common in clinical practice, ranking second only to cirrhosis as a cause of fatal liver disease.[119] The liver is uniquely vulnerable to invasion by tumour cells, but a clear understanding of this property does not exist: its size, high rate of blood flow, and double perfusion by hepatic artery and portal vein combine to make the liver the most common site of metastases except for regional lymph nodes. In addition, local tissue factors or endothelial membrane characteristics appear to enhance metastatic implants. Virtually all types of neoplasms may metastasize to the liver.

The most common origin of liver metastases are tumours from the gastrointestinal tract, lung, breast, and melanoma. Less common sites of origin include prostate, thyroid and skin. Most metastatic carcinomas respond poorly to all forms of treatment. The drugs used for liver metastases do not differ in general with respect to the site of the primary tumour. Usually, chemoresponsivity of liver metastases may be considered 'moderate' when there is objective a response rate of 30–40% and a prolonged survival time.

Therapy for advanced tumours has not improved significantly in recent years and remains strictly palliative. Nevertheless, efficacy of treatment in general depends on the chemosensitivity of the primary tumour.

Literature data report that good response rates are obtained in several tumours and in particular breast, ovarian, pulmonary and testicular primaries.

Table 10.11 Systemic chemotherapy in liver metastases: a case list of S. Carlo Borromeo Hospital, Milan (from 1972 to 1983)

Primary tumour site	Patients (n)	Evaluable patients (n)	Percentage complete + partial response	Median units to progression (months)	Advantage in survival
Unknown site	43	17	17.6%	4	no
Breast	30	18	38.8%	14	yes
Ovary	19	5	20	8	no
Small cell lung carcinoma	11	5	20%	7+	no
Non-small cell lung carcinoma	9	4	0%	–	no
Soft tissue Sarcomas	6	3	33.3%	5	no
Melanoma	5	1	0%	–	no
Others (three testicular)	13	6	83.3%	7	no
Total	136	59	30.5%	7.5+	

Unfortunately a realistic advantage in survival is reached only in patients affected with advanced breast cancer. Results from an audit of chemotherapy for differing types of liver metastases from S. Carlo Borromeo Hospital of Milan (from 1972 to 1983) are given in Table 10.11.[120]

Advanced breast cancer represents a demonstrative example of a chemosensitive tumour, which frequently metastatizes to liver. Many available cytotoxic agents are active in metastatic breast cancer; of these, anthracyclines, alkylating agents, purine base analogues and vinca alkaloids result in mean object response rates of 30%. An alternative approach to improve the results is the introduction of new active cytotoxic drugs for example docetaxel (Taxotere®).

Results from a recent European phase II trial[121] performed in patients affected with advanced breast cancer, indicated that docetaxel represent a new effective therapeutic option as a single agent as first-line chemotherapy. The objective response was 67.7%. Response rates according to site of tumour are listed in Table 10.12. A particularly noteworthy point is the high response rate of measurable liver metastases: 12 of 16 responded.

It remains to be determined whether newer drugs or combination chemotherapy will eventually improve the results in terms of objective response and survival. Nevertheless, the management of advanced disease still remains a much-debated topic: there are too many variables involved in the choice of the most efficacious treatment and it is important to stress that efficacy of chemotherapy, when used as a second or third line option, is difficult to demonstrate. This is due to the fact that responses are less likely to occur due to lower performance status, decreased marrow reserves, acquired multidrug resistance, often high tumour burden, reduced quality of life due to the treatment and subsequent poor compliance of patients.

Table 10.12 Docetaxel in breast cancer: responses according to assessable tumour sites (WHO criteria)

Site of disease	Response (patients, n)				
	CR	PR	SD	PD	Total
Primary tumour	2	2	4	2	10
Metastatic nodes	3	1	3	3	10
Skin	1	2	0	3	6
Lung	2	0	0	1	3
Liver	4	8	4	0	16

CR = complete response; PR = partial response; SD = stable disease; PD = progression disease.

References

1. Heidelberg C, Chaudhuri NK. *Nature*, 1957; **179**:663.
2. Heidelberg C. Pyrimidine and pyrimidine nucleoside antimetabolites. In *Cancer Medicine*, Holland J, F, Frei E, (eds), 1973; 768. Philadelphia, *Lea & Febiger*.
3. Mandel HG. Incorporation of 5-fluorouracil into RNA and its molecular consequences. *Prog Mol Subcell Biol* 1969; **1**:82–135.
4. Schuetz JD, Collins JM, Wallace HJ Alteration of the secondary structure of newly synthesized DNA from murine bone marrow cells by 5-fluorouracil. *Cancer Res* 1986; **46**:119–123.
5. Lokich JJ, Ahlgren JD, Gullo JJ. A prospective randomized comparison of continuous infusion fluorouracil with a conventional bolus schedule in metastatic colorectal carcinoma: A Mid-Atlantic Oncology Program study. *J Clin Oncol* 1989; **7**:425–432.

6. Weinerman B, Shah A, Fields A. Systemic infusion versus bolus chemotherapy in measurable colorectal cancer. *Am J Clin Oncol* 1992; **15**:518–523.

7. Rougier P, Paillot B, Lapplanche A. End result of multicenter randomized trial comparing 5-FU in continous systemic infusion to bolus administration in measurable metastatic colorectal cancer. *Proc ASCO* 1992; **11**:465.

8. Hansen R, Ryan L, Anderson T, Quebberman E, Haller D. A phase III trial of bolus 5-FU versus protracted infusion 5-FU cisplatin in metastatic colorectal cancer. An Eastern Cooperative Oncology Group study (EST 2286). *Proc ASCO* 1992; **11**:499.

9. Leichman CG, Fleming TR, Muggia FM. Phase II study of fluorouracil and its modulation in advanced colorectal cancer: a Southwest Oncology Group study. *J Clin Oncol* 1995; **13**:1303–1311.

10. Ardalan B, Chua L, Tian EM. A phase II study of weekly 24-hour infusion with high-dose fluorouracil with leucovorin in colorectal carcinoma. *J Clin Oncol* 1991; **9**(4):625–630.

11. Weh HJ, Wilke HJ, Dierlamm J. Weekly therapy with folinic acid and high-dose 5-fluorouracil 24-hour infusion in pretreated patients with metastatic colorectal carcinoma. *Ann Oncol* 1994; **5**:233–237.

12. Jaeger E, Klein O, Wachtter B, Muller B, Braun U, Knuth A. A second line treatment with high dose 5-fluorouracil and folinic acid in advanced colorectal cancer refractory to standard-dose 5-fluorouracil treatment. *Oncology* 1995; **52**:470–473.

13. Loeffler, Personal comunication, 1995.

14. Lorenz, Personal comunication, 1996.

15. Petrelli N, Herrera L, Rustum Y. A prospective randomized trial of 5-fluorouracil versus 5-fluorouracil and high dose leucovorin versus 5-fluorouracil and methotrexate in previously untreated patients with advanced colorectal carcinoma. *J Clin Oncol* 1987; **5**:1559–1565.

16. Valone FH, Friedman MA, Wittlinger PS. Treatment of patients with advanced colorectal cancer with fluorouracil alone, high dose leucovorin plus fluorouracil, or sequential, methotrexate, fluorouracil and leucovorin: a randomized trial of the Northern California Oncology Group. *J Clin Oncol* 1989; **7**:1427–1436.

17. Di Costanzo F, Bartolucci R, Sofra M. 5-fluorouracil alone vs. high dose folinic acid and 5-FU in advanced colorectal cancer. A randomized trial of the Italian Oncology Group for Clinical Research (GOIRC). *Proc ASCO* 1989; **8**:410.

18. Labianca R, Pancera G, Aitini E. Folinic acid + 5-fluorouracil (5-FU) versus equidose 5-FU in advanced colorectal cancer. Phase III study of GISCAD (Italian Group for the Study of Digestive Tract Cancer) *Ann Oncol* 1991; **2**:673–679.

19. Nobile MT, Vidili MG, Sobrero A. 5-fluorouracil alone or combined with high-dose folinic acid in advanced colorectal cancer patients. *Proc ASCO* 1988; **7**:371.

20. Erlichman C, Fine S, Wong A. A randomized trial of fluorouracil and folinic acid in patients with metastatic colorectal carcinoma. *J Clin Oncol* 1988; **6**:469–475.

21. Doroshow JH, Multauf P, Leong L *et al.* Prospective randomized comparison of fluorouracil versus fluorouracil and high dose continuous infusion leucovorin calcium for the treatment of advanced measurable colorectal cancer in patient previously unexposed to chemotherapy. *J Clin Oncol* 1990; **8**:491–501.

22. Petrelli N, Douglass HO, Herrera. The modulation of fluorouracil and leucovorin in metastatic colorectal cancer: A prospective randomized phase III trial. *J Clin Oncol* 1989; **7**:1419–1426.

23. Cricca A, Martoni A, Guaraldi M. Randomized clinical trial of 5-FU and folinic acid in advanced gastrointestinal cancers. *Proc ESMO* 1988; **13**:427.

24. Poon MA, O'Connell MJ, Moertel CG. Biochemical modulation of fluorouracil. Evidence of significant improvement of survival and quality of life in patients with advanced colorectal carcinoma. *J Clin Oncol* 1989; **7**:1427–1436.

25. Advanced Colorectal Cancer Metaanalysis Project: Modulation of fluorouracil by leucovorin in patients with advanced colorectal cancer. *J Clin Oncol* 1992; **10**:869–903.

26. Buroker TR, O'Connell MJ, Wieand HS. Randomized comparison of two schedules of fluorouracil and leucovorin in the treatment of advanced colorectal cancer. *J Clin Oncol* 1994; **12**:14–20.

27. Jaeger E, Klein O, Bernhard H: Weekly high-dose folinic acid (FA)/5-fluorouracil (FU) versus low-dose FA/FU in advanced colorectal cancer. Results of a randomized multicentric trial. *Proc ASCO* 1994; **13**:556.

28. Poon MA, O'Connell MJ, Wieand HS. Biochemical modulation of fluorouracil with leucovorin: confirmatory evidence of improved therapeutic efficacy in advanced colorectal cancer. *J Clin Oncol* 1991; **9**:1967–1972.

29. Valsecchi R, Labianca R, Cascinu S. High-dose versus low-dose L-leucovorin as a modulator of 5 days 5-fluorouracil in advanced colorectal cancer: a GISCAD phase III study. *Proc ASCO* 1995; **14**:457.

30. DeGramont A, Bosset JF, Milan C. A prospective randomized trial comparing 5-FU bolus with low-dose folinic acid (FUFOLId) and 5-FU bolus plus continuous infusion with high-dose folinic acid (LV5FU2) for advanced colorectal cancer. *Proc ASCO* 1995; **14**:455.

31. Marsh JC, Bertino JR, Katz KH. The influence of drug interval on the effect of methotrexate and fluorouracil in the treatment of advanced colorectal cancer. *J Clin Oncol* 1991; **9**:371–380.

32. Hermann R, Knuth A, Kleeberg U. Sequential methotrexate and 5-fluorouracil (FU) vs. FU alone in metastatic colorectal cancer. *Ann Oncol* 1992; **3**:539–543.

33. Machiavelli M, Leone BA, Romero A. Advanced colorectal carcinoma: a prospective randomized trial of sequential methotrexate, 5-fluorouracil, and leucovorin versus 5-fluorouracil alone. *Am J Clin Oncol* 1991; **14**:211–217.

34. Nordic Gastrointestinal Tumor Adjuvant Therapy Group: Superiority of sequential methotrexate, fluorouracil and leucovorin to fluorouracil alone in advanced symptomatic colorectal carcinoma. A randomized trial. *J Clin Oncol* 1989; **7**:1437–1446.

35. Piedbois P, Buyse M, Blijham G *et al.* Meta-analysis of randomized trial testing the biochemical modulation of fluorouracil by methotrexate in metastatic colorectal cancer. *J Clin Oncol* 1994; **12**:960–969.

36. Wadler S, Wiernik PM. Clinical update on the role of fluorouracil and recombinant interferon alpha-2a in the treatment of colorectal carcinoma. *Semin Oncol* 1990; **17**:16.

37. Fornasiero A, Daniele O, Ghiotto C. Alpha-2 interferon and 5-fluorouracil in advanced colorectal cancer. *Tumori* 1990; **76**:385–389.

38. Kemeny N, Younes A, Seiter K, *et al.* Interferon alfa-2a and 5-fluorouracil for advanced colorectal carcinoma. Assessment of activity and toxicity. *Cancer* 1990; **66**:2470–2475.

39. Pazdur R, Ajani JA, Patt YZ, Winn R, Jackson D, Shepard B. Phase II study of fluorouracil and recombinant interferon alpha-2a in previously untreated advanced colorectal carcinoma. *J Clin Oncol* 1990; **8**:2027–2031.

40. Wadler S, Goldman M, Lyver A, Wiernik PH. Phase I trial of 5-fluorouracil and recombinant alpha (2a)-interferon in patients with advanced colorectal carcinoma. *Cancer Res* 1990; **50**:2056–2059.

41. Wadler S, Wiernik PH. Clinical update on the role of fluorouracil and recombinant interferon alpha-2a in the

treatment of colorectal carcinoma. *Semin Oncol* 1990; **17**(Suppl 1):16–21.

42. Wadler S, Lembersky B, Atkins M. Kirkwood J, Petrelli N. Phase II trial of fluorouracil and recombinant interferon alfa-2a in patients with advanced colorectal carcinoma: an Eastern Cooperative Oncology Group Study. *J Clin Oncol* 1991; **9**:1806–1810.

43. Ajani JA, Rios AH, Ende K. Phase I and II studies of the combination of recombinant human interferon gamma and 5-fluorouracil in patients with advanced colorectal carcinoma. *J Biol Response Mod* 1989; **8**:140–146.

44. Huberman M, Mc Clay E, Atkins M. Phase II trial of 5-fluorouracil (5-FU) and recombinant interferon alpha 2-a (IFN) in advanced colorectal cancer. *Proc ASCO* 1991; **10**:478.

45. Donillard JY, Leborgne J, Danielou JY. Phase II trial of 5-fluorouracil (5-FU) and recombinant alpha interferon (R-IFN) (INTRON A) in metastatic, previously untreated colorectal cancer (CRC). *Proc ASCO* 1991; **10**:422.

46. John W, Neef J, Smith M. 5-fluorouracil (5-FU) and interferon-alpha (IFN) in advanced colon cancer: the University of Kentucky experience. *Proc ASCO* 1992; **11**:570.

47. Dufour P, Husseini F, Cure P. Randomized study of 5-fluorouracil (5-FU) versus 5-FU + alpha 2a interferon (IFN) for metastatic colorectal carcinoma (MCRC). *Proc ASCO* 1992; **11**:583.

48. York M, Greco FA, Einhorn L. A randomized phase III trial comparing 5-FU with or without interferon alpha-2a for advanced colorectal cancer. *Proc ASCO* 1993; **12**:200 (Abstr 590).

49. Hill M, Norman A, Cunningham D. Royal Marsden phase III trial of fluorouracil with or without interferon alpha-2b in advanced colorectal cancer. *J Clin Oncol* 1995; **13**:1297–302.

50. Grem JL, McAtee N, Murphy RF *et al.* A pilot study of interferon alpha-2a in combination with fluorouracil plus high dose leucovorin in metastatic gastrointestinal carcinoma. *J Clin Oncol* 1991; **9**:1811–1820.

51. Piedbois P, Gimonet JF, Fenilhade F *et al.* 5-FU, folinic acid and alpha-2a interferon combination in advanced gastrointestinal cancer. *Proc ASCO* 1991; **10**:430.

52. Taylor C, Modiano M, Alberts D *et al.* Combination therapy with 5-fluorouracil (5-FU), leucovorin (LCV) and interferon-alpha (IFN-alpha) in patients with adenocarcinoma. *Proc ASCO* 1991; **10**:432.

53. Punt CJA, de Mulder PHM, Burghouts JM. A phase I-II study of high-dose 5-fluorouracil (5-FU), leucovorin (LV) and alpha interferon (alpha-IFN) in patients with advanced colorectal cancer. *Proc ASCO* 1991; **10**:465.

54. Inoshita G, Yalavarthi P, Murthy S. Phase I trial of 5-FU, leucovorin (LV) and IFN-alpha 2a in metastatic colorectal cancer. *Proc ASCO* 1991; **10**:475.

55. Kohne-Wompner CH, Schmoll HJ, Hiddemann W *et al.* 5-fluorouracil (5-FU), leucovorin (LV), alpha-2b interferon (IFN) in advanced colorectal cancer (CC): a phase I-II study. *Proc ASCO* 1991; **10**:503.

56. Labianca R, Pancera G, Tedeschi L. High dose alfa-2b interferon + folinic acid in the modulation of 5-fluorouracil. A phase II study in advanced colorectal cancer with evidence of an unfavorable cost/benefit ratio. *Tumori* 1992; **78**:32.

57. Cascinu S, Fedeli A, Luzi Fedeli S. Double biochemical modulation of 5-fluorouracil by leucovorin and cyclic low dose interferon alpha 2b in advanced colorectal cancer patients. *Ann Oncol* 1992; **3**:489.

58. Labianca R, Giaccon G, Pancera G. Low dose alpha 2b interferon (IFN) + folinic acid (FA) + 5-fluorouracil (5-FU) in advanced colorectal cancer (ACC): a phase II study of GISCAD (Italian Group for the Study of Gastrointestinal Cancer). *Proc ASCO* 1992; **11**:523.

59. Moore MJ, Kaizer L, Erlichman C. A phase II clinical and pharmacological study of 5-fluorouracil (5-FU) + leucovorin + interferon in advanced colorectal cancer. *Proc ASCO* 1992; **11**:548.

60. Van Hazel GA, Buck M, Byrne MJ. Phase II study of the combination of 5-fluorouracil (5-FU), folinic acid (FA) and alpha interferon (IFN) in metastatic colorectal adenocarcinoma cancer (CC). *Proc ASCO* 1992; **11**:594.

61. Recchia F, Nuzzo A, Lombardo M. 5-fluorouracil (5-FU) and high dose folinic acid (hdFA) chemotherapy (CT) with or without alpha 2b interferon (IFN) in advanced colorectal cancer (ACC). Preliminary report of a randomized trial. *Proc ASCO* 1992; **11**:461.

62. Brunetti I, Falcone A, Bertuccelli M. Double 5-fluorouracil (5-FU) modulation with folinic acid (FA) and recombinant alpha 2b interferon (IFN) in patients with metastatic colorectal carcinoma. *Proc ASCO* 1992; **11**:514.

63. Schmoll HJ, Kohne-Wompner CH, Hiddemann W. Bolus 5-fluorouracil (FU), folinic acid (FA) and alpha-2b Interferon (IFN) in advanced colorectal cancer (CRC): a multicenter phase II trial. *Proc ASCO* 1992; **11**:535.

64. Cortesi E, D'Aprile M, Di Palma M. Advanced colorectal cancer: a phase II study chemoimmunotherapy with IFN alpha 2b + 5-FU C.I. or 5-FU + FA. *Proc ASCO* 1992; **11**:545.

65. Lembersky B, Koff H, Miketic L *et al.* Phase II trial of 5-fluorouracil (FU), leucovorin (LV) and interferon alpha-2b (IFN) in the treatment of metastatic colorectal cancer (CRC). *Proc ASCO* 1992; **11**:559.

66. Kreuser ED, Hilgenfeld RU, Matthias M. Final update on a phase II trial of interferon alpha-2b with folinic acid and 4-hour infusion of 5-fluorouracil in advanced colorectal carcinoma. *Proc ASCO* 1992; **11**:581.

67. Grem JL, Jordan R, Robson M. A phase II study of interferon alpha-2a in combination with 5-fluorouracil and leucovorin in advanced colorectal cancer. *Proc ASCO* 1993; **12**:600.

68. Corfu-A study group. Phase III randomized study of two combinations with either interferon alfa-2a or leucovorin for advanced colorectal cancer. *J Clin Oncol* 1995; **13**:921–928.

69. Fujii S, Okuda H, Toide H. Studies on the fate of FT-207, an antitumor agent. Absorption, tissue distribution, and excretion. *Pharmacokinetics* 1974; **8**:589–595.

70. Mukherjee K, Heidelberger C. Studies on fluorinated pyrimidines. IX. The degradation of 5-fluorouracil-6-C.[14] *J Biol Chem* 1960; **235**:433–437.

71. Taguchi T, Hanano Y, Jikuya K, Fujii S. Effect of uracil on the antitumor activity of ftorafur. *Jpn J Cancer Chemother* 1978; **5**:1161–1165.

72. Ota K, Taguchi T, Kimura K. Report on nationwide pooled data and cohort investigation in UFT Phase II studies. *Cancer Chemother Pharmacol* 1988; **22**:333–338.

73. Ikenaka K, Shirasaka T, Kitano S. Effect of uracil on metabolism of 5-fluorouracil *in vitro*. *Gann* 1979; **70**:353–359.

74. Ho DH, Covington WP, Pazdur R *et al.* Clinical pharmacology of combined oral uracil and ftorafur. *Drug Metab Dispos* 1992; **20**:936–940.

75. Au JL, Sadee W. Activation of ftorafur [*R,S*-1-(tetrahydro-2-furanyl)-5-fluorouracil] to 5-fluorouracil and gamma-butyrolactone. *Cancer Res* 1980; **40**:2814–2819.

76. El Sayed YM, Sadee W. Metabolic activation of *R,S*-1-(tetrahydro-2-furanyl)-5-fluorouracil (ftorafur) to 5-fluorouracil by soluble enzymes. *Cancer Res* 1983; **43**:4039–4044.

77. Pazdur R, Lassere Y, Rhodes V, Ajani JA, Sugarman SM, Patt YZ, Jones DV, Markowitz AB, Abbruzzese JL, Bready B, Levin B. Phase II trial of uracil and tegafur plus oral leucorovin: an effective oral regimen in the treatment of

metastatic colorectal carcinoma. *J Clin Oncol* 1994; **12**:2296–2300.

78. Saltz LB, Leichman CG, Young CW, Muggia FM, Conti JA, Spies T, Jeffers S, Leichman LP. A fixed-ratio combination of uracil and ftorafur (UFT) with low dose leucorovin. *Cancer* 1995; **75**:782–785.

79. Bollag W, Hartmann HR. Tumor inhibitory effects of a new fluorouracil derivative: 5-deoxy-5-fluorouridine. *Eur J Cancer* 1979; **16**:427–432.

80. Alberto P, Mermillod B, Germano G *et al.* Randomized comparison of doxifluorouridine and fluorouracil in colorectal carcinoma. *Eur J Cancer (Clin Oncol)* 1988; **24**:559–563.

81. Trave F, Canobbio L, Lai-Sim Au J *et al.* Role of administration route in the therapeutic efficacy of doxifluorouridine. *J Natl Cancer Inst* 1987; **78**:527–532.

82. Yoshimori K, Hasegawa K. Study on efficacy and safety of 5-deoxy-5-fluorouridine (5′-dFUR) with intermittent administration. *Prog Antimicrob Anticancer Chemother* 1987; **3**:493–495.

83. Alberto P, Winkelmann JJ, Pashoud N *et al.* Phase I study of oral doxifluridine using two schedules. *Eur J Cancer (Clin Oncol)* 1989; **25**:905–908.

84. Bajetta E, Colleoni M, Di Bartolomeo M. Doxifluridine (dFUR) and leucovorin: an oral treatment combination in advanced colorectal cancer. *J Clin Oncol* 1995; **13**:2613–2619.

85. Jones TR, Calvert AH, Jackman AL. A potent antitumor quinazoline inhibitor of thymidylate synthase: synthesis, biological properties and therapeutic results in mice. *Eur J Cancer* 1981; **17**:11–19.

86. Jones TR, Thornton TJ, Flinn A. Quinazoline antifolates inhibiting thymidylate synthase: 2-desamino derivates with enhanced solubility and potency. *J Med Chem* 1989; **32**:847–852.

87. Hughes LR, Jackman AL, Oldfield J. Quinazoline antifolate thymidylate synthase inhibitors: alkyl, substituted alkyl, and aryl substituents in the C2 positions. *J Med Chem* 1990; **33**:3060–3067.

88. Jackman AL, Taylor GA, O'Connor BM. Activity of the thymidylate synthase inhibitor 2-desamino-N⁰-propargyl-5,8-dideazafolic acid and related compounds in murine (L1210) and human (W1L2) systems *in vitro* and in L1210 *in vivo*. *Cancer Res* 1990; **50**:5212–5218.

89. Jackman AL, Marsham PR, Moran RG, Kimbell R, O'Connor BM, Hughes LR, Calvert AH. Thymidylate synthase inhibitors: the *in vitro* activity of a series of heterocyclic benzoyl ring modified 2-desamino-2-methyl-N10-substituted-5,8-dideazafolates. *Adv Regul* 1991; **31**:13–27.

90. Jackman AL, Brown M, Kelland L, Gibson W, Abel G, Boyle FT, Judson I. *Proc AACR* 1991; **32**:326.

91. Jodrell DI, Newell DR, Calvete JA, Stephens TC, Calvert AH. Pharmacokinetic and toxicity studies with the novel quinazoline thymidylate synthase inhibitor, D1694. *Proc AACR* 1990; **31**:341.

92. Judson I, Clarke S, Ward J, Planting A, Verweii J, M de Boer, Spiers J, Smith R, Sutcliffe F. A phase I trial of the thymidylate synthase inhibitor ICI D1694. *Ann Oncol* 1992 (Suppl 5; Abstr 201); **3**:51.

93. Sorensen JM, Jordan E, Grem JL *et al.* Phase I trial of ZD1694 ('Tomudex'), a direct inhibitor of thymidylate synthase. *Ann Oncol* 5: 1994 (Suppl 5; Abstr 241).

94. Zalcberg JR, Cunningham D, Van Custem E *et al.* ZD1694: A novel thymidylate synthase inhibitor with substantial activity in the treatment of patients with advanced colorectal cancer. *J Clin Oncol* 1996; **14**(3):716–729.

95. Cunningham D, Zalcberg JR, Rath U, Olver I, Van Custem E, Svensson C, Seitz JF, Harper P, Kerr D, Perez-Manga G, Azab M, Seymour L, Lowery K and the Tomudex Colorectal Cancer Study Group. Tomudex (ZD1694): results of a randomised trial in advanced colorectal cancer demonstrate efficacy and reduced mucositis and leucopenia. *Eur J Cancer* 1995; **31**(12):1945–1954.

96. Wall ME, Wani MC, Cook CE. Plant anti-tumor agents. The isolation and structure of camptothecin, a novel alkaloidal leukemia and tumor inhibition from *Camptotheca acuminata. J Am Chem Soc* 1966; **88**:3888–3890.

97. Kawato Y, Aonima M, Hirota Y. Intracellular roles of SN-38, a metabolite of the camptothecin derivative CPT-11, in the antitumor effect of CPT-11. *Cancer Res* 1991; **51**:4187–4191.

98. Tanizawa A, Fujimori A, Fujimori Y. Comparison of topoisomerase I inhibition, DNA damage, and cytotoxicity of camptothecin derivatives presently in clinical trials. *J Natl Cancer Inst* 1994; **86**:836–842.

99. Shimada Y, Rothenberg M, Hilsenbeck SG. Activity of CPT-11 (irinotecan hydrochloride), a topoisomerase I inhibitor, against human tumor colony-forming units. *Anticancer Drugs* 1994; **5**:202–206.

100. Funakoshi S, Aiba K, Shibata H. Enhanced antitumor activity of SN-38, an active metabolite of CPT-11, and 5-fluorouracil combination for human colorectal cancer cell lines. *Proc ASCO* 1994; **12**:1607–1611.

101. Abigerges D, Chabot GG, Armand J. Phase 1 and pharmacologic studies of the camptothecin analogue irinotecan administered every 3 weeks in cancer patients. *J Clin Oncol* 1995; **13**:210–221.

102. Abigerges D, Armand JP, Chabot GG. Irinotecan (CPT-11) high-dose escalation using intensive high-dose loperamide to control diarrhea. *J Natl Cancer Inst* 1994; **86**:446–449.

103. Shimada Y, Yashino M, Wakui A. Phase II study of CPT-11, a new camptothecin derivative, in metastatic colorectal cancer *J Clin Oncol* 1993; **11**:909–913.

104. Conti JA, Kemeny N, Saltz L, Irinotecan (CPT-11) is an active agent in untreated patients with metastatic colorectal cancer (CRC). *Proc ASCO* 1994; **13**:195.

105. Pitot HC, Wender D, O'Connell MJ. A phase II trial of CPT-11 (irinotecan) in patients with metastatic colorectal carcinoma: A North Central Treatment Group (NCCTG) study. *Proc ASCO* 1994; **13**:197.

106. Rothenberg ML, Eckardt JR, Burris HA III. Irinotecan (CPT-11) as second line therapy for PTS with 5-FU-refractory colorectal cancer. *Proc ASCO* 1994; **13**:198.

107. Rougier P, Bugat R, Brunet P. Clinical efficacy of CPT-11 in patients with inoperable advanced colorectal cancer (CRC): Results of a multicentric open phase II study. *5th International Congress of Anti-cancer Chemotherapy, Paris, France, 31 January–3 February 1995.*

108. Bugat R CPT-11 in the treatment of colorectal cancer (CRC): Safety profile. *5th International Congress of Anti-cancer Chemotherapy, Paris, France, 31 January–3 February 1995.*

109. Shimada Y, Sasaki Y, Sugano K. Combination phase I study of CPT-11 (irinotecan) combined with continuous infusion 5-fluorouracil (5-FU) in metastatic colorectal cancer *Proc ASCO* 1993; **12**:196.

110. Kidani Y, Noji M, Tashiro T. Antitumor Activity of platinum (II) complexes of 1,2-diaminocyclohexane isomers. 1980; **71**:637–643.

111. Jennerwein MM, Eastman A, Khokhar AR. The role of DNA repair in resistance of L1210 cells to isomeric 1,2-diaminocyclohexane platinum(II) complexes. *Chem-Biol Interactions* 1989; **70**:39–49.

112. Silvestro L, Anal H, Sommer F, Trincal G, Tapiero H. Comparative effects of a new platinum analog (*trans-l*-1,2-diaminocyclohexane oxalatoplatinum; L-OHP) with CDDP on various cells: Correlation with intracellular

accumulation. *3 International Conference Anticancer Research*, October 1990.

113. Mathé G, Kidani Y, Noji M, Maral R, Bourut C, Chenu E. Antitumor activity of L-OHP in mice. *Cancer Lett* 1985; **27**:135–143.

114. Machover D, Diaz-RubioE, de Gramont A. Two consecutive phase II studies of oxaliplatin (*l*-OHP) for treatment of patients with advanced colorectal carcinoma who were resistant to previous treatment with fluoropyrimidines. *Ann Oncol* 1996; **7**:95–98.

115. Diaz-Rubio E, Zaniboni A, Gastiaburu J. Phase II multicentrc trial of chemotherapy in metastatic colorectal carcinoma (MCRC). *Proc ASCO* 1996; **15**:207 (Abstr 468).

116. Lèvi F, Perpoint B, Garufi C *et al*. Oxaliplatin activity against metastatic colorectal cancer: a phase II study of 5-day continuous venous infusion at circadian-rhythm modulated rate. *Eur J Cancer* 1993; **29A**:1284–1293.

117. De Gramont A, Gastiaburu J, Tournigand C *et al*. Oxaliplatin with high dose folinic acid and 5-fluorouracil

48 h infusion in pretreated metastatic colorectal cancer. *Proc ASCO* 1994; **13**: Abstract 666.

118. Levi F, Misset JL, Brienza S *et al*. A chronopharmacologic Phase II clinical trial with 5-fluorouracil, folinic acid, and oxaliplatin using an ambulatory multichannel programmable pump. *Cancer* 1992; **69**:893–900.

119. Wilson JD, Braunwald E, Isselbacher KJ, Petersdorf RG, Martin JB, Fauci AS, Root RK. *Harrison's Principles of Internal Medicine*, 12th edn. *Neoplasm of the Liver. Metastatic Tumors*, 1991: 1350–1352.

120. Luporini G, Labianca R, Locatelli MC, Beretta G. *Chemioterapia Locoregionale e Sistemica dei Tumori Epatici*. '*I Tumori Gastroenterici*', 1984: 303–315. Milan, CEA Casa Editrice Ambrosiana.

121. Chevallier B, Fumoleau P, Kerbrat P *et al*. Docetaxel is a major cytotoxic drug for the treatment of advanced breast cancer: a Phase II trial of the clinical screening cooperative group of the European Organization for Research and Treatment of Cancer. *J Clin Oncol* 1995; **13**(2):314–322.

Regional Infusion Therapy

Riccardo A. Audisio, H. Stephan Stoldt and James G. Geraghty

11

Introduction

Surgical resection is presently the only therapeutic option that provides patients with liver neoplasms a chance of cure. Nonetheless, at the time of diagnosis, the majority of patients with liver tumours present with unresectable hepatic disease.[1] The need for new forms of treatment aimed at improving survival in patients with liver neoplasms while preserving quality of life is thus quite apparent.

Systemic treatment of liver metastases with intravenous chemotherapy has been employed extensively when surgery has been rendered inappropriate, either because of extent of the disease or because of the poor condition of the patient (see Chapter 10. Nevertheless, a substantial number of patients have irresectable disease confined to the liver and this has led to the most widespread use of local hepatic infusional chemotherapy.

Theoretical Basis of Hepatic Infusional Chemotherapy

Early metastatic liver seedings, like normal hepatocytes, derive their principal nutrients from the portal vein. However, once tumour metastases are >1 cm in size, they develop their own blood supply derived mainly from the hepatic artery.[2] Wang *et al.*[3] have been able to show that portal blood flow contributes ≤16% of tumour blood in small lesions and ≤4% in larger tumours. There is also evidence that hepatic arterial infusion of antineoplastic drugs may reduce the development of experimental micrometastasis by approximately two-thirds. These observations have enhanced the interest in hepatic arterial infusion on the basis of the following:

- The concept of a stepwise pattern of metastatic progression was defined as 'metastatic inefficiency'.[4] Since tumour spread to the liver is delivered through the portal flow, followed eventually by other steps including involvement of lung and other organs, there is a place for interrupting the progression at the first step with adequate liver treatment (surgery or infusional chemotherapy).

- Both animal and human studies using labelled fluorodeoxyuridine (FUDR)[5,6] have shown that liver metastases establish their neovascularity directly from the hepatic arterial circulation. Liver and tumour biopsies indicated that patients with metastatic disease, when given FUDR into the portal vein, had the same liver parenchymal FUDR level when compared to those who had hepatic arterial infusion with the same drug. In these studies the mean tumour FUDR levels following hepatic artery or portal vein infusion were 12.4 and 0.8 nmol/g, respectively[6] ($P < 0.001$), thus indicating that hepatic arterial infusion increases the relative exposure of drug to tumour cells compared to normal hepatocytes.

- High intrahepatic drug levels can be obtained by hepatic arterial infusion chemotherapy. A high drug concentration gradient created between the drug level in the artery and the tumour[7] is important for those drugs showing a steep dose–response curve such as the fluoropyrimidines (FUDR and 5-fluorouracil).[8] Those drugs which are not rapidly cleared by the liver circulate in the bloodstream repeatedly and minimize the advantage of hepatic arterial infusion over

Table 11.1 Drugs used in hepatic arterial infusion chemotherapy

Drug	Half-life (min)	Total body clearance (ml/min)	Estimated increased exposure by hepatic arterial infusion	Plasma clearance (ml/min)
5-FU	10	4 000	5–10-fold	4800
FUDR	<10	25 000	100–400-fold	500–1300
Mitomycin C	<10	1 000	6–8-fold	600–1100
Doxorubicin	60	900	2-fold	500
Methotrexate	–	–	6–8-fold	110
BCNU	<5	1 000	6–8-fold	1000
Cisplatin	20–30	400	4–7-fold	42

systemic chemotherapy administration. The high regional exchange rate is typical of the hepatic arterial blood flow (≤1500 ml/min) hence drugs with an elevated clearance rate are better employed. FUDR is the most frequently used drug due to its high extraction rate (94–99% at first liver passage) (Table 11.1).[9]

- The high hepatic extraction rate of some compounds allows the use of high dose chemotherapy with less drug related systemic toxicity. Tumours with a low response to intravenous chemotherapy may respond better to intra-arterial infusion of the same drug at the same concentration.[10,11] Although it is unlikely that increased tumour concentrations of chemotherapeutic drugs alone might achieve a marked therapeutic benefit, those tumours which do respond to intravenous chemotherapy, might do so with a slight therapeutic advantage when the same drug is administered intra-arterially at even higher doses.

Indications

Hepatic arterial infusion for liver metastases was first performed 50 years ago,[12] but gained increasing interest only in the 1960s when percutaneous intra-arterial catheters with external pumps became widely available.[13,14] The method has been popularized more recently through improvements in instrumentation and surgical technique in the placement of the required catheters and pumps, as well as through a gain in the understanding of pharmacokinetics. The indications for hepatic arterial infusion chemotherapy are:

- unresectable liver neoplastic disease;
- adjuvant treatment after resection.

Patients with liver metastases from colorectal cancer, carcinoid and occasionally other histological types should be considered for hepatic arterial infusion when they have been excluded as candidates for surgical resection. Cholangiocarcinoma involving the liver is almost always associated with jaundice, and this is a contraindication to treatment with such infusion. Metastases from gallbladder, gastric and renal carcinomas, as well as metastases from melanomas and sarcomas have been treated by hepatic arterial infusion.[15,16] Most experience in the use of this modality has been gained from patients with colorectal liver metastasis as a consequence of the high prevalence of colorectal carcinoma from which approximately 60% of patients develop metastatic disease in the liver.[17]

Carcinoid tumour is a rare neuroendocrine neoplasm, most frequently originating from the appendix (40%), small bowel (27%) or large bowel (7%). Carcinoid tumours are unfortunately being diagnosed with a mean lead time of four years, and 90% of patients have stage IV disease by the time of presentation. For the above-mentioned reasons, only 7% metastatic neuroendocrine tumours are surgical candidates.[18]

By far the most common site of metastasis from ocular melanoma is the liver, either as the sole site or in association with disseminated disease; extrahepatic metastasis will occur in <50% of the patients.[19] There have been isolated reports of hepatic surgery, including liver transplant, for such tumours and hepatic arterial infusion has been employed in the management of a limited number of such patients. Preliminary results are encouraging with a 3–10% complete response rate and partial response in 43% of cases.[20]

Appropriate staging (abdominal/thoracic computed tomography, double contrast enema/colonoscopy) is an essential prerequisite to hepatic arterial infusion, aimed at minimizing the number of patients with macroscopic extrahepatic disease. Patients with no evidence of extrahepatic disease are considered to be the most appropriate candidates for infusion,[21,22] although patients with minimal extrahepatic involvement might also be considered. This is due to the fact that the presence of minimal extrahepatic disease may not influence outcome.[23]

The disease-free interval from resection of the primary has also been proposed as a selection criterium: Shumata et al.[24] has suggested that metastases discovered on follow-up may be suitable for hepatic arterial infusion when this interval exceeds one year. Intravenous chemotherapy might be a more prudent treatment for patients with shorter disease-free intervals. These same authors have suggested that hepatic arterial infusion can be started after six months of intravenous chemotherapy, by which time extrahepatic dissemination will have declared itself.

The potential benefit of hepatic arterial infusion in an adjuvant setting after radical liver resection for metastatic colorectal cancer is presently being addressed with prospective studies (such as the EORTC #40911 trial). Sure it has been suggested that the probability of local recurrence is higher in those patients with larger hepatic involvement.[25] In a preliminary prospective study, better survival and a longer disease-free interval was reported by Ligidakis, when surgical resection was followed by adjuvant immunochemotherapy, as compared to surgery alone.[26] These results are consistent with a previous report from Japan. Seven patients who had hepatic arterial infusion of mitomycin-C, 5-fluorouracil (5-FU), doxorubicin and lipiodol emulsion enjoyed a prolonged disease-free interval and survival, when compared to 16 cases without hepatic arterial infusion in an adjuvant setting.[27] The experience of Sugarbaker's group supports the policy of a cytoreductive approach in the treatment of liver metastases. They used induction chemotherapy with the purpose of achieving a response, or of stabilizing liver disease, following which patients could be selected for surgery. This aggressive policy increased the median survival in a limited number of cases when compared to intraarterial chemotherapy alone.[28]

Contraindications to hepatic arterial infusion are poor performance status (<60 Karnofsky or Performance Status > grade 2 according to the World Health Organization), nutritional impairment, portal hypertension, neoplastic ascites, vitamin K-resistant clotting abnormality, high

Table 11.2 Contraindications for the use of hepatic arterial infusion chemotherapy

- Performance Status >2
- Proven extrahepatic spread
- Extensive liver involvement >75%
- Available effective systemic treatment
- Portal hypertension, jaundice, ascites
- Metabolic impairment
- Nutritional impairment
- Cardiovascular failure
- Renal failure
- Active infection
- Complex hepatic arterial anatomy
- Poor compliance
- Geographical location
- History of drug allergy

serum bilirubin level (>4 mg%), poor hepatic synthesis (serum albumin <2.5 g%) and renal failure (serum creatinine level >2 mg%). Cardiovascular and respiratory failure are relative contraindications, as well as previous radiotherapy in the upper right abdominal region. Good intellectual function is required to ensure adequate treatment compliance (Table 11.2).

Technical Details

Materials

Numerous systems are presently available for locoregional chemotherapy and newer ones are being developed on an ongoing basis.

Access Ports

These allow intra-arterial infusion and require external instrumentation for perfusion. Costs are limited although an external pump is necessary and the patient must attend or keep close contact with the hospital for several days each month of treatment. A further disadvantage is the high risk of catheter clotting when the flow is interrupted at the end of every infusion and thus experienced nursing care is required. There is also a reduction in the therapeutic efficacy of those drugs which cannot be delivered by continuous infusion. A variety of delivery systems is presently available. Studied plastic chambers, including Delvin and Polysulphon, are lighter and cheaper than titanium varieties which theoretically last longer. Patients may become cachectic with disease progression and the thickness of the overlying subcutaneous fat tissue may become reduced, thus increasing the risk of ulceration onto the chamber from repeated puncture. 'Low profile' devices have been designed to reduce this risk, although it may be difficult to locate them for needle puncture when they are first implanted.

Totally Implantable Pumps

These are battery powered or gas powered and can store almost 20 ml of the relevant drug and deliver it by a continuous infusion. Some devices contain a microprocessor-based programmable circuitry with varying infusional modes (bolus, multistep bolus, continuous flat, continuous complex, bolus delay). The choice of the infusional system is not complex and can be made predominantly on an economical basis, but also upon issues such as therapeutic scheduling, drug toxicity, availability of maintainance and ease of access. Newer devices with chambers of $\leqslant$100 ml are being produced.

Both access ports and totally implantable pumps deliver the drug through catheters of different composition (polyethylene, silicone, Teflon and others). Unfortunately all catheters are thrombogenic to varying extents and thrombosis occurring in the main hepatic artery or its branches is one of the most frequent complications. Teflon catheters are reported to be more thrombogenic than their polyethylene counterparts, but the latter are more frequently dislodged. The ideal catheter has yet to be found and existing devices carry their own advantages and disadvantages. There are still many technical hurdles to overcome before the optimal device is identified.

Surgical Technique

A midline incision is often used, although the incision which often provides the best exposure for hepatic artery cannulation and proper placement of the subcutaneous port or pump is a right subcostal or right paramedian incisions. The small and large bowel as well as the retroperitoneal areas including periaortic and celiac nodes can normally be explored adequately through these incisions. Careful inspection for extrahepatic disease is essential and any suspicious lesions require frozen section histological diagnosis since most of these

patients are unlikely to benefit from hepatic arterial infusion.[29] This opinion, however, is not universally shared.[30]

Anatomical variations in arterial blood supply to the liver are common[31] and the regional anatomy must be defined pre-operatively by angiography. This study will also identify atherosclerotic disease which may interfere with proper positioning of the intra-arterial catheter. For these reasons, many surgeons prefer to delay the insertion of an infusional system, at the time of accidental discovery of liver metastasis during laparoromy for malignant primary disease, to a second intervention following adequate angiographic evaluation.

Careful dissection and complete vascular isolation is required for adequate catheter placement and prevents drug misperfusion and the potentially severe complications such as gastritis, cholecystitis, duodenitis, possible necrosis and perforation. For this reason, the right gastric artery is identified and tied in continuity.

Cholecystectomy is mandatory to prevent chemotherapy-induced cholecystitis from gallbladder chemoperfusion. This complication has occurred in one-third of cases in which cholecystectomy was not performed. This part of the operation is best undertaken initially and begun at the porta hepatis to allow proper identification of the regional anatomy. The hepatic artery which usually crosses the common bile duct dorsally (85% cases) is dissected proximally towards the gastroduodenal artery. Segmental areas of the hepatic and gastroduodenal arteries ($\geqslant$1.5 cm in length) must be freely dissected proximal to their junction in order to allow arteriotomy and catheter placement.

Normal anatomical arterial supply to the liver is encountered in approximately 60% of the population.[31,32] In this setting, an angled vascular clamp is placed precisely to occlude the gastroduodenal artery at its junction with the hepatic artery, while maintaining hepatic flow. The gastroduodenal artery is ligated 1.5–2 cm distal to its origin. A small longitudinal arteriotomy is performed proximal to the ligature and the beaded catheter is introduced into the gastroduodenal arteriotomy and advanced to the point of the vascular clamp. The tip should not protrude into the hepatic artery since it might alter hepatic artery flow and result in thrombosis. Double ligation of the catheter to the vessel prevents advancement of the catheter into the hepatic artery or its retraction from the gastroduodenal artery. The sutures should not be tightened too firmly as the lumen of the catheter may be narrowed and patency must be checked immediately.

Anatomical Variations

A wide range of anatomical variations are commonly seen in hepatic arterial supply and may render the procedure technically more complex. Furthermore, it has been suggested that patients with variant anatomy may have a poorer response to hepatic arterial infusion than those with conventional anatomy.[33] Conversely, if care is taken to ensure that both lobes of the liver are perfused, no significant difference in response to regional chemotherapy in this group of patients compared to those with normal anatomy can be demonstrated.[32]

In the most frequent variant (30%), a *left hepatic artery* takes origin from the left gastric artery. This vessel may be ligated and transected close to the gastrohepatic ligament or, when this variant vessel is responsible for most of the liver perfusion (as shown by angiography), it should be utilized for catheter placement. Its proximal end is ligated together with the right gastric and gastroduodenal arteries. Also frequently seen (20%) is a *right hepatic artery* taking origin from the superior mesenteric artery. This variant artery usually follows a retroduodenal course, where it should be identified and ligated allowing delivery of hepatic arterial infusion through the left hepatic artery. When the gastroduodenal artery originates from the left hepatic artery, two separate infusional systems or one system with two catheters may be implanted to administer bilateral infusion. The left hepatic artery is cannulated as previously described through the gastroduodenal artery, and the right hepatic artery is cannulated at the porta hepatis.

Trifurcation of the common hepatic artery is a frequent variant. The left hepatic artery can be safely ligated in this setting and the catheter placed via the gastroduodenal artery. If both hepatic arteries originate from the splenic artery, proper mixing of the drug is achieved with cannulation of the splenic artery. The catheter tip is inserted into the origin of the common hepatic artery and the proximal stump ligated. Overall, the approach to variants with double arterial supply has not been uniform. Implantable devices accommodating double catheterization are uncommon and, as a result, some surgeons have elected to transpose the right hepatic artery arising from the superior mesenteric

on to the proper or left hepatic artery.[34,35] Ligation of the variant vessel has been accepted more widely and is supported by anatomical and radiological appraisal that interlobar and intersegmental arterial anastomoses are vascularised immediately following ligation of the vessel, so that the entire liver flow is provided by the parent artery.[36,37]

Patients with anatomical variations of the hepatic arterial system do represent a high risk group for misperfusion during chemotherapy. It has been shown that despite attempts to correct for arterial abnormalities, only a small proportion (8%) will show the expected hepatic perfusion on postoperative studies. The majority will show additional perfusion of extrahepatic organs such as spleen, stomach, bowel or pancreas, as well as unsatisfactory perfusion of the liver. Postoperative complications are also more frequent in patients with arterial anomalies compared to those who have normal postoperative scintigraphic findings.[38,39]

Insertion of Pump

During insertion of a hepatic arterial infusion pump and catheter, a separate transverse incision over the right anterolateral costal area, characteristically 5–8 cm from the incision line, is used to conceal the pump. A separate incision is also advisable if the pump is being inserted at the time of colonic resection to reduce the risk of contamination. The flap overlying the infusional device should be properly tailored so that it is thick enough (generally 1.5 cm) to prevent cutaneous erosion, but sufficiently thin to allow proper needle insertion.

Haemostasis in the formed pocket is essential as haematoma in the presence of an implantable device increases the risk of sepsis. The pump is filled with heparinized saline, inserted into the pocket and fixed with four non-absorbable stitches to the underlying fascia. The catheter is subsequently tunnelled through fascia, muscle and peritoneum. The length of the catheter should be sized carefully to avoid redundant loops, kinking, undue tension or dislocation, taking into consideration the possible volume variations of the peritoneal cavity due to gas and bowel shifts. Injection of a bolus of fluoroscein dye or methylene blue will allow assessment of adequate catheter placement, completeness of liver perfusion and recognition of unwanted vascular branches to nearby structures such as the lesser curvature of the stomach and duodenum. Infusion of agents can be started immediately, although post-operative scintigraphic control of the implanted system, using ^{99m}Tc-microspheres or ^{99m}Tc-macroaggregated albumin, may be carried out within one week and before treatment is started.[38,40]

Literature Review and Results

Despite recent advances in the understanding and management of metastatic liver disease, the prognosis of patients with unresectable liver tumours has not been significantly modified. Despite the strong theoretical support for the use of hepatic arterial infusion,[41] a clear-cut survival advantage has not been established in patients undergoing this form of therapy. Although data from phase II studies in patients treated with hepatic arterial infusion and FUDR[29] have demonstrated a high objective response rate in patients with colorectal metastases with a median survival of 17 months, such favourable results have also been reported in subjects receiving intravenous chemotherapy. Nevertheless, skeptics are justified in their plea for

this treatment modality to remain within the confines of controlled clinical trials, since only 654 patients have been randomized into Phase III trials.[42]

Few reports on hepatic arterial infusion for liver metastases other than those from colorectal cancer are available. Preliminary reports of experience from Germany recorded a 39% partial remission rate and a five-month mean survival among 59 breast cancer patients with liver secondaries.[43] Conclusive prospective studies are still required for treatment of liver metastasis by hepatic arterial infusion in all of these histological subtypes.

While sporadic reports on hepatic arterial infusion should be considered with great caution,[44] several prospective and two meta-analysis studies have been conducted comparing intra-arterial FUDR and intravenous chemotherapy in metastatic liver disease of colorectal origin (Tables 11.3 to 11.5).[30,45–51] Therapeutic advantages have been shown when hepatic arterial infusion with FUDR infusion is compared to non-uniform control groups either receiving chemotherapy, other palliative or no treatment at all. Although one-third of the treatment limb in the French trial, received both hepatic arterial infusion and systemic 5-FU.[48] Crossover designs have occurred in 40–60% of cases

Table 11.3 Randomized studies comparing hepatic arterial infusion (HAI) with intravenous chemotherapy (IVC)

Author	Patients (n)	Response rate (%)		Median survival (months)		survival (%) (HAI/IVC)	
		HAI	IVC	HAI	IVC	One year	Two years
Kemeny (1994)[49]	163	52	20	17	12	60/50	35/18
Hohn (1989)[46]	143	42	10	17	16	60/42	30/30
Chang (1987)[45]	64	62	17	20	11	85/40	44/13
Martin (1990)[47]	74	48	21	12.6	10.5	60/42	18/10

Table 11.4 Randomized studies comparing hepatic arterial infusion (HAI) with control groups of supportive care with or without intravenous chemotherapy (IVC)

Author	Patients (n)	Response rate (%)		Median survival (months)		survival (%) (HAI/IVC)	
		HAI	IVC	HAI	IVC	One year	Two years
Rougier (1992)[48]	166	41	12	15	10	64/44	23/11
Allen-Mersh (1994)[30]	100	–	–	13.4	7.5	50/42*	18/17*

* Data computed from graphs by the authors.

Table 11.5   Results of the meta-analysis group in Cancer (1996): hepatic arterial infusion (HAI) versus intravenous chemotherapy (IVC)

Patients (n)	Response rate (%)		Median survival (months)		survival (%) (HAI/IVC)	
	HAI	IVC	HAI	IVC	One year	Two years
654	41	14	17*	11*	65/45*	25/20*

* Data computed from graphs by the authors.

and have therefore produced confusing results.[46,52] Furthermore, patients unable to undergo hepatic arterial infusion because of extrahepatic disease found at laparotomy or because of intraoperative technical problems were apparently considered as treatment failures in the control arms of two studies.[45,48] An equally important issue is that these trials were designed to answer different questions, and comparison, as well as final conclusions, are difficult to draw. When prospective trials are analysed in detail, a number of observations can be drawn. The first concerns *tumour response*. Treatment with hepatic arterial infusion using FUDR generally yields tumour response rates at least three times as high as intravenous chemotherapy. The overall response rate in reported studies averaged 41% for hepatic arterial infusion (range 31–50%; complete response 3%; partial response 38%) and only 14% for intravenous chemotherapy (complete response 2%; partial response 12%), suggesting a significant advantage of hepatic arterial infusion over intravenous chemotherapy. The time to disease progression was also superior in the hepatic arterial infusion group, with an average of 38 vs. 32 weeks for the chemotherapy. Furthermore, treatment modality was found to be the only significant prognostic factor for tumour response.

No individual trial comparing hepatic arterial infusion with intravenous chemotherapy nor their combination by meta-analysis[50] has shown a statistically significant advantage for hepatic arterial infusion in terms of *survival*. The median survival time in the reviewed trials was 16 months for the infusion-treated group compared to 12.2 months for the intravenous chemotherapy-treated group. A statistically significant advantage for hepatic arterial infusion in terms of overall survival was detected only when this treatment group was compared to an *ad libitum* control group analysis,[50] including observation only with supportive care at the onset of symptoms. The median survival time for the hepatic

artery infusion-treated group was 14.5 months compared to 10.1 months for the *ad libitum* treatment group analysis.[50] A second meta-analysis was recently published[51] which included the large study by Hohn *et al.*[46] A survival advantage was only observed at one year for those patients treated by regional infusion therapy. The one-year survival difference being 12.9% (95% confidence interval, 4.8–20.9%; $P = 0.002$). This effect was not maintained at two years where the survival difference was 7.5% (95% confidence interval, 0.9–14.2%; $P = 0.026$).

Local *toxicity* from the use of hepatic arterial infusion, include chemical hepatitis (26–79%), hyperbilirubinaemia and biliary sclerosis. These may become life threatening as a consequence of sclerosing cholangitis (8–35%) and inflammation or ulceration of the stomach or duodenum (Table 11.6) (30–40%). In this setting such ulceration generally does not respond to H_2-receptor blockade. Careful ligation of the minor gastric and duodenal branches originating from the hepatic artery may reduce such gastroduodenal morbidity,[53] but biliary toxicity is unpredictable. Diarrhoea, which can be severe enough to require hospitalization, occurs in 50–60% of patients receiving intravenous chemotherapy but is not found in patients treated with hepatic arterial infusion chemotherapy. The frequent toxicity of this method necessitates treatment interruption in a large proportion of patients (52%),[46] but temporary cessation or dose reduction[48] is often sufficient to control these side-effects. The administration of dexamethasone at a total dose of 20 mg for 14 days,

Table 11.6   Toxicity of hepatic arterial infusion chemotherapy

Complication	Range (%)
Gastritis	17–56
Ulcer	4–40
Diarrhoea	0–23
Biliary sclerosis	0–29
Increased serum glutamate-oxaloacetate transaminase	23–80
Increased bilirubinaemia	13–78

together with FUDR, is effective in preventing hyper-bilirubinaemia while increasing the response rate to 71%.[54] Early recognition and treatment of toxicity is mandatory and liver function should be frequently checked by measuring serum levels of lactate dehy-drogenase, which has proved to be a highly useful marker.[55,56] The toxicities of at least 20 chemothera-peutic agents have been experimentally shown to be dependent on the time of the day administered[57] and the anticancer efficacy of many of these agents has also been shown to have a circadian dependence. Circadian scheduled chemotherapy is feasible both with a totally implantable and with an external pump, but the large amount of infusional fluids required often necessitate more than one external pump. Since the results of non randomized clinical studies are so far available,[55,56] further investigation is needed to support this therapeutic approach.

As previously mentioned, many reports have failed to discriminate between technical and chemotherapeutic complications, which range from 30 to 79%. Nonetheless, it is apparent that approx-imately half of these are related to technical factors alone. In this clinical setting, life threatening com-plications affect 1 out of 5 patients. In addition, it has been shown that a two- to threefold increase in complications exists when the infusion system is implanted by an inexperienced surgeon.[39]

Quality of life is an important issue when dis-cussing treatment options in patients with liver metastasis. Unfortunately this topic has been addressed only by one group[30] utilizing hepatic arte-rial infusion chemotherapy. In this study it was con-cluded that survival can be prolonged and an adequate quality of life can be attained when hepatic arterial infusion is delivered. Nonetheless, this group of treated patients was highly selected and matched against all groups who did not receive hepatic arterial infusion, including those undergo-ing intravenous chemotherapy, palliation only or no treatment at all. No significant difference in post-randomization symptoms, anxiety or depression scores between hepatic arterial infusion and control groups was recorded.

The need to take into account patient preference as well as treatment efficacy and side-effects when con-sidering hepatic arterial infusion chemotherapy has been elegantly pointed out in an editorial by Cole.[58] While regretting the lack of a standard methodology, he stressed that several methods now available to evaluate favourable or unfavourable treatment effects in clinical trials strongly advocated their adoption.

Cost analysis has become an important factor when considering new treatment modalities. Charges that encompass hospitalization, diagnostic work-up, surgical procedures, consultations, drug administration, outpatient visits and nursing, as well as costs associated with time lost from work, should be considered. Only by taking account of all of these factors can the costs be quantified more appropriately than has been previously available when cost-effectiveness analysis was performed. The cost-effectiveness of hepatic arterial infusion could then be determined by calculating the ratio of the incremental cost of such infusion to the average quality-adjusted time gained.[58]

Other Therapeutic Options

Selective means of delivering radiation and biologi-cal therapy are further alternatives to the non-surgi-cal locoregional management of hepatic metastasis. Experimental studies demonstrate that angiotensin II and somatostatin analogues have some effect in redirecting hepatic flow by increasing the volume of flow towards liver metastases. Albumin micros-pheres have been effectively used to enhance intra-arterial drug delivery to tumour tissue in animal models and in preliminary clinical studies.[59] Eighteen Japanese patients with colorectal liver metastasis were treated in one study with de-gradable starch microspheres (DSM).[60] Tumour response rates (11% complete response and 66% partial response) were proportional to the degree of arterial blood flow blockage. The pharmacokinetic properties of arterially infused cisplatin adminis-tered with or without starch microspheres in patients with liver metastasis were extensively inves-tigated by Civalleri.[61] In that study, patients were given intra-arterial cisplatin (25 mg/m^2) with or without 600 mg degradable starch microspheres during intraoperative placement of a catheter. Mean plasma levels of platinum peaked at 2 min and were significantly lower after injection of platinum with DSM than after platinum alone. No differences in urine excretion, total body clearance or plasma protein binding of platinum were observed between the two groups. Tumour platinum concentrations, evaluated by tissue biopsies, were significantly higher after injection of the drug together with

DSM. These results indicate that DSM administration together with the chemotherapeutic agent redistributes the blood flow and induces the extraction of the drug from the liver. In further clinical Phase II studies from Japan,[62,63] response rates of 41% and 69% for colorectal and gastric cancer metastasis respectively were reported with a response duration of 42 days. However, adverse reactions were recorded in 69% of cases (pain 49%, nausea and vomiting 33%, fever 31%, anorexia 6%). Phase III prospective trials are required to assess the use of these agents.

Transcatheter chemoembolization is an alternative locoregional treatment aimed at prolonging contact time of the drug and provoking ischaemia in the neoplastic tissue. This can be achieved by the injection of embolic material such as lipiodol in association with emulsified chemotherapeutic agents. Lipiodol is a lipid compound which has long been used as a lymphatic contrast agent, and recently reintroduced into chemoembolization regimens. By means of a percutaneous femoral arterial approach, selective or even superselective catheterization is possible in experienced hands, using 3Fr gauge angiographic catheters. The procedure may be concluded with the injection of Gelfoam powder, to obstruct the large supplying portal vessels. This obstruction is often temporary and may need to be repeated often. Transcather chemoembolization is generally well tolerated, although various complications have been reported in two-thirds of the patients. Fever, nausea, vomiting or abdominal and back pain represent the so-called 'postembolization syndrome'. Most of these complications either resolve spontaneously or with appropriate medical treatment.[64] It is an effective technique in the management of hepatocellular carcinoma, but there is little evidence to support its role in the treatment of liver metastases.

Intra-arterial chemoinfusion, with complete hepatic venous and extracorporeal chemofiltration, has been developed to increase regional exposure of the drug while reducing systemic toxicity. This consists of percutaneous selective catheterization of the proper hepatic artery for chemoinfusion and placement of a dual-balloon positioned transfemorally within the inferior vena cava to obtain complete hepatic venous isolation. Preclinical evaluation showed that extracorporeal chemofiltration reduced post filter and systemic levels of doxorubicin by >90% compared with prefilter levels.[65] Preliminary experiences have been reported in the treatment of hepatocellular carcinoma, and these experimental studies provide evidence of a possible theoretical advantage also in the treatment of metastatic liver disease.

Finally, the association of regional perfusion with cryotherapy or other treatment modalities, opens further therapeutic perspectives.[66]

Conclusions

Despite the enthusiasm for hepatic arterial infusion chemotherapy by some workers, only very small and selected groups of patients appear likely to benefit from this approach. Although colorectal cancer is highly prevalent in Western societies, only 5% of patients are detected at a time when the liver is the sole site of metastases. Of these, one-half are candidates for liver resection.[67] The resulting low candidacy for hepatic arterial infusion would also apply to patients with liver metastases from other primary tumours.

The therapeutic option of hepatic arterial infusion is expensive. According to the charges of a private Italian institution, pump implantation including pre-operative angiography, laparotomy, surgeon's fees, hospitalization and scintigraphy, cost US$ 5300. Furthermore, the cost of one year of treatment is calculated at US$ 9700 compared to the overall one year cost of 5-FU and folinic acid intravenous chemotherapy of US$ 8800.

Hepatic arterial infusion is associated with not inconsiderable morbidity and consequently cannot be employed as a standard treatment for every patient with metastatic liver disease. Therapeutic infusions are not yet standardized and a variety of drug combinations, modulators, biological response modifiers and steroids have been proposed and administered using different regimens. Furthermore, survival and toxicity have been evaluated using markedly different criteria.[30,44,49,52,68–72]

Although locoregional treatment of the hepatic remnant after surgical resection of metastatic disease has also been attempted, no significant improvement in survival has so far been achieved.[72] This is not to suggest that this complex and highly technological procedure should be withdrawn from the surgical oncologist's armamentarium, but its use should be confined to prospective clinical studies. In the future the administration of systemic treatment together with HAI might decrease the high observed extrahepatic recurrence rates. Ongoing trials should help to address these problems.[74]

It is the physician's responsibility, when approaching a patient with unresectable liver metastases, to explain the option of hepatic arterial infusion chemotherapy as well as other treatment modalities in a realistic manner which is evidence-based. The efficacy as well as the complications of hepatic arterial infusion must be explained in full detail to the patient and family. Treatment goals must include not only an improvement in survival rates, but also in quality of life in this poor prognosis patient population.

References

1. De Brauw LM, Van de Velde CJH, Bouwhuis-Hoogerwerf ML, Zwaveling A. Diagnostic evaluation and survival analysis of colorectal cancer patients with liver metastasis. *J Surg Oncol* 1997; **34**:81–86.
2. Breedis C, Young G. The blood supply of neoplasms in the liver. *Am J Pathol* 1954; **30**:969–985.
3. Wang Li-Qing, Persson BG, Bergquist L, Bengmark S. Influence of dearterialization on distribution of absolute tumor blood flow between hepatic artery and portal vein. *Cancer* 1994; **74**:2454–2459.
4. Weiss L. Metastatic inefficiency and regional therapy for liver metastases from colorectal carcinoma. *Reg Cancer Treat* 1989; **2**:77–81.
5. Cohen A, Schaeffer N, Higgins J. Treatment of metastatic colorectal cancer with hepatic artery combination chemotherapy. *Cancer* 1986; **57**:1115–1117.
6. Sigurdson ER, Ridge JA, Kemeny N, Daly JM. Tumor and liver drug uptake following hepatic artery and portal vein infusion. *J Clin Oncol* 1987; **5**:1936–1940.
7. Collins JM. Pharmacologic rationale for regional drug delivery. *J Clin Oncol* 1984; **2**:498–504.
8. Chen HS, Gross JF. Intra-arterial infusion of anticancer drugs: theoretic aspects of drug delivery and review of responses. *Cancer Treat Rep* 1980; **64**:31–40.
9. Ensminger WD, Rosowsky A, Raso V. A clinical-pharmacological evaluation of hepatic arterial infusion of 5-fluoro-2'-deoxyuridine and 5-fluorouracil. *Cancer Res* 1978; **38**:3784–3792.
10. Oberfield RA, Mc Cahney JA *et al.* Prolonged and continuous percutaneous intraarterial hepatic infusion chemotherapy in advanced metastatic liver adenocarcinoma from colorectal primary. *Cancer* 1979; **44**:414.
11. Ansfield FJ, Ramirez G. Intrahepatic arterial infusion with 5-FU. *Cancer* 1971; **28**:1147–1151.
12. Klopp CT, Alford TC, Bateman J *et al.* Fractionated intra-arterial cancer chemotherapy with methylbisamine hydrochloride: a preliminary report. *Ann Surg* 1950; **132**:811–832.
13. Clarkson B, Young C, Dierick W, Kuehn P, Kim M, Berrett A, Clapp P, Lawrence W Jr. Effects of continuous hepatic artery infusion of antimetabolites on primary and metastatic cancer of the liver. *Cancer* 1962; **15**:472–488.
14. Brennan MJ, Talley RW, Drake EH *et al.* 5-fluorouracil treatment of liver metastases by continuous hepatic artery infusion via catheter. *Ann Surg* 1963; **158**:405–419.
15. Ohya T, Fukunaga J, Kitahama H *et al.* Clinical evaluation and problem of intra-arterial infusion chemotherapy of liver metastases from digestive organ cancer. *Gan To Kagaku Ryoho* 1990; **17**:1808–1810.
16. Taguchi T. Proceedings: International Conference on Regional Chemotherapy for Liver Cancer. *Reg Cancer Treat* 1992; **5**:1–170.
17. Kemeny N. The systemic chemotherapy of hepatic metastases. *Sem Oncol* 1983; **10**:148–158.
18. McEntee GP, Nagorney DM, Kvols LK *et al.* Cytoreductive hepatic surgery for neuroendocrine tumors. *Surgery* 1990; **108**:1091–1096.
19. Kath R, Hayungs J, Bornfeld N *et al.* Prognosis and treatment of disseminated uveal melanoma. *Cancer* 1993; **72**:2219–2123.
20. Mavligit GM, Charsangavej C, Carrasco CH *et al.* Regression of ocular melanoma metastatic to the liver after hepatic chemoembolization with cisplatin and polyvinyl sponge. *J Am Med Ass* 1988; **260**:974–976.
21. Niederhuber JE, Ensminger W, Gyves J, Thrall J, Walker S, Cozzi E. Regional chemotherapy of colorectal cancer metastatic to the liver. *Cancer* 1984; **53**(6):1336–43.
22. Barone RM, Byfield JE, Goldfarb PB, Frankel S, Ginn C, Greer S. Intra-arterial chemotherapy using an implantable infusion pump and liver irradiation for the treatment of hepatic metastases. *Cancer* 1982; **50**(5), 850–62.
23. Patt YZ, Boddie AW Jr, Charnsangavej C, Ajani JA, Wallace S, Soski M, Claghorn L, Mavligt GM. Hepatic arterial infusion with floxuridine and cisplatin: overriding importance of antitumor effect versus degree of tumor burden as determinants of survival among patients with colorectal cancer. *J Clin Oncol* 1986; **4**(9):1356–64.
24. Shumata CR. Colorectal cancer hepatic metastases: the surgeons role. *Alabama Medical* 1994; **63**:15–8.
25. Bozzetti F, Doci R, Bignami P *et al.* Patterns of failure following surgical resection of colorectal cancer liver metastases: rationale for a multimodal approach. *Ann Surg* 1987; **204**:264–270.
26. Ligidakis NJ, Ziras N, Parissis J. Resection versus resection combined with adjuvant pre- and post-operative chemotherapy–immunotherapy for metastatic colorectal liver cancer. *Hepato-gastroenterology* 1995; **42**:155–161.
27. Endo Y, Tani T, Kawaguchi A *et al.* Prevention of postoperative recurrence after hepatic resection for metastatic colorectal cancer by adjuvant locoregional chemotherapy. *Gan To Kagaku Ryoho* 1993; **20**(11):1535–1537.
28. Sugarbaker PH, Steves MA. A cytoreductive approach to treatment of multiple liver metastases. *J Surg Oncol* (Suppl) 1993; **3**:161–165.
29. Kemeny N. Role of chemotherapy in the treatment of colorectal carcinoma. *Sem Surg Oncol* 1987; **3**:190–214.
30. Allen-Mersh TG, Earlam S, Fordy C *et al.* Quality of life and survival with continuous hepatic-artery floxuridine infusion for colorectal liver metastases. *Lancet* 1994; **344**:1255–1260.
31. Michels NA. Newer anatomy of the liver and its variant blood supply and collateral circulation. *Am J Surg* 1996; **112**:337–347.
32. Doughty JC, Warren H, Anderson JH *et al.* Response to regional chemotherapy in patients with variant hepatic arterial anatomy. *Br J Surg* 1995; **83**:652–653.
33. Burke D, Earlam S, Fordy C, Allen-Mersh TG. Effect of aberrant hepatic arterial anatomy on tumour response to hepatic artery infusion of floxuridine for colorectal liver metastases. *Br J Surg* 1995; **82**:1098–1100.
34. Hughs KS, Villella ER. An improved technique for regional perfusion chemotherapy in the presence of a replaced right hepatic artery using a single implantable pump. *Surgery* 1984; **95**:355–357.
35. Watkins E Jr, Khazei AM, Nahra KS. Surgical basis for arterial infusion chemotherapy of disseminated carcinoma of the liver. *Surg Gynecol Obstet* 1970; **130**:581–605.

36. Healey JD, Schroy PC. The intrahepatic distribution of the hepatic artery in man. *Intern Coll Surg* 1953; **20**: 133.

37. Chuang VP, Wallace S. Hepatic artery redistribution for intraarterial infusion of hepatic neoplasm. *Radiology* 1980; **135**:295–9.

38. Civelek AC, Sitzmann JV, Chin BB et al. Misperfusion of the liver during hepatic artery infusion chemotherapy: value of postoperative angiography and postoperative pump scintigraphy. *AJR* 1993; **160**:865–870.

39. Campbell KA, Burns RC, Sitzmann JV et al. Regional chemotherapy devices: effect of experience and anatomy on complications. *J Clin Oncol* 1993; **11**:822–826.

40. Kaplan WD, Ensminger WD, Come SE et al. Radionuclide angiography to predict patient response to hepatic artery chemotherapy. *Cancer Treat Resp* 1980; **64**:1217–1222.

41. Patt YZ. Regional hepatic arterial chemotherapy for colorectal cancer metastatic to the liver: the controversy continues. *J Clin Oncol* 1993; **11**:815–819.

42. Durand Zaleski I, Roche B, Buyse M, Carlson R, O'Connell MJ. Economic implications of hepatic arterial infusion chemotherapy in treatment of nonresectable colorectal liver metastasis. Meta-Analysis Group in Cancer. *J National Cancer Inst* 1997; **89**(11):790–5.

43. Zimmerman T, Padberg W, Kelm C et al. Locoregional chemotherapy in the treatment of liver metastasis of breast carcinoma. *Zentralbl Chir* 1992; **117**(4):226–230.

44. Sugihara K. Continuous hepatic arterial infusion of 5-fluorouracil for unresectable colorectal liver metastases: Phase II study. *Surgery* 1995; **117**:624–628.

45. Chang AE, Schneider PD, Sugarbaker PH. A prospective randomized trial of regional versus systemic continuous 5-fluorodeoxyuridine chemotherapy in the treatment of colorectal liver metastases. *Ann Surg* 1987; **206**:685–693.

46. Hohn DC, Stagg RJ, Friedman MA et al. A randomized trial of continuous intravenous versus hepatic intraarterial floxuridine in patients with colorectal cancer metastatic to the liver: The Northern California Oncology Group trial. *J Clin Oncol* 1989; **7**:1646–1654.

47. Martin JK, O'Connel MJ, Wienand HS et al. Intra-arterial floxuridine versus systemic fluorouracil for hepatic metastases from colorectal cancer: a randomized trial. *Arch Surg* 1990; **125**:1022–1027.

48. Rougier P, Laplache A, Hugier M et al. Hepatic arterial infusion of fluxuridine in patients with liver metastases from colorectal carcinoma: long-term results of a prospective randomized trial. *J Clin Oncol* 1992; **10**:1112–1118.

49. Kemeny N. Current approach to metastatic colorectal cancer. *Sem Oncol* 1994; **21**:67–75.

50. Meta-Analysis Group in Cancer. Reappraisal of hepatic arterial infusion in the treatment of nonresectable liver metastases from colorectal cancer. *JNCI* 1996; **88**(5):252–258.

51. Harmantas A, Rotstein LE, Langer B. Regional versus systemic chemotherapy in the treatment of colorectal carcinoma metastatic to the liver – is there a survival difference? Meta-analysis of the published literature. *Cancer* 1996; **78**:1639–1645.

52. Kemeny b N, Daly J, Reichman B et al. Intrahepatic or systemic infusion of fluorodeoxyuridine in patients with liver metastases from colorectal carcinoma: a randomized trial. *Ann Intern Med* 1987; **107**:459–465.

53. Hohn DC, Stagg RJ, Price DC, Lewis BJ. Avoidance of gastroduodenal toxicity in patients receiving hepatic arterial 5-fluoro-2'-deoxyuridine. *J Clin Oncol* 1985; **3**:1257.

54. Kemeny N, Seiter K, Niedzwiecki D et al. A randomized trial of intrahepatic infusion of fluorodeoxyuridine with dexamethasone versus fluodeoxyuridine alone in the treatment of metastatic colorectal cancer. *Cancer* 1992; **69**:327–334.

55. Hrushesky WJM. Infusional chronochemotherapy for cancer. *J Infusional Chemotherapy* 1992; **2**:64–65.

56. Hrushesky WJM. Theoretical and practical implications of circadian pharmacodynamics. *J Infusional Chemotherapy* 1992; **2**:66–68.

57. Hrushesky WJ, Bjarnason GA. Circadian cancer therapy. *J Clin Oncol* 1993; **11**:1403–1417.

58. Cole BF. Trade-offs of hepatic arterial infusion. *JCNI* 1996; **88**(5):223–224.

59. McCulloch P. Nonsurgical treatment of liver metastases. *Curr Opin Gen Surg* 1994; **151**:5.

60. Yamada T. Experimental and clinical trial of degradable starch microspheres (DSM) in treatment of hepatic neoplasm. *Nippon Igaku Hoshasen Gakkai Zasshi* 1995; **55**(11):732–738.

61. Civalleri D, Esposito M, Fulco RA et al. Liver and tumor uptake and plasma pharmacokinetic of arterial cisplatin administered with and without starch microspheres in patients with liver metastases. *Cancer* 1991; **68**(5):988–994.

62. Taguchi T, Tanikawa K, Sano K et al. Multi-center cooperative Phase II study of combined infusion of PJ-203 (degradable starch microspheres) into hepatic artery in metastatic liver cancer. *Gan To Kagaku Ryoho* 1993; **20**(13):2015–2025.

63. Taguchi T, Kondo M, Tanikawa K et al. Comparative clinical study in metastatic liver cancer between intra-arterial infusion of mitomycin-C alone and intra-arterial infusion of mitomycin-C combined with PJ-203 (degradable starch microspheres). *Gan To Kagaku Ryoho* 1993; **20**(13):2027–2035.

64. Audisio RA, Doci R, Mazzaferro V, Bellegotti L et al. Hepatic arterial embolization with microencapsulated mitomycin C for unresectable hepatocellular carcinoma in cirrhosis. *Cancer* 1990; **66**:228–236.

65. Curley SA, Chase JL, Roh MS et al. Technical considerations and complications associated with the placement of 180 implantable hepatic arterial infusion devices. *Surgery* 1993; **114**:928–935.

66. Krentz A, Mayer D, Olliff S, Bailey C, Libman L, Nattrass M. Cryotherapy of hepatic metastases and regional perfusion with low-dose streptozocin in the management of metastatic malignant insulinoma. *Endocrine-Related Cancer* 1996; **3**:3411–345.

67. Begos DG, Ballantyne GH. Regional chemotherapy for colorectal liver metastases: thirty years without patient benefit. *J Surg Oncol* 1994; **56**:139–144.

68. Kemeny N, Cohen A, Bertino JR et al. Continuous intrahepatic infusion of floxuridine and leucovorin through an implantable pump for the treatment of hepatic metastases from colorectal carcinoma. *Cancer* 1990; **65**:2446–2450.

69. Kemeny N, Cohen A, Seiter K et al. Randomized trial of hepatic arterial floxuridine, Mitomycin C and carmustine vs. floxuridine alone in previously treated patients with liver metastases from colorectal cancer. *J Clin Oncol* 1993; **11**:330–335.

70. Stagg RJ, Venook AP, Chase JL et al. Alternating hepatic intra-arterial floxuridine and Fluorouracil: a less toxic regimen for treatment of liver metastases from colorectal cancer. *JNCI* 1991; **83**:423–428.

71. Klotz HP, Weder W, Largiader F. Local and systemic toxicity of intra-hepatic arterial 5-FU and high-dose or low-dose leucovorin for liver metastase of colorectal cancer. *Surg Oncol* 1994; **3**:11–16.

72. Mavligit GM, Zukiwski AA, Charsangavej C et al. Regional biologic therapy. Hepatic arterial infusion of recombinant human tumor necrosis factor in patients with liver metastases. *Cancer* 1992; **69**:557–561.

73. Wagman LD, Kemeny MM, Leong L et al. A prospective, randomized evaluation of the treatment of colorectal cancer metastatic to the liver. *J Clin Oncol* 1990; **8**:1885–1893.

74. Kemeny MM. Hepatic resection: when, what kind, and for which patients? *J Surg Oncol* (Suppl) 1991; **2**:54–58.

Radiotherapy

Carlo Greco and Bruce D. Minsky

12

Introduction

Until recently, radiation therapy has had a relatively limited role in the management of patients with liver metastases from solid tumours. Two broad approaches of radiation therapy in the treatment of liver metastasis can be considered. It can be employed as a palliative modality in patients with painful metastasis or secondly as a potentially curative therapy for patients with medically or technically unresectable metastasis and who have no evidence of extrahepatic disease.

In the palliative setting, whole liver radiation has been beneficial in patients with symptomatic disease. With doses of 20–30 Gy, 55–90% of patients had improvement in liver function tests and pain and 50% had a decrease in liver size.[1-5]

Unfortunately, the tolerance of the normal liver is 30 Gy which considerably restricts the dose of radiation that can be safely administered to the whole liver. This dose is inadequate to control gross disease of solid tumours and therefore limits the role of radiation as a curative modality.[6] In order to address this limitation, research has been directed both at methods of amplifying the effects of radiation on the tumour relative to normal liver parenchyma such as hypoxic cell sensitizers and chemotherapy, as well as methods of delivering radiation more selectively to the tumour while sparing surrounding normal liver such as intraoperative brachytherapy, radiolabelled microspheres, and three-dimensional conformal radiation therapy. To date, the theoretical advantages of hypoxic cell radiation sensitizers such as misonidazole have not translated into improved responses in clinical trials.[7] More promising results have been obtained with the addition of systemic and/or intra-hepatic chemotherapy, however, randomized trials are needed before this is known with certainty.

The availability of three-dimensional treatment planning with dose volume histogram (DVH) analysis as well as the development of conformal techniques of radiation delivery has made it feasible to concentrate high doses of radiation to tumour-bearing areas of the liver while not exceeding normal liver tissue tolerance. These techniques allow the escalation of radiation doses to limited portions of the liver. When combined with chemotherapy, this approach offers the most promising results in selected patients with liver metastases not amenable to surgical resection.[8-10]

This chapter will review the tolerance of the liver to radiation therapy, the results of treatment with conventional radiation techniques, and the rationale and preliminary results with the use of newer radiotherapeutic approaches. The discussion is limited to patients with liver metastasis from solid tumors, the majority of which derive from colorectal cancer.

Radiation Tolerance of the Liver

The ability to deliver therapeutic doses of radiation to the liver is significantly restricted by its radiosensitivity. The clinical syndromes and the associated pathologic changes associated with liver radiation have been well described.

Clinical Appearance of Radiation Hepatitis

The clinical syndrome of acute radiation hepatitis may develop 2–24 weeks after radiation and clinically resembles the Budd–Chiari syndrome. It is characterized by rapid weight gain, increased abdominal girth, tender hepatomegaly and ascites.[11] Serum alkaline phosphatase is usually elevated, while other liver function tests may be only slightly abnormal. The treatment of acute radiation hepatitis is similar to the medical management of hepatic insufficiency. The majority of patients recover within three months.

Clinicopathologic Features of Radiation Hepatitis

The primary histological feature of radiation hepatitis is central vein thrombosis at the lobular level resulting in hepatocyte changes due to obstruction in small efferent veins. This veno-occlusive mechanism of tissue damage is unique to the liver and is unlike the more typical fine arteriolar-capillary damage observed in most other radiation-induced normal tissue injuries. It may represent an endothelial platelet agglutination phenomenon.[12] Thrombocytopenia frequently accompanies the onset of radiation hepatitis.

Sufficient revascularization usually occurs within four months from the onset of radiation hepatitis, allowing restoration of the normal hepatic architecture and function. However, if severe acute histological changes have occurred, they often lead to progressive fibrosis and/or cirrhosis with subsequent liver failure. Cell-to-cell interactions mediated by cytokines such as transforming growth factor (TGF-β_1) may play an important role in radiation-induced liver injury.[13]

Ingold et al. published a landmark report in the 1960s describing 40 patients who received whole-liver irradiation during the course of abdominal radiation therapy for Hodgkin's disease or ovarian carcinoma. Total doses ranged between 13 Gy in 18 days to 51 Gy in 40 days.[11] Four to six weeks following radiation therapy, 13 patients developed symptoms of liver damage, consisting of anorexia, tender hepatomegaly, jaundice and ascites. Liver biopsies revealed abnormalities in the centrolobular zone with severe sinusoidal congestion and dilated central veins. Repeat biopsies obtained three to four months later showed changes in the central veins ranging from minimal hyaline endothelial thickening to complete occlusion of the vein. Of the 13 patients, 3 died from radiation-induced liver failure.

A similar study by Reed and Cox outlined the temporal sequence of histological changes following liver radiation.[14] Twelve patients underwent multiple sequential liver biopsies following hepatic irradiation. A characteristic progression of changes were observed during the first four months following radiation. These consisted of hyperaemia, centrolobular cell necrosis and occlusion of efferent veins. With further follow-up, these changes were replaced by either centrolobular fibrosis with cirrhotic reconstruction of liver architecture, or more commonly, by eventual restoration of normal liver parenchyma.

Normal Liver Tolerance to Radiation

As seen with other organs, the risk of developing radiation hepatitis is related to total dose and fractionation schedule. Following whole-liver radiation with conventional fractionation (1.8–2.0Gy/fraction), radiation hepatitis is uncommon at total doses between 20 and 30 Gy, but there is a marked increase in incidence with total doses >35 Gy. The hepatocyte is a highly differentiated cell with low repair capacities and an estimated α/β ratio of 1.5 Gy.

The tolerance dose for whole-liver radiation with conventional fractionation for a 5% incidence of radiation hepatitis (TD_5) is 25 Gy, while the dose for a 50% incidence (TD_{50}) is 35 Gy. The accepted tolerance doses in adults for whole-liver irradiation with non-conventional fractionation schedules vary from 21 to 24 Gy at 3 Gy/fraction, 24 Gy at 2.5 Gy/fraction and 30 Gy at 1.5 Gy/fraction.[15]

Since the publication of the data from Ingold et al., most radiation oncologists have been reluctant to treat the liver with doses >30 Gy. However, since normal liver tolerance depends, in part, on the volume of radiated tissue, small volumes of the liver can be safely treated to higher doses. The use of DVH analysis, which produces a graphic display of the distribution of dose over specifically defined volumes, has greatly contributed to the definition of normal tissue complication probabilities (NTCPs) of liver irradiation.[8,16] Using a conformal radiation therapy approach, the incorporation of DVH analysis in the treatment-planning process may enable an escalation of the dose to the tumour within a prescribed NTCP. A cumulative DVH of the normal liver (normal liver volume minus tumour volume) receiving a dose not >50% of the prescribed dose can be used as a safe criterion to establish the total dose to the target volume. For example, if the amount of normal liver treated to >50% of the prescribed dose is <33%, then the target volume dose can be escalated to 66 Gy. If the DVH reveals that the amount of liver receiving >50% of the prescribed dose falls between 33% and 66%, then a total dose of 48 Gy should not be exceeded.[9]

The Impact of Other Modalities on Liver Tolerance

Although the combination of therapies may improve the results of radiation therapy, they may (also) increase its toxicity. This increase has been reported with the addition of both surgery and/or chemotherapy.

Radiation hepatitis occurs more commonly following partial hepatectomy. Clinical data suggest that a lower dose threshold should be applied for liver radiation in the immediate postresection period.[17] However, if a sufficient amount of time (usually about one month) is allowed for liver parenchyma regeneration after partial hepatectomy, normal liver tolerance is found.[6]

The concomitant use of radiation therapy plus chemotherapy may result in greater liver toxicity. However, there appears to be a considerable variation of normal tissue damage depending on the drug and its sequencing with radiation. Clinical experience in children treated for Wilms' tumour reveals that actinomycin D results in higher liver toxicity when it is delivered concomitantly with radiation than would be expected by either agent alone.[18] Due to impaired liver metabolism, actinomycin D and vincristine have a longer half-life in patients who receive liver radiation. The concomitant use of Adriamycin and liver irradiation may also increase liver toxicity.[19] However, the combination of radiation therapy and fluorinated pyrimidine infusion has not been reported to result in significantly enhanced liver toxicity.[6]

Whole Liver Radiation Therapy

Conventional Fractionation

Five studies have examined the effectiveness of whole-liver external beam radiation therapy in the management of patients with liver metastases

Table 12.1 Response rate and survival following external beam radiation therapy for hepatic metastases

Author	Patients (n)	Dose (Gy)	Response (%)	Survival (months)
Phillips[2]	36	20–37.5	72%	NK
Turek Masicheider[5]	11	16–25	90%	NK
Prasad[3]	20	19–31	95%	4
Sherman[1]	50	21–30	89%	4.5
Borgelt[4]	103	21–30	55%	2.8

NK = not known.

(Table 12.1).[1-5] Most of the patients included in these studies had liver metastases from colorectal primaries had failed systemic chemotherapy, and were treated with total doses of 20–30 Gy at 1.5–3.0 Gy/fraction. 'Significant' palliation (pain relief) was achieved in 55–95% and up to 49% experienced a decrease in liver size and improvement in liver function tests. The median survival was short (3–9 months) and death was usually due to progression of disease. Sherman et al. reported a one year actuarial survival of 21% and pain relief usually lasting for the duration of the patient's survival.[1]

Hyperfractionation

Hyperfractionated radiation therapy involves multiple small fractions (two or more a day) separated by 4–6 hours to allow for normal tissue repair. The rationale is to improve local control by reducing the opportunity for tumour repopulation by rapidly proliferating tumour clonogens.[20] The goal is to decrease long-term morbidity while increasing the total dose of radiation that can be safely delivered in a shorter overall treatment time. This approach has been tested by the Radiation Therapy Oncology Group (RTOG) in a dose-escalation study for palliation of patients with symptomatic liver metastases (RTOG 8405).

In order to determine if there is a palliative benefit from this treatment a favorable subset of patients with a median survival of at least six months must be identified. Leibel et al. assessed clinical data from previous RTOG studies and determined that patients presenting with the following clinical characteristics have a predicted survival of 50% at six months: total bilirubin <1.5 mg/dl Karnovsky Performance Score >80, and no extrahepatic metastases.[21] When examined by primary site, patients with colorectal primaries had a significantly better prognosis than those with either lung or breast cancer. There was no significant survival difference between patients with solitary versus multiple liver metastases.

Patients selected for the RTOG 8405 dose-escalation study were treated with 1.5 Gy/fraction twice a day to total doses of 27, 30 and 33 Gy. Further dose escalation to 36 Gy was not possible since two patients developed clinical radiation hepatitis at the 33 Gy dose level. However, both patients died of progression of disease rather than toxicity. The median survival was approximately four months and dose had no significant impact on survival.[22]

Radiation Combined with Misonidazole

As tumours enlarge, they tend to outgrow their blood supply resulting in focal and diffuse areas of necrosis surrounded by a zone of cells with borderline oxygen tension. Well-oxygenated cells are up to three times more sensitive to the effects of radiation compared with hypoxic cells.

A group of compounds known as the nitroimidazoles selectively sensitize hypoxic tumour cells both in vitro and in vivo. The hypoxic cell sensitizer misonidazole was introduced into clinical trials by the RTOG in 1977.[7] The initial trial was a phase I/II study assessing the safety and efficacy of misonidazole combined with whole-liver irradiation (3.0 Gy/fraction $\times$ 7) in patients with liver metastasis.[23] Of the 42 evaluable patients who presented with abdominal pain, 63% had complete pain relief. The median survival was 4.2 months and patients continued in either a mild pain or pain-free status for 80% of their remaining life. There were no cases of radiation hepatitis.

Based on these preliminary data, the RTOG conducted a randomized prospective trial to determine if the combination of whole liver irradiation (3.0 Gy/fraction $\times$ 7) plus misonidazole (1.5 g/m^2 orally, daily 4–6 h before each treatment) was superior to whole-liver radiation therapy alone. Of 187 evaluable patients, 94 were randomized to radiation therapy alone and 93 received the combination of radiation and misonidazole. Endpoints included hepatic pain, Karnovsky Performance Score, alkaline phosphatase liver and tumour size, and overall survival.

Although there was a trend towards an improved response rate with misonidazole, it did not improve

significantly any of the endpoints studied. In symptomatic patients, liver radiation was effective in relieving pain in 80% and in 54%, the pain disappeared completely. Pain was relieved more frequently in patients treated in the combined radiation plus misonidazole arm compared to radiation alone (87% vs. 74%). The majority of patients who experienced clinical improvement did so within three weeks and the median duration of response was 13 weeks. The median survival of patients treated with radiation therapy plus misonidazole was similar to radiation therapy alone (4.2 months vs. 4.3 months, respectively). Liver radiation was well tolerated, with 22% of patients in both treatment groups developing only mild nausea. There were no documented cases of radiation-induced hepatitis. Although there were no life-threatening complications with misonidazole, neurotoxicity was noted. Seventeen patients developed peripheral neuropathy and three developed central nervous system toxicity. For the total patient group the one-year survival was 12%.[7]

Radiation Combined with Chemotherapy

In an attempt to increase the effectiveness of radiation therapy, a number of trials have been designed to evaluate the combination of conventional external beam radiation therapy and chemotherapy. In these trials, chemotherapy was given by intrahepatic infusion, intravenous infusion or a combuation of both. The intrahepatic route is preferred since the blood supply of both primary and metastatic liver tumours is primarily derived from the hepatic artery. This is in contrast to the normal liver parenchyma which obtains 75–80% of its blood supply from the portal vein.[24]

The rationale for the combined modality approach is based on in vivo animal tumour models. They suggest a synergistic effect with the combination of radiation with certain drugs, particularly the halogenated pyrimidines.[25,26] 5-Fluorouracil (5-FU), 5-fluorodeoxyuridine (FUDR), and other halogenated pyrimidines have been shown to sensitize selectively tumour cells to radiation, probably through synchronization at the G_1–S interphase.

Several studies have been performed using whole-liver external beam radiation in combination with 5-FU and/or FUDR (Table 12.2).[27–33] FUDR and 5-FU are ideal agents for regional chemotherapy delivered by hepatic artery infusion, since they are actively

Table 12.2 Clinical studies of combined radiation and chemotherapy for hepatic metastases

Author	Year	Patients (n)	Dose (Gy)	Drug	Response (%)	Survival (months)
Herbsman[28]	1978	13	25–30	IAH FUDR	68	16
Webber[31]	1978	25	25	IAH FUDR	72	12.3
Friedman[27]	1979	21	13.5–21	IAH 5-FU/Doxo	55	3.4
Lokich[29]	1981	16	25–30	IAH 5-FU or FUDR	62	NA
Barone[32]	1982	18	30	IAH FUDR	67	8
Rotman[30]	1986	23	27.25	i.v. 5-FU	83	6.9
Raju[33]	1987	12	21 HF	IAH FUDR or 5-FU	83	>18

Abbreviations: IAH, intra-arterial hepatic; 5-FU, 5-fluorouracil; FUDR, 5-fluorodeoxyuridine; Doxo, doxorubicin; HF, hyperfractionated RT; NA, data not available.

extracted by the liver leading to reduced systemic drug levels. Hepatic extraction of FUDR in particular, was found to be 97–99% when administered by hepatic artery infusion, compared to 25–30% extraction of 5-FU, suggesting that FUDR is a more selective drug for this route of administration.[34,35]

In general, patients have received whole-liver radiation to total doses of 20–30 Gy at 2.0–3.0 Gy/fraction with concomitant intra-arterial FUDR or systemic continuous infusion 5-FU. In one study, both Adriamycin and 5-FU were concomitantly administered by intra-arterial hepatic infusion.[27] In the study by Raju et al., 12 patients with liver metastases from colorectal cancer were treated with hyperfractionated whole-liver radiation therapy at 1.5 Gy/fraction to a total dose of 21 Gy. Four patients received concurrent intrahepatic FUDR and 8 received concurrent continuous infusion 5-FU. Symptomatic relief of symptoms was seen in all patients and 83% had an objective response confirmed by CT scan. Two patients were alive at two years. There were no significant differences in the quality, degree or duration of palliation in patients treated with intrahepatic FUDR compared with continuous infusion 5-FU.[33]

Most studies report that the combined modality therapy is well tolerated with acceptable acute and late toxicity. However, Byfield et al. reported a case of treatment related fatal hepatic necrosis in one of 28 patients who received intrahepatic FUDR and concomitant whole-liver radiation therapy (2.5 Gy × 4, every 2–3 weeks to a total dose of 30 Gy.[36]

The mean response rates of combined modality therapy (68%, range: 55–83%) are similar if not superior to those reported in studies using intravenous chemotherapy alone (approximately 30%) or intra-arterial chemotherapy alone (approximately 60%), and suggest an improvement when retrospectively compared with whole liver irradi-

ation alone. Unfortunately, few prospective randomized data exist. Wiley et al. performed a randomized trial of intraarterial 5-FU alone versus intra-arterial 5-FU plus sequential 25.5 Gy whole-liver radiation. The response and survival rates were similar in the two treatment arms. It should be emphasized, however, that the sequential design (rather than concurrent) may not have offered the ideal method of radiosensitization by 5-FU.[37]

Innovative Radiation Therapy Techniques

Innovative methods of delivering radiation to the liver include intra-operative brachytherapy, intrahepatic yttrium-90 labelled microspheres, radiolabelled antibodies, and three-dimensional conformal therapy.

Intra-operative Brachytherapy

Intra-operative brachytherapy has the dosimetric advantage of delivering a high radiation dose within the tumour volume with a corresponding rapid dose fall-off to allow for normal tissue tolerance. The availability of modern ultrasonography techniques for needle placement has made this approach technically feasible for percutaneous application. DriTschilo et al. reported the results of a pilot study in which patients with technically inoperable liver metastases were treated with an afterloading interstitial high activity (10 Ci) lr-192 source delivering 20 Gy in a single fraction. The number of lesions treated in each patient ranged from two to eleven.

With a median follow-up of 8 months (range: 3–18 months), there were no radiation-related complications.[38] In an update of this approach reported by Thomas et al. doses of up to 30 Gy were delivered. Of 24 interstitial irradiation procedures at a median follow up of 11 months, no acute or late radiation toxicity was observed.[39] Tumours were locally controlled for a median of 8 months. Two patients underwent a second procedure and a biopsy of the previously treated lesions revealed a complete pathologic response.

Intrahepatic Yttrium-90 Labelled Microspheres

Yttrium-90 is a pure beta emitter with an average energy of 0.94 MeV and an average half-life of 64 h. Following injection into the hepatic artery, the microspheres are selectively entrapped within the tumour capillary bed. Calculated tumour doses of 50–100 Gy can be delivered resulting in a 65% response rate in selected patients.[40,41] Yttrium-90 microsphere therapy has received approval for use as a conventional therapy in Canada.[42]

Radiolabeled Antibodies

The monoclonal antibody I-131 labelled anti-carcinoembryonic antigen (CEA) lgG has been used by Order et al. in patients with metastatic colorectal cancer to the liver. There were no significant responses and dosimetric studies showed that the tumour concentration achieved was not significantly different than normal liver parenchyma.[43] CEA may not be the ideal target antigen. Antibodies against other antigens and new isotopes are being investigated. Further experience in the use of monoclonal antibodies is detailed in Chapter 14.

Three-Dimensional Conformal Radiation Plus Chemotherapy

While it is accepted that normal liver tissue tolerance to radiation depends on the volume of tissue treated, the tools to evaluate this relationship have only recently become available. Lawrence et al., from the University of Michigan have designed a series of protocols for the treatment of liver malignancies which use DVH analysis to determine the total dose of radiation that could be delivered safely to reduced portions of the liver. Their initial experience included 36 patients with liver metastasis from colorectal cancer who received hyperfractionated whole-liver radiation (1.5 Gy/fraction twice a day separated by at least 4 h plus concomitant intra-arterial FUDR. Of the 36, 21 (58%) had disease that could be delineated on computed tomography scan, and received an additional boost. The total dose was determined by the DVH and was based on the volume of normal tissue treated to a dose >50% of the prescribed dose in the process of treating the tumour volume. The normal liver volume was defined as the volume of apparently uninvolved liver remaining after the tumour volumes were subtracted from the entire liver volume. The patients whose boost plan DVH indicated that ⩽25% of the normal liver would be treated during the boost received an additional of 30–36 Gy. If the DVH indicated that a patient could receive a boost while still sparing >50% of the normal liver, an additional dose of 15–18 Gy was given. A minimum treatment volume of 1000 cm^3 was required to be eligible for boost treatment. Only two patients developed significant radiation hepatitis.[8]

In a more recent report from the University of Michigan group using a similar treatment regimen, 11% (9 of 79) of patients developed radiation hepatitis.[44] However, all 9 had received whole liver irradiation as all or part of their treatment, thereby resulting in a mean total whole-liver dose of at least 37 Gy. Patients treated with the high dose three-dimensional conformal radiation therapy have had better response rates compared with those treated by whole-liver radiation therapy alone.[44,45] In an effort to further improve the results of high-dose three-dimensional conformal radiation therapy for metastatic colorectal cancer, a clinical trial using intra-arterial bromodeoxyuridine, a thymidine analog radiosensitizer, is currently in progress.[9]

Robertson et al. from the University of Michigan group, reported the results of a dose escalation study in 22 patients[4]. Based on the treatment related liver toxicity seen in the previous studies, the practice of whole-liver radiation as the first portion of the treatment was avoided, except in 3 of the 22 patients. The total dose to the target volume was based on the DVH analysis which examined the percentage volume of normal liver treated to >50% of the prescribed dose. If the amount of normal liver treated to >50% of the dose was <33%, the target volume received 66 Gy, whereas if the amount of normal liver treated to >50% of the prescribed dose was 33–66%, then the dose was limited to 48 Gy. The radiation was administered twice a day at 1.5 Gy/fraction with concomitant intra-arterial FUDR (0.2 mg/kg/day). The total dose of radiation was escalated by 10% (52.8 Gy and 72.6 Gy respectively) after at least 3 patients, for each of the two dose values, had completed treatment and had been observed for at least two months. In order to maintain the same overall treatment time, the 10% dose escalation was achieved by increasing the fraction size to 1.65 Gy/fraction. Of the 22 patients treated with this regimen, 2 of the 3 who had received whole-liver irradiation as a portion of their treatment developed radiation hepatitis. Of the patients who did not receive whole liver irradiation, none developed radiation hepatitis. The objective response rate was 50% (2 complete responses, 9 partial responses). The median survival was 20 months, which compares favourably with published results for whole-liver radiation combined with intra-arterial chemotherapy as well as for continuous intraarterial FUDR alone.[46]

Similar findings have been reported by Mohiuddin et al.[10] They performed a retrospective analysis of patients treated with whole-liver radiation to a median dose of 21 Gy (range: 8–31 Gy) versus whole-liver irradiation followed by a boost (total dose 33–60 Gy). All but one patient received concomitant 5-FU based chemotherapy. Patients who received the higher doses had a longer medial survival compared with those who received whole liver irradiation alone (14 months versus 4 months, respectively).

In summary, the three-dimensional conformal approach offers the most promising results in combination with chemotherapy. With the use of DVH analysis and three-dimensional conformal radiation delivery, radiation therapy may offer a curative approach in selected patients with liver metastases from colorectal cancer.

References

1. Sherman DM, Weichselbaum R, Order SE, Cloud L, Trey C, Piro AJ. Palliation of hepatic metastasis. *Cancer* 1978; 41:2013–2017.
2. Phillips R, Darnofsky DA, Hamilton LD, Nichson JJ. Roentgen therapy of hepatic metastases. *Am J Roentgen* 1954; 71:826–834.
3. Prasad B, Lee M, Hendrickson FR. Irradiation of hepatic metastases. *Int J Radiat Oncol Biol Physics* 1977; 2:129–132.
4. Borgelt BB, Gelber R, Brady LW, Griffin T, Hendrickson FR. The palliation of hepatic metastases. Result of the Radiation Therapy Oncology Group pilot study. *Int J Radiat Oncol Biol Physics* 1987; 7:587–591.
5. Turek-Masicheider M, Kazem I. Palliative irradiation of liver metastases. *J Am Med Ass* 1975; 232:625–628.
6. Kinsella TJ. the role of radiation therapy alone and combined with infusion chemotherapy for treating liver metastases. *Semin Oncol* 1983; 10:215–222.
7. Leibel SA, Pajak TF, Massullo V, Order SE, Komaki RU, Chang CH, Wasserman TH, Phillips TL, Lipshutz RN, Durbin LM. A comparison of misonidazole sensitized radiation therapy to radiation therapy alone for the palliation of hepatic metastases: results of a Radiation Therapy Oncology Group randomized prospective trial. *Int J Radiat Oncol Biol Physics* 1987; 13:1057–1064.
8. Lawrence TS, Tesser RJ, Ten Haken RK. An application of dose volume histograms to the treatment of intrahepatic malignancies with radiation therapy. *Int J Radiat Oncol Biol Physics* 1990; 19:1041–1047.
9. Robertson JM, Lawrence TS, Walker S, Kessler ML, Andrews JC, Ensminger WD. The treatment of colorectal liver metastases with conformal radiation therapy and regional chemotherapy. *Int J Radiat Oncol Biol Physics* 1995; 32:445–450.
10. Mohiuddin M, Chen E, Ahmad N. Combined liver radiation and chemotherapy for palliation of hepatic metastases from colorectal cancer. *J Clin Oncol* 1996; 14:722–728.
11. Ingold JA, Reed GB, Kaplan HS, Bagsjaw MA. Radiation hepatitis. *Am J Roentgen* 1965; 93:200–208.
12. Rubin PP, Constine LS, Nelson DF. Late effects of cancer treatment: radiation and drug toxicity. In: Perez CA, Brady LW (eds), 1992: 124–161. *Principles and Practice of Radiation Oncology*. Philedelphia, JB Lippincott.
13. Anscher MS, Crocker IR, Jirtle RL. Transforming growth factor-beta-1 expression in irradiated liver. *Radiat Res* 1990; 122:77–85.
14. Reed GB, Cox AJ. The human liver after radiation injury. *Am J Pathol* 1966; 46:597–611.
15. Minsky BD, Leibel SA. The treatment of hepatic metastases from colorectal cancer with radiation therapy alone or combined with chemotherapy or misonidazole. *Cancer Treat Rev* 1989; 16:213–219.
16. Jackson A, Ten Haken RK, Robertson JM, Kessler ML, Kutcher GJ, Lawrence TS. Analysis of clinical complication data for radiation hepatitis using a parallel architecture mode. *Int J Radiat Oncol Biol Physics* 1995; 31:883–891.
17. Tefft M, Mitus A, Vawter GF, Filler RM. Irradiation of the liver in children: review of experience in the acute and chronic phases, and in the intact normal and partially resected. *Am J Roentgen Rad Ther Nucl Med* 1971; 111:165–173.
18. Tefft M. Radiation related toxicities in national Wilms' tumor study 1. *Int J Radiat Oncol Biol Physics* 1977; 2:455–464.
19. Kun LE, Camitta B. Hepatopathy following irradiation and Adriamycin. *Cancer* 1978; 42:81–84.
20. Thamses HD, Peters LJ, Withers RH, Fletcher GH. Accelerated fractionation vs. hyperfractionation. Rationales for several treatments per day. *Int J Radiat Oncol Biol Physics* 1983; 9:127–138.
21. Leibel SA, Guse C, Order SE, Hendrickson FR, Komaki RU, Chang CH, Brady LW, Wasserman TH, Russel KJ, Asbell SO, Phillips TL, Russel AH, Pajak TF. Accelerated fractionation radiation therapy for liver metastases: selection of an optimal patient population for the evaluation of late hepatic injury in RTOG studies. *Int J Radiat Oncol Biol Physics* 1989; 18:523–528.

22. Russel AH, Clyde C, Wasserman TH, Turner SS, Rotman M. Accelerated hyperfractionated hepatic irradiation in the management of patients with liver metastases: results of the RTOG dose escalating protocol. *Int J Radiat Oncol Biol Physics* 1993; **27:**117–123.

23. Leibel SA, Order SE, Rominger CJ, Asbell SO. Palliation of liver metastases with a combined hepatic irradiation and misonidazole. *Cancer Clin Trials* 1987; **4:**285–293.

24. Bierman HR,. Byron RL, Kelley KH, Grady A. Studies on blood supply of tumours in man. III. Vascular patterns of liver by hepetic arteriography *in vivo*. *J Nat Cancer Inst* 1952; **12:**107–131.

25. Heidelberger C, Griesbach L, Montag BJ. Studies on fluorinated pyrimidines. II. Effects on transplated tumours. *Cancer Res* 1958; **18:**305–317.

26. Phillips TL, Wharam MD, Margolis LW. Modification of radiation injury to normal tissues by chemotherapeutic agents. *Cancer* 1977; **35:**1678–1685.

27. Friedman M, Cassidy M, Levine M, Phillips T, Spivack S, Resser KJ. Combined modality therapy of hepatic metastasis. *Cancer* 1979; **44:**906–913.

28. Herbsman H, Haasan A, Gardner B, Bohorquez J, Alfonso A, Newman J. Treatment of hepatic metastases with a combination of hepatic artery infusion chemotherapy and external radiotherapy. *Surg Gynecol Obstet* 1979;**147:**13–17.

29. Lokich JJ, Kinsella T, Perri J, Malcolm A, Clouse M. Concomitant hepatic radiation and fluorinated pyrimidine therapy. Correlation of liver scan, liver function tests and plasma CEA with tumor response. *Cancer* 1982; **48:**2569–2574.

30. Rotman M, Kuruvilla AM, Choi KC, Bhutiani I, Rosenthal J, Braverman A, Marti J, Brandys M. Response of colorectal hepatic metastasis to concomitant radiotherapy and intravenous infusion 5-fluorouracil. *Int J Radiat Oncol Biol Physics* 1986; **12:**2179–2187.

31. Webber BM, Soderberg CH, Leone LA, Rage VB, Glicksman AS. A combined treatment approach to management of hepatic metastases. *Cancer* 1978; **42:**1087–1095.

32. Barone RM, Byfield JE, Goldfarb PB, Frankel S, Ginn C, Greer S. Intra-arterial chemotherapy using an implantable infusion pump and liver irradiation for the treatment of hepatic metastases. *Cancer* 1982; **50:**850–862.

33. Raju PI, Maruyama Y, DeSimone P, MacDonald J. Treatment of liver metastases with a combination of chemotherapy and hyperfractionated external radiation therapy. *Am J Clin Oncol* 1987; **10:**41–43.

34. Ensminger WD, Rosowsky A, Raso V *et al.* A clinical–pharmacological evaluation of hepatic arterial infusion of 5-fluoro-2′-deoxyuridine and 5-fluorouracil. *Cancer Res* 1978; **38:**3784–3792.

35. Sigurdson ER, Ridge JA, Kemeny N, Daly JM. Tumor and liver drug uptake following hepatic artery and portal vein infusion. *J Clin Oncol* 1987; **5:**1836–1840.

36. Byfield JF, Barone RM, Frankel SS, Sharp TR. Treatment with combined intra-arterial 5-FUDR infusion and whole liver radiation for colon carcinoma metastatic to the liver. *Am J Clin Oncol* 1984; **7:**319–325.

37. Wiley AL, Wirtanen GW, Stephenson JA, Ramirez G, Demets D, Lee JW. Combined hepatic artery 5-fluorouracil and irradiation of liver metastases. A randomized study. *Cancer* 1989; **64:**1783–1789.

38. DriTschilo A, Harter KW, Thomas D, Nauta R, Holt R, Lee TC, Rustgi S, Rodgers J. Intraoperative radiation therapy of hepatic metastses: technical aspects and report of a pilot study. *Int J Radiat Oncol Biology Physics* 1988; **14:**1007–1011.

39. Thomas DS, Nauta RJ, Rodgers JE, Popescu GF, Nguyen H, Lee TC, Petrucci PE, Harter WK, Holt RW, DriTschilo A. Intraoperative high-dose rate interstitial irradiation of hepatic metastases from colorectal carcinoma. *Cancer* 1993; **71:**1977–1981.

40. Grady P. Internal radiation therapy of hepatic cancer. *Dis Colon Rectum* 1979; **22:**371–375.

41. Herba MJ, Illescas FF, Thirlwell MP, Boos GJ, Rosenthall L, Atri M, Bret PM. Hepatic malignancies: improved treatment with intraarterial Y-90. *Radiology* 1988; **169:**311–314.

42. Niederhuber JE, Ensminger WD. Treatment of metastatic cancer to the liver. In: *Cancer: Principles and Practice of Oncology.* De Vita VT, Hellman S, Rosenberg SA, (eds), **1:** 1993:2201–2225.

43. Order SE, Klein JL, Leichner PK, Ettinger DS, Kopher K, Finney K, Surdyke M, Leibel SA. Radiolabeled antibody treatment of primary and metastatic liver malignancies. *Recent dv Cancer Res* 1986; **100:**307–314.

44. Lawrence TS, Ten Haken RK, Kesseler ML, Robertson JM, Lyman JT, Lavigne ML, Brown MB, DuRoss DJ, Andrews JC, Ensminger WD, Lichter AS. The use of 3-D dose volume analysis to predict radiation hepatitis. *Int J Radiat Oncol Biol Physics* 1992; **23:**781–788.

45. Lawrence TS, Dworzanin LM, Walker-Andrews SC, Andrews JC, Ten Haken RK, Wollner IS, Lichter AS, Ensminger WD. Treatment of cancers involving the liver and porta hepatis with external beam irradiation and intraarterial hepatic fluorodeoxyuridine. *Int J Radiat Oncol Biol Physics* 1991; **20:**555–561.

46. Rougier P, Laplanche A, Huguier M, Hay JM, Ollivier JM, Escat J, Salmon R, Julien M, Audy JR, Gallot D, Gouzi JL, Pailler JL, Elisa D, Lacaine F, Roos S, Rotman N, Luboinski M, Lasser P. Hepatic arterial infusion of floxuridine in patients with liver metastases from colorectal carcinoma: long term results of a prospective randomized trial. *J Clin Oncol* 1992; **10:**1112–1118.

Gene Therapy for Primary and Metastatic Cancer to the Liver

13

M. Wayne Flye and Katherine Parker Ponder

Introduction

The term 'gene therapy' applies to all approaches involving the introduction of genetic material into a patient's cells to produce a therapeutic protein or inhibit gene function. This therapy is possible because viruses, bacteria, plants and mammals all share the same interchangeable genetic code. Gene therapy is currently being employed in an attempt to cure or ameliorate the growth of various malignancies.[1,2] The potential experimental gene therapies used for treating cancer may (1) transfer 'suicide genes' whose protein products converts a non-toxic precursor to a toxic molecule that kills the cancer cells (2) inhibit or regulate oncogenes (3) transfer tumour suppressor genes, such as *p53* (4) promote or reinforce an immunological response to the tumour (5) inhibit proteins necessary for promoting metastases (6) inhibit tumour angiogenesis or (7) transfer drug resistance genes for bone-marrow protection from high-dose chemotherapy. This area of potential therapy is in its infancy and most approaches have yet to pass even the most preliminary clinical tests demonstrating their overall safety and efficacy. Common issues that are applied to the gene therapy of all diseases involves gene transfer, gene regulation, vector efficiency and safety.

Hepatocellular carcinoma (HCC) is one of the most common malignant tumours in man, causing over one million deaths annually worldwide.[3] Conventional chemotherapy and radiotherapy are ineffective and surgical resection is appropriate for only a small percentage of patients. Therefore, innovative therapeutic approaches are warranted. Furthermore, the liver is the most frequent site of metastasis from gastrointestinal cancers. While partial hepatectomy remains the best available therapy for localized hepatic disease, <15% of patients have isolated hepatic metastases that can benefit from surgical resection.[4] The results of chemotherapy and immunotherapy have been disappointing. Their treatment with gene therapy may prove to be a promising new approach.

Gene Transfer

Efficient delivery of foreign genes into the appropriate target cells is a major hurdle facing all gene therapy approaches today. Delivery systems can be divided into viral (e.g. retrovirus, adenovirus and adeno-associated virus (AAV) and non-viral (e.g. plasmid DNA, which is a circular piece of DNA that can be propagated in bacteria, or oligodeoxynucleotides) (Table 13.1).[1,5] Major considerations determining the optimal vector and delivery system are (1) the target cells and their accessibility to the vector used to deliver the DNA and (2) whether or not treatment requires long-term expression of the gene.

Choice of Target Cells

The cells targeted for gene therapy vary according to which mechanism of gene therapy is being used. In the case of suicide genes, it is necessary to transfer the gene into a high fraction of cancer cells *in vivo*, but not into normal cells. Access to the tumour cells by the transfecting gene can pose a significant hurdle

Table 13.1 Summary of the relative advantages and disadvantages of vectors frequently used for gene therapy

Delivery vehicle	Advantages of vector	Disadvantages of vector
Retroviral Vectors	Medium capacity (7 kb) Easy production Efficient transfer Less likely to produce immune response Stable expression	Transduces only dividing cells Random DNA insertion Titers moderately low Risk of generating wild-type virus
Adenovirus	Large capacity (7–10 kb) Transduces non-dividing cells Efficient transfer	Possible host immune reactions Risk of generating wild-type virus Transient expression
Adeno-associated virus (AAV)	Less likely to produce immune response Transduces non-dividing cells Stable expression	Risk of generating wild-type virus Small capacity (5 kb)
Plasmid DNA	No size limitation Easy to produce No risk of wild-type virus Less likely to produce immune responses	Low efficiency of transfer Transient expression

in the case of solid tumours, where the cells are not easily accessed by intravascular injection. For example, adenoviral vectors can transfect the cells surrounding HCC but are inefficient at transferring the gene into the cancer cells themselves. [6,7] Other approaches to gene therapy do not require transfer into the cancer itself. For example, gene therapy designed to stimulate immunity to the cancer can be effective by transferring genes into cancer cells or normal antigen-presenting cells. Since the therapy stimulates an immunological response against the cancer, it is not necessary to transfer the gene into a high fraction of cells. Thus, the genes can be delivered *in vivo* to the animal. Alternatively, transduction of cells *in vitro* followed by *in vivo* infusion of these modified cells can be used.

Duration of Gene Expression Required

The second major factor that influences the optimal vector for gene therapy is the duration of required expression. Since suicide genes result in the rapid death of transfected cells, it is not necessary to achieve long-term expression for this approach. Similarly, immunotherapy should be effective after a relatively short period of immune system priming. In contrast, some approaches will require long-term expression of the transferred gene. For example, expression of a tumour suppressor gene or inhibition of an oncogene would need to be maintained indefinitely. Retroviral and AAV vectors integrate in the host cell chromosome, resulting in long-term expression, while adenoviral and non-viral vectors

generally result in short-term expression and, therefore, would only be effective where short-term gene expression is sufficient.[2,5,8]

Viral Vectors

Most viral vectors are disabled so that they may deliver DNA into the target cell but not undergo replication once inside the target cell, i.e. they are replication incompetent. Features that distinguish the different viral vectors include the size of the gene insert accepted, whether or not the virus infects non-dividing cells, the duration of expression and possible host immune responses to viral proteins.

Adenoviral vectors

Adenoviral-based systems are the most efficient for transient transfection and have been most frequently used as vectors for localized *in vivo* gene delivery, such as delivery of the cystic fibrosis transmembrane receptor (*CFTR*) gene for the treatment of cystic fibrosis (Figure 13.1). Adenoviruses deliver extremely high numbers of viral particles and achieve high-level expression. It is especially advantageous that these vectors can infect non-dividing cells, which retroviral vectors require cellular proliferation. Jones and Shank[9] demonstrated that the *E1* region adenoviral gene products could be supplied in trans by a packaging cell, thus allowing the production of replication defective vectors with foreign genes of interest replacing the *E1* region.

A. Wild–type Adenovirus

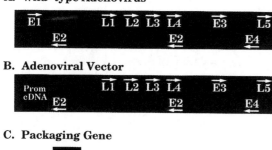

B. Adenoviral Vector

C. Packaging Gene

Figure 13.1. Adenoviral vectors for gene therapy. (A) Wild-type adenovirus. Adenoviruses contain a double-stranded linear DNA genome of ~36 kilobases. The inverted terminal redundancies of 100 basepairs at either end are necessary for replicating the DNA. Multiple early (*E*) and late (*L*) genes encode for proteins that are necessary for replicating the DNA and producing an infectious adenoviral particle. (B) Adenoviral vector. Most adenoviral vectors have deleted the *E1* gene and replaced it with a promoter and therapeutic gene (shown in blue). This results in a vector that still contains most of the adenoviral genes (shown in red). Some adenoviral vectors have deleted additional adenoviral genes. (C) Packaging cells. The adenoviral vector alone cannot produce adenoviral particles because it does not contain the *E1* gene. Packaging cells that express *E1* and contain the adenoviral vector sequences are necessary for producing adenoviral particles that can transmit information to a new cell.

However, a major limitation is that adenoviral vectors generally result in short-term gene expression because the immunological response to the remaining viral proteins results in rapid elimination of the transduced cells. This immunological response can result in severe inflammation at the site of delivery and associated organ dysfunction. Furthermore, the vigorous host immune response to the surface proteins rapidly clears the adenovirus and diminishes the efficacy of repeat administration. The deletion of some adenoviral genes (such as *E4* and *E2a*) has led to increased stability, while the presence of other adenoviral genes may act to stabilize the vectors. For example, the *E3* region is normally involved in helping the virus to avoid the immune system of the host by blocking class I major histocompatibility complex (MHC) presentation of viral antigens and thus adenoviral vector expression is prolonged.[10] Studies in immunodeficient mice have demonstrated that in the absence of antigen-specific immunity, gene expression is prolonged. Ongoing studies to identify the immunogenicity of adenoviral vector proteins will help to further improve the persistence of these vectors. The use of immunosuppressive therapy could also allow persis-

tent gene expression following adenovirus-mediated gene transfer. For example, temporary inhibition of the CD28/B7 T-lymphocyte costimulatory response with a soluble form of murine CTLA4 immunoglobulin has led to prolonged gene expression.[11]

In order for adenoviral vectors to be used for gene therapy in the treatment of primary and metastatic liver cancer, it is necessary to be able to deliver them to the liver. Potential routes for delivering these vectors to liver tumours include portal vein or hepatic artery injection, or direct injection into the tumour. Up to 100% of hepatocytes in normal animals can be transduced with adenoviral vectors after portal vein or peripheral vein injection, if a sufficient number of particles are injected. However, adenoviral vectors are not very efficient at transducing the tumour cells themselves in the liver after vascular injection, although the cells surrounding the tumour are readily transduced.[6,7] This may be due to the fact that the tumour blood vessels contain a continuous layer of endothelial cells that may block egress of the large adenoviral vector particle,[12,13] while the normal liver sinusoids have fenestrations that allow direct contact of blood with hepatocytes. Thus, intrahepatic tumour cells are less accessible to intravenous injection of adenoviral vectors than are normal hepatocytes. However, the direct tumour injection of adenoviral vector has successfully resulted in gene transfer into the cells of small tumours *in vivo*.[14,15]

In summary, adenoviral vectors result in high-level, but transient, expression of the transduced gene. Modification of the adenoviral vector to decrease its immunogenicity or the suppression of the recipient's immune response may prolong expression and/or allow repeated delivery in patients.

Retroviral Vectors (RV)

Retroviral vectors currently are the system of choice for strategies in which persistent expression is desired (Figure 13.2). Most vectors are based on the Moloney murine leukemia virus. The development of packaging cells which provide the viral *gag, pol* and *env* genes in the trans position has allowed the construction of stable production systems which do not generate replication competent virus. There are fewer problems with immune stimulation than with adenoviral vectors because all the coding sequences are removed from the retroviral vector. Because they integrate into the host cell chromosome, retro-

A. Wild–type Retrovirus

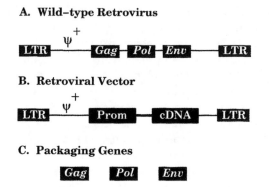

B. Retroviral Vector

C. Packaging Genes

Figure 13.2. Retroviral vectors for gene therapy. (A) Wild-type retrovirus. Retroviruses contain a single-stranded RNA genome of 5–7 kilobases. Long-terminal repeats (LTRs) are present at both ends and are necessary for reverse transcription of the RNA into a double-stranded DNA copy, and for integration of the DNA into the chromosome. The packaging signal (ψ^+) is necessary for the RNA to bind to the inside of a viral particle. The retroviral packaging genes *gag, pol,* and *env* code for proteins that are necessary for producing a viral particle. All retroviral sequences are shown in red. (B) Retroviral vector. Retroviral vectors have deleted the retroviral coding sequences and replaced them with a promoter and therapeutic gene, which are shown in blue. The vector still contains the LTR and ψ^+ (shown in red), which are necessary for the vector to transmit its genetic information into a target cell. (C) Packaging cells. The retroviral vector alone cannot produce a retroviral particle because the retroviral coding sequences are not present. These packaging genes, which are shown in red, need to be present in a packaging cell line along with the vector in order to produce a retroviral vector that can transfer genetic information into a new cell.

viral vectors can result in expression for months to years. However, a number of factors ultimately limit their clinical usefulness. Most relevant is the requirement for target cell replication in order for proviral integration to occur. A second drawback to retroviral vectors is that only a low concentration of infectious particles can be achieved, making it difficult *in vivo* to transfer the gene into all cancer cells. A third problem is that expression of genes with a RV vector can sometimes be shut off in animals due to poorly understood mechanisms. This problem can be circumvented, however, by using appropriate organ specific promoters, such as the liver specific albumin or α_1-antitrypsin promoter, to activate the gene.[16–18]

In order for retroviral vectors to be used for the gene therapy of primary and metastatic liver cancer, it is necessary to be able to deliver them to the liver. Both *ex vivo* and *in vivo* methods have been used to transfer retroviral vectors into normal hepatocytes. The *ex vivo* method of transfer involves isolation of hepatocytes, *in vitro* gene transfer, and reinfusion of

the modified cells. This approach can result in the establishment of the modified cells in the liver.[19,20] For example, this *ex vivo* approach could be used for the transfection of cytokine genes that would result in stimulation of the host's immune response. In contrast, the *in vivo* approach involves injection of retroviral vector into the portal vein during liver regeneration. Liver regeneration is necessary because hepatocytes are normally quiescent and retroviral vectors only transduce dividing cells.[21] Liver regeneration has been stimulated in the rat by performing a 70% partial hepatectomy,[16,22] by occluding the portal vein branches that serve 70% of the liver (which induces compensatory replication of the remaining liver.[23] or by injection of a hepatotrophic factor that induces replication of liver cells.[24]

Although some methods for retroviral cancer gene therapy, such as immunostimulation, might be effective by delivery of a gene into the surrounding hepatocytes, other methods will require transfer of the gene into proliferating cells of the tumour itself. In one study, injection of a retroviral vector alone into the portal venous circulation was inefficient at transferring genes into tumour cells into the liver, although injection of the entire packaging cells themselves into the portal venous system was effective.[25] The fact that cancer cells are already dividing because of their malignant growth properties might abrogate the need to induce normal hepatocyte replication. Alternatively, a small percentage partial hepatectomy, portal vein branch occlusion, or a small dose of a hepatic growth factor, might dramatically increase the percentage of the tumour cells that replicate while having little effect upon the normal liver, thus achieving selective transfer to the tumour. However, since alterations in the blood supply to liver tumours might limit the ability of vector delivered via the portal vein or hepatic artery (as was found for adenoviral vectors), it may be necessary to inject retroviral vector directly into the tumour.

In summary, retroviral vectors can result in stable gene expression but the efficacy of delivery is limited by the need for cell replication and the relatively low concentrations of vector that can be prepared.

Adenovirus-Associated Virus (AAV) Vectors

Adenovirus-associated virus vectors have only been utilized for gene therapy for a short period of time.[5]

A. Wild–type Adenovirus–associated Virus (AAV)

B. AAV Vector

C. Packaging Genes

Figure 13.3. Adenovirus-associated virus (AAV) vectors for gene therapy. (A) Wild-type AAV. AAV contain a single-stranded DNA genosome of 4.6 kilobases. The inverted terminal repeats (ITRs) are necessary for conversion of the single-stranded genome to double stranded DNA, and for integration into the chromosome. The protein products of the *rep* and *cap* genes are necessary for replicating the AAV genome and for producing an AAV particle. (B) AAV vectors. AAV vectors have deleted the AAV coding sequences and replaced them with a promoter and therapeutic gene, which are shown in blue. They still contain the ITRs (shown in red), which are necessary for the vector to transmit its genetic information into a target cell. (C) Packaging cells. The AAV vector alone cannot produce an AAV particle because the *rep* and *cap* genes are not present. These AAV genes, which are shown in red, need to be present in a packaging cell line along with the AAV vector in order to produce an AAV particle that can transfer genetic information into a cell. In addition, another virus such as an adenovirus needs to be present for the production of infectious particles.

They are similar to retroviral vectors in that all of the coding sequences have been deleted and replaced with a promoter and coding sequence of interest, as shown in Figure 13.3. This eliminates the problem of an immune response to the viral proteins, as occurs for adenoviral vectors. A major advantage of AAV vectors is that they integrate into the host cell chromosome of non-dividing cells. However, this process appears to be slow, since peak expression from an AAV vector in the liver or muscle requires approximately 2 months to be achieved. In addition, it is difficult to produce large amounts of AAV vectors for use in clinical studies.

In summary, although AAV vectors have not yet been used in gene therapy trials for cancer, their use in the future is likely to increase since they can result in stable, long-term gene expression in non-dividing cells after an initial lag period.

Non-Viral Vectors

Non-viral vectors include any method of gene transfer that does not involve production of a viral parti-

A. Oligodeoxynucleotides.

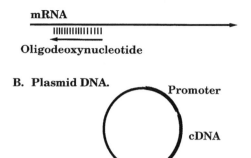

B. Plasmid DNA.

Figure 13.4. Non-viral vectors for gene therapy. Non-viral vectors are any type of vector that does not involve a viral particle that can alter gene expression in a cell. (A) Oligonucleotide vectors. Oligonucleotides, or the more stable phosphorothioate analog, contain 10–25 bases and can hybridize with RNA or form a triple helix with DNA. They alter expression of the gene or RNA with which they associate. Alternatively, oligodeoxynucleotides can serve as a decoy by binding to transcription factors, which prevents the transcription factor from binding to chromosomal DNA and activating expression of cellular genes. Oligodeoxynucleotides can enter cells much more efficiently than large pieces of DNA. (B) Plasmid DNA. Plasmids are double-stranded circles of DNA that replicate efficiently in bacteria. They can contain up to 20 kilobases of genetic information. They generally contain a promoter and coding sequence which results in expression of a therapeutic protein. Although plasmid DNA does not enter cells efficiently because of its large size, cationic liposomes or receptor-mediated targeting can be used to facilitate its entry into cells.

cle. Non-viral vectors (Figure 13.4) provide no opportunity for possible replication of competent viruses. Plasmid DNA vectors can deliver large pieces of DNA and the use of liposomes can generally increase the efficacy of an otherwise inefficient transfer.[26] The relatively short-term expression obtained with these plasmid vectors may be acceptable or even preferable in the treatment of some tumours, for example, with the expression of a potent toxin or a conditionally lethal gene in a localized cancer. Alternately, antisense oligodeoxynucleotides of 15–25 nucleotides can be used to alter gene expression. They can hybridize to a critical tumour mRNA and block its translation into a protein, or bind to a transcription factor and prevent it from activating certain cellular genes.[1]

In summary, while plasmid DNA and oligodeoxynucleotides can be used for gene therapy and are relatively safe, their efficacy of transfer and longevity of gene transfer remain problematic.

Gene Regulation

While gene delivery is currently the greatest limitation in the field of gene therapy, regulation of gene expression may be the next greatest problem. A promoter is an upstream sequence of DNA that activate expression of a gene. Promoters function by binding to transcription factors that reroute RNA polymerase to the gene, which is copied into messenger RNA (mRNA). For many gene therapy approaches, the ideal promoter would only be expressed in the cancer that is being treated. For example, one would want to limit expression of a suicide gene only to the cancer in order to avoid killing normal cells. For other approaches, such as immunotherapy, cancer-specific expression is not necessary.

One of the characteristics of several cancers is the reactivation of genes that are normally expressed only during fetal development. For example, the alpha-fetoprotein (AFP) gene is normally transcriptionally silent in adult liver but is often abnormally reactivated in HCC (hepatoma). Hepatoma-specific expression of a gene has been achieved *in vivo* and *in vitro* by constructing a recombinant retroviral[27] or adenoviral vector[7,15] containing transcriptional elements from rat AFP.

A second fetal gene is the carcinoembryonic antigen (CEA) which is expressed in many tumours arising in the gastrointestinal tract. Targeting of therapeutic genes via the CEA regulatory sequence has been used to achieve expression of a suicide gene in colorectal cancer cells *in vitro* and *in vivo*.[28]

Alternatively, a promoter could be used that is activated by cancer directed therapy, such as radiation. Weichselbaum *et al.* (29) attempted to selectively deliver tumour necrosis factor (TNF-α) to tumour cell deposits by using a radiation-inducible promoter. Radiation induced the Egr-1–TNF construct to produce a 2.7–3.2-fold increase in TNF-α *in vitro* and *in vivo* and increased tumour regression in animals treated with irradiation.

Similarly, γ-irradiation and topoisomerase inhibitors dramatically increased the number of fibroblasts that expressed a gene from an AAV vector in liver cells in animals.[30] Since the copy number of the AAV vector in the liver was not increased by the treatment, the increased number of cells that expressed the gene was probably due to activation of the viral promoter.[30] Thus radiation or chemotherapeutic drugs may serve as an on/off switch for cancer therapy.

In summary, tumour-specific promoters can result in selective expression of genes in the cancer, but not in normal tissue, while radiation can activate certain promoters. Further refinements in the promoters should limit the toxicity of the vectors for normal cells.

Basic Mechanisms of Gene Therapy

Several different approaches have been taken in attempts to treat cancer with gene therapy: (1) transfer of a 'suicide gene' whose protein product converts a non-toxic precursor into a toxic molecule; (2) inhibition or regulation of oncogenes; (3) transfer of a tumour suppressor gene; (4) promotion of an immunological response to the tumour; (5) inhibition of the potential for metastases; (6) inhibition of angiogenesis; and (7) transfer of drug resistance genes to allow the administration of high doses of chemotherapy. A summary of attempts to use some of these methods to treat primary and metastatic cancer to the liver follows.

Transfer of a Suicide Gene into Cancer Cells

The principle of suicide gene therapy is to transfer a gene encoding a metabolically active enzyme into a cancer cell. This enzyme metabolizes a nontoxic product to a compound that is highly toxic for dividing cancer cells but not for non-dividing normal cells.[31] To achieve selectivity, the suicide gene must be introduced into as many cancer cells as possible while limiting transfer or expression in normal cells. The fact that many tumour cells are proliferating make them susceptible to the toxic metabolite. In some cases, there is a so-called 'bystander' effect that confers cytotoxicity to neighboring non-transduced cells. This probably occurs by diffusion of the toxic product into adjacent cells. This 'bystander' effect alleviates the necessity to deliver the suicide gene to every tumour cell.[32]

The most widely used suicide gene to date is the gene encoding herpes simplex type 1 thymidine kinase (TK) (Figure 13.5). In contrast to the kinases of most mammals, this enzyme can efficiently phosphorylate nucleoside analogs such as acyclovir or ganciclovir (Cytovene) into a monophosphorylated form. This substrate is then converted by cellular kinases into triphosphate metabolites which are incorporated into elongating DNA during cellular division, causing chain termination and cell death. TK-expressing cells are killed by *in vitro* concentrations of ganciclovir that are 1 000 to 10 000-fold lower than that required to kill parental cells. The *TK* gene predisposes transfected tumour cells to killing with the subsequent *in vivo* systemic administration of ganciclovir.[33]

A second suicide gene is the cytosine deaminase (*CD*) gene which converts 5-fluorocytosine (5-FC) to the highly toxic 5-fluorouracil (5-FU) (Figure 13.6). Expression of *CD* in cancer cells has resulted in killing when 5-FC is administered. A 'bystander effect' was observed in that non-transduced tumour cells could also be killed. Gap junctions between malignant cells allow the transfer of molecules between cells. Because gap junctions do not extend into normal tissue, the rest of the body is not affected. This 'bystander effect' may, therefore, be due to diffusion of 5-FU into adjacent cells. Alternatively, the bystander effect could be due to the fact that *CD*-treated cancer cells resulted in the migration of cytolytic lymphocytes or antibodies into hepatic metastases.[34]

An alternative method for suicide gene therapy is to develop a vector that replicates selectively in cancer cells with resulting cell lysis. An adenoviral vector that replicates selectively in cancer cells that lack functional *p53* was demonstrated to lead to tumour regression[35] and to increase the sensitivity of the cells to standard chemotherapeutic agents in animals.[36]

Inhibition or Regulation of Oncogenes

Proto-oncogenes are normally involved in regulating cellular replication. They become oncogenes when they are expressed inappropriately or when they are mutated so that the protein produced is constitutively active. The *p21-Ras* genes encode a family of proteins that function in signal transduction.[37] *p21-Ras* is normally activated when insulin or growth factors, such as transforming growth factor-β (TGF-β) bind to their cognate receptors on the cell surface. The activated *p21-Ras* activates downstream signaling molecules, such as mitogen

activated protein kinase, which phosphorylates transcription factors such as Fos and Jun family members. The mutation of *Ras* genes to encode a constitutively active protein occurs in a variety of tumours, including liver cancers.[37] When the *Ras* gene that encoded a constitutively active Ras protein was transduced into rat hepatocytes and animals were treated with a low dose of the liver carcinogen diethyl nitrosamine, liver cancers developed in 40% of the rats by 6 months.[38] This suggests that activation of *Ras* can contribute to liver cancer.

Inhibition or regulation of oncogenes is one approach to gene therapy for cancer. Antisense oligonucleotide technology has been used in an attempt to inhibit replication of cells that expressed a mutant *Ras* gene. Cells were transduced with a plasmid or retroviral vector that produced an antisense RNA complementary to the *Ras* gene that blocked the production of protein. This reduced the growth rate of human lung cancers *in vitro* and *in vivo* in immunodeficient mice.[39-41] This approach has not yet been used in an attempt to cure liver cancer in animals.

Transfer of a Tumour Suppressor Gene

Tumour suppression genes, such as *p53*, function to inhibit cellular replication. Transfer of a tumour suppressor gene could theoretically inhibit cellular replication in cells that have lost the expression of that suppressor gene through mutation or deletion. *p53* was initially considered to be an oncogene because mutant forms could cooperate with activated *Ras* to transform primary rat cells. However, it was subsequently discovered that wild-type *p53* is a tumour suppressor gene. *p53* is a nuclear phosphoprotein with a strong transactivation domain which binds to DNA in a sequence-specific manner. DNA damage induced by ionizing radiation, metabolic stress or chemotherapeutic agents results in stabilization and nuclear accumulation of wild-type p53 protein, which in turn induces either apoptosis or arrest at the G1/S phase of the cell cycle. Thus, *p53* has a direct role in controlling a cell-cycle checkpoint for DNA damage. *p53* activates other genes such as the cyclin-dependent kinase inhibitor p21 which, in turn, inhibits cell-cycle progression and thus prevents replication. *p53* also increases expression of the angiogenesis inhibitor, thrombospondin.[42] Because the induction of angiogenesis is critical for the growth and metastasis of tumours, this *p53*-regulated pathway may be important in tumour suppression.

The function of *p53* can be lost by genetic mutation or formation of complexes with other cellular or viral proteins.[43] *p53* is mutated in 50–70% of unselected primary colorectal adenocarcinomas.[44] Allelic loss of genetic markers in the 17p13 region is found in approximately 70% of these cases, usually in concert with mutation of the remaining allele, which yields tumour cells that completely lack wild-type *p53*. These two 'hits' leading to elimination of wild-type *p53* are usually tightly coincident with transition from colonic adenomas to invasive cancer, a late step in the genesis of colorectal carcinoma.[45] Mutations of *p53* have also been detected in up to 60% of HCC, especially in geographic areas with epidemiologic association with hepatitis B infection and dietary aflatoxin B exposure and is associated with a more advanced clinical stage. Functional inactivation of wild-type *p53* also occurs when bound to hepatitis B protein X.

Gene therapy has been attempted for a variety of cancers using vectors that express *p53*.[1] Gene therapy for colorectal and HCC using a vector that expresses *p53* is appealing since replication of most tumour cell lines is inhibited by the introduction of wild-type *p53*. The results of studies that use *p53* gene therapy to treat HCC or metastatic liver cancer are discussed below. Others have expressed p21 cyclin-dependent kinase inhibitor in an effort to inhibit growth of tumours *in vivo*.[46]

Promotion of an Immunological Response to the Tumour

Immunotherapy involves stimulation of the patient's immune response to the cancer, resulting in the eradication of primary and metastatic cancer cells. The identification of tumour-specific antigens, the effects of cytokines and the separation of T cells into subsets, has improved our understanding of tumour immunology. Multiple approaches have developed to trigger an effective immune response against tumour cells. The cells transduced can be either the tumour cells or cells of the immune system that are capable of presenting appropriate antigen(s). Transduction can be performed *in vitro*, with subsequent transplantation of the transduced cells (the *ex vivo* approach) or directly *in vivo*. Two approaches predominantly have been used to stimulate the immune response: stimulation of cytokines that

result in activation of lymphocytes; and introduction of molecules that promote antigen presentation.

Cytokines

A variety of cytokine genes have been used to promote tumour cell rejection, including IL-2, IL-4, IFN-γ, TNF-α, IL-1, IL-3, IL-6, IL-7, IL-12, and granulocyte colony-stimulating factor.[1,47–49] Forni *et al.*[50] pioneered the injection of the cytokine, interleukin-2 (IL-2) directly into an existing tumour to induce lymphocytes to mediate a local antitumour effect. IL-2 not only led to rejection of the growing tumour but, in some cases, protection against subsequent challenge with live tumour. These and subsequent studies indicated that defects in cytokine production either locally, at the site of growing tumour, or in the draining lymph node were related to tumour progression and suggested that these defects might be amenable to therapeutic intervention.[51] Tumour cells engineered to secrete a particular cytokine (such as IL-2 or TNF-α) more profoundly influenced the host anti-tumour response than did local injections of recombinant cytokine. Retroviral mediated transfer of TNF-α and IL-2 into tumour-infiltrating lymphocytes has also been used in patients with metastatic melanoma, although there is yet no clear evidence of efficacy.[47]

Antigen Presentation

A second approach to stimulate the immune system is to promote the presentation of tumour cell antigens. T-lymphocytes can recognize a foreign protein only after it has been processed by an antigen presenting cell (e.g. dendritic cells, macrophages, B-cells, etc.) and presented with its own class I or class II MHC surface molecules. The lymphocyte's T-cell receptor (TCR) can then be stimulated by the peptide presented by the antigen-presenting cell. When antigen is presented with class I MHC in conjunction with β_2-microglobulin, CD8$^+$ surface-positive lymphocytes (i.e. cytotoxic T-lymphocytes (CTL)) are stimulated to proliferate. Antigen plus class II MHC activates CD4$^+$ T-cells (i.e. helper cells which facilitate the activation of CD8$^+$ cells by the production of cytokines such as the interleukins 2, 4, 10, etc.). In order for lymphocyte activation to occur, a second signal (costimulation) must occur by the interaction of molecules on the antigen presenting cell (e.g. B7 family) and T-lymphocyte (e.g. CD28/CTLA4).[52] The relatively poor immune response to tumours may reflect a deficiency of lymphocyte costimulation by the tumour cells.[53]

A variety of approaches have been used to promote antigen presentation or to enhance the response to antigen in order to stimulate the immune system to reject a tumour. For example, the gene encoding the heat shock protein-65 (HSP-65) has been transfected into tumour cells with the intent of enhancing the loading of antigenic peptides onto tumour MHC molecules.[54] Recombinant β_2-microglobulin has been used to stabilize the tertiary complex of MHC class I, β_2-microglobulin and tumour peptide(s).[55] Transfection with the B7-1 molecule has been used to increase the tumour cell immunogenicity by providing a costimulatory signal with MHC antigen for effector T-lymphocytes.[26] Cytotoxic lymphocytes can also be targeted to tumours by the induction of specific immune receptors by gene transfer. For example, the TCR recognizing the MART-1 melanoma antigen has been cloned and expressed in Jurkat cells.[56] The expression of T-cell receptors that recognize tumour antigens could then be used to redirect cytotoxic lymphocytes to the tumour.

Inhibition of the Potential for Metastases

Cancer metastases are due to the movement of cancer cells from the primary site of occurrence to another region of the body such as the lung or liver. Two events are necessary for metastasis to occur: (1) the malignant cells fail to adhere tightly to adjacent cells or to the extracellular matrix, allowing single cells or clusters to be released from the cancer into the circulation;[57] and (2) the malignant cells express proteases that degrade the extracellular matrix that normally encases them and prevents their movement.[58] Gene therapy could potentially prevent metastases by expressing integrin molecules or inhibitors of metalloproteases, although this approach has not yet been used successfully.

Inhibition of Angiogenesis

All mammalian cells, including those with malignant growth properties, are dependent upon a nearby blood supply to receive nutrients and oxygen. Cancers, therefore, need to stimulate the production of new blood vessels in order to con-

tinue to enlarge. This angiogenesis is dependent upon growth factors that stimulate the replication of blood vessel cells. Antisense targeting of basic fibroblast growth factor and fibroblast growth factor receptor-1 blocked tumour angiogenesis and the growth of melanoma cells in mice.[59] In addition, peptides have been identified that experimentally inhibit angiogenesis in animals, and slow or prevent the occurrence of metastatic cancers.[60,61] The use of angiostatic genes is thus another promising approach for the future.

Transfer of Drug Resistance Genes for Bone-Marrow Protection

The dose of chemotherapy that can be used to treat a cancer is often limited by toxicity to other organs, such as the bone marrow. Higher doses could be tolerated if the bone marrow could be made more resistant to the chemotherapeutic drugs.[1] The multiple drug resistance gene (MDR1) produces P-glycoprotein, which functions to pump drugs out of cells and is responsible for resistance to some hydrophobic compounds. Similarly, the O-methylguanidine-DNA-methyltransferase can protect cells from nitrosourea-induced toxicity, while a methotrexate-resistant dihydrofolate reductase protects cells from methotrexate. Although drug resistance genes are currently being used to allow higher doses of chemotherapeutic agents to be administered in patients with breast and ovarian cancer, this approach has not yet been used for liver cancer.

Trials of Gene Therapy for Liver Cancer in Animals

Gene therapy has been used to treat HCC or cancers that have metastasized from sources to the liver. Numerous studies[1] have demonstrated that a variety of cancer cell types can be completely killed in vitro by introducing wild-type p53 expression,[62] by expressing TK in conjunction with the administration of ganciclovir[63] or by expressing CD in conjunction with the administration of 5-FC.[64] Gene therapy is usually highly efficient in vitro because cultured cells grow in a monolayer and can be transduced with either retroviral or adenoviral vectors. In

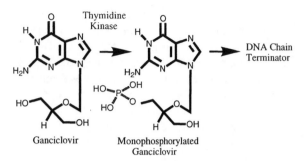

Figure 13.5. Mechanism of action of thymidine kinase Ganciclovir contains a guanine base attached to a structure that resembles deoxyribose. It has no biological activity in normal cells. Mammalian cells that have been engineered to express the herpes simplex virus 1 thymidine kinase (TK) by gene therapy can phosphorylate ganciclovir to the monophosphorylated ganciclovir. Monophosphorylated ganciclovir gets converted to triphosphorylated ganciclovir by cellular enzymes, which then gets incorporated into newly synthesized DNA. Further DNA synthesis is blocked because the ganciclovir prevents further elongation of the DNA. This results in cell death due to the inability to replicate DNA. Thymidine kinase, therefore, functions as a suicide gene in cancer cells when ganciclovir is administered. Non-replicating cells that contain TK are not killed because the ganciclovir does not get incorporated into the DNA.

contrast, it is much more difficult to efficiently deliver a vector *in vivo* because the cancer cells are less accessible to gene transfer. Thus, gene therapy in animals has been less successful than that achieved *in vitro*.

Suicide Genes

Thymidine Kinase

Studies in Transgenic Mice

The mechanism of the killing of replicating cells with *TK* gene transfer combined with ganciclovir treatment is shown in Figure 13.5. The efficacy of this approach for treating HCC was first established using transgenic mice.[65] Mice that express the SV40 T antigen with the albumin promoter developed HCC and died within 125 days after birth. The SV40 T-antigen-expressing animals then were bred with transgenic mice that expressed the *TK* gene. When these double transgenic mice were treated with continuous ganciclovir starting at 4 weeks of age, some animals survived for 200 days. Although the cause of death was not clear, many animals had grossly observable tumour nodules at the time of death. However, the expression of the SV40 T antigen in all liver cells may have contributed to eventual death due to liver insufficiency. These data demonstrate

that expression of TK in conjunction with ganciclovir treatment can delay the development of HCC and prolong life.

Transplantation of Genetically Modified Cancer Cells
Since cancer is a clonal disease in which one abnormal cell originates upon a background on non-malignant cells, it is more appropriate to determine if a cancer can be treated when the background liver cells are normal. Several studies have implanted HCC cells genetically modified *in vitro* with a retroviral vector or plasmid DNA expressing TK and tested the effect of ganciclovir on survival and the appearance of cancer in animals. Kuriyama *et al.*[63] demonstrated that when TK-transduced HCC cells were implanted and the animals were treated with ganciclovir for 2 weeks, the majority of the animals were cured of their cancer, while all animals that received untransduced parental HCC cells develop progressive cancer. In addition, the TK/ganciclovir treatment exerted a 'bystander effect', upon cells that did not express TK. This was demonstrated by mixing TK-transduced murine HCC cells with an equal number of non-transduced HCC cells. When ganciclovir was given, all animals were cancer free at 3 months. When only 25% of the cells were transduced with TK, 22% of the animals developed HCC. These data suggest that a relatively high percentage (>25%) of cells need to be transduced in order to efficiently achieve this bystander effect *in vivo*.

In vivo Administration of Gene Therapy to Established Cancer
Although these experimental data are encouraging, gene therapy in humans will require that the vector be efficiently delivered to the cancer *in vivo*. Ultimately, *in vivo* gene therapy will need to cure cancers that are already established at the time of diagnosis.

Wills *et al.*[14] injected an adenoviral vector that expressed TK with the CMV promoter into established subcutaneous (SQ) hepatoma cell line Hep3B tumours and demonstrated that treatment with ganciclovir could decrease the tumour volume by 90% at 2 months. The tumours were directly injected with the three doses of the adenoviral vector over a 5-day period when they were ~1 mm in diameter and the mice were treated with 10 days of ganciclovir beginning 1 day after the first injection. After 2 months, the tumours that received a control virus not expressing TK were ~5 mm in diameter, while the tumours in mice that received the *TK* gene were

~2 mm. Although the differences in tumour size were significant, animal survival was not reported. Kaneko *et al.* [27] also injected an adenoviral vector that expressed TK with either the Rous sarcoma virus (RSV) promoter or the AFP promoter into established tumours of 2–3 mm in diameter and demonstrated a decrease in tumour size after 3 weeks.

Two hepatoma cell lines were injected SQ and allowed to replicate for 5 (HuH7) or 9 (SK-Hep1) days before an adenoviral vector was injected directly into the tumour for two successive days, and ganciclovir was started one day after the last injection of adenovirus. After 10 days of ganciclovir, the tumour size in experimental animals was only 25% that of animals that received a control adenoviral vector (did not express TK) or that received the TK-expressing adenoviral vectors but did not receive ganciclovir.

When Caruso *et al.*[34] directly injected a packaging cell line that produced retroviral vector particles expressing TK into liver metastases established with the colon carcinoma cell line DHDK12, regression of the tumours resulted when animals were treated for 5 days with ganciclovir. The tumour diameter was 2–3 mm at the time of injection. In the treated animals, the mean tumour volume was 10% that of animals that received retroviral vector packaging cells that expressed a control *β-gal* gene. Pathological examination suggested that the residual tumour mass was actually a fibrotic scar devoid of cancer cells.

In summary, these studies demonstrate that expression of TK from either retroviral or adenoviral vectors in a tumour can result in regression when the animals are treated with ganciclovir. However, in most of these studies, the tumours were very small at the time of treatment, and long-term

evaluation was not reported. The clinical experience in humans has been limited. Among 12 patients with inoperable brain tumours, there were 2 complete responses and 2 partial responses to TK transfection and ganciclovir treatment. The complete responders were alive 52 and 47 months after treatment.[66]

Cytosine Deaminase (CD)

Transplantation of Genetically Modified Cancer Cells (5-Fluorouracil) (5-FU), is a chemotherapeutic drug commonly used to treat metastatic colon cancer or HCC. CD converts (5- fluorocytosine (5-FC) to 5-FU (Figure 13.6). Huber *et al.*[67] demonstrated that tumours derived from the CD-transduced human colorectal carcinoma cell line WiDr regressed in all mice when the animals were treated daily with 5-FC between day 10 and day 20 after SQ injection of the cells. Thirty percent of the tumours were cured, although the remainder relapsed at approximately 3 weeks after the 5-FC was discontinued. A similar tumour regression followed by relapse was observed when the colorectal carcinoma cell line NCI H508 cells were transfected with a plasmid expressing CD with the CEA promoter and animals were treated with 5-FC.[28]

Huber *et al.*[64] demonstrated that CD-transduced cells can exert a bystander effect upon nearby non-transduced cells from a human colorectal cell line after 5-FC therapy. Seven days after CD-transduced cells mixed with non-transduced cells at varying ratios were administered to mice, half the animals were started on daily 5-FC for the first 2 weeks, then three times a week for 10 weeks. When all of the implanted cells contained the *CD* gene, 80% of the animals that received 5-FC were tumour free at 10 weeks, and the remaining 20% had tumours that were considerably smaller than in control animals.

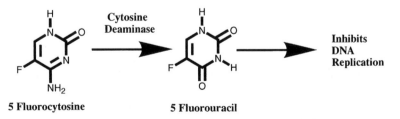

5 Fluorocytosine   **5 Fluorouracil**

Figure 13.6. Mechanism of action of cytosine deaminase (CD). 5-fluorocytosine (5-FC) is a cytosine analog that has no biological activity in normal mammalian cells. Mammalian cells that are engineered to contain the bacterial enzyme CD by gene therapy convert 5-FC to 5-fluorouracil (5-FU). 5-FU is a chemotherapeutic agent that is commonly used to treat colon and other cancers. 5-FU gets converted by cellular enzymes to 5-fluoro-23-deoxyuridine-53-phosphate, which is a potent inhibitor of thymidylate synthetase. This results in cell death due to inhibition of DNA synthesis. CD, therefore, functions as a suicide gene in cancer cells when 5-FU is administered.

Some animals receiving a mixture of transduced and non-transduced cells were also cured. When as few as 2% of the tumour cells expressed CD, significant regression in all tumours was observed when the host mouse was treated with non-toxic levels of 5-FC. These data demonstrate that expression of CD in combination with 5-FC treatment can lead to cure or regression of a cancer, and that a bystander effect occurs when transduced cells are mixed with non-transduced cells.

In vivo Administration of Gene Therapy to Established Cancer

The above data clearly establish the principle that 5-FC can kill CD-expressing cells injected into animals. However, treatment of patients will also require efficient delivery of the vector to an established tumour. Kanai et al.[15] demonstrated that the injection of 10 million PLC/PRF/5 mouse hepatoma cells SQ resulted in tumours measuring ~3 mm in diameter after 3 weeks. The direct tumour injection with an adenoviral vector expressing CD from the AFP transcriptional elements resulted in regression of tumour to about one-third their original size during a 2-week period of 5-FC treatment, while the tumours in control animals doubled in size. These data demonstrate that in vivo administration of a CD-expressing adenoviral vector can lead to regression of small established HCC in mice.

Administration of a Tumour Suppressor Gene

The wild-type tumour suppressor gene, p53, has been delivered to metastatic colorectal cancers or HCC in an attempt to lead to tumour regression. Since malignant liver tumours derive nearly 100% of their blood supply from the hepatic artery, hepatic artery infusion of the recombinant adenoviral p53 has been used to selectively target the tumour blood supply. Overexpression of wild-type p53 in both quiescent or regenerating livers after a partial hepatectomy does not affect normal hepatocyte metabolism or regeneration. In addition, p53 replacement may increase the effectiveness of chemotherapy.

Bao et al.[6] demonstrated that an adenoviral vector that expressed wild-type p53 from the CMV promoter had no effect upon established tumour growth that developed in transgenic mice. HCC–SV40 T-antigen-expressing animals were treated with portal vein injection of adenoviral

vector at 8 weeks, when they had occasional small tumours. While the majority of the SV40 T-antigen-expressing mice died from the toxicity of the adenoviral vector, there was no evidence of regression of the tumours in surviving animals. They attributed this failure at least in part to the fact that the adenoviral vector only transduced cells at the periphery of the tumour but not within the center of the tumour. Their failure to transduce the majority of the cancer cells with the adenoviral vector is similar to the results that were observed by Arbuthnot et al.[7] and represents a significant limitation for this treatment in larger tumours.

A Phase I clinical gene therapy protocol for administering p53 via the hepatic artery for both primary and metastatic tumours of the liver has been initiated at the University of California, San Francisco but results are not yet available.

Immunotherapy

Immunotherapy involves stimulation of the immune system to kill an established cancer. Some cures of HCC or liver metastases have been achieved in mice after transfer of an IL-2 or IL-4 gene. Treatment with an IL-2 expressing adenoviral vector of mice with established hepatomas of ~2 mm in diameter obtained after injection of the hepatocellular cell line, MH134, resulted in a cure rate of >50%. The development of systemic antitumour cellular immunity protected against a subsequent challenge with tumour cells implanted at distant sites.[68] Hurford et al.[25] also demonstrated that immunotherapy with a retroviral vector that expressed IL-2 or IL-4 could reduce the size of hepatic metastases. Three days after hepatic micrometastases were established by injection of sarcoma cells into the spleen, animals were injected with retroviral vector-producing cells into the portal system, and the number of micrometastases was quantitated 6 days later. The IL-2-expressing retroviral packaging cells resulted in a >90% reduction in the number of observable metastases as compared with controls that received retroviral vector packaging cells that contained a non-functional IL-2 molecule, while the IL-4-expressing retroviral vector packaging cells resulted in a 75% decrease in the number of nodules. Caruso et al.[69] demonstrated that an adenoviral vector expressing IL-12 could also increase survival time and lead to cure of 25% of animals after intratumoral injection.

In summary, these data suggest that immunotherapy is a promising approach for treating liver cancer.

Conclusions

In summary, several studies have demonstrated the efficacy of suicide gene therapy at curing cancers *in vivo* when all of the cells express the suicide gene. In some cases, a bystander effect has been observed when non-transduced cells are mixed with transduced cells, although the percentage of cells that need to be transduced for effective tumour treatment is probably approximately 25%. However, efficient delivery of a vector into an established tumour is more difficult, and has achieved only mixed success. In the studies that reported a positive effect of the gene therapy on an established tumour, the tumours have generally been small at the initiation of the study (1–3 mm), and relatively short-term evaluation (<1 month) was reported. It is likely that large tumours will be harder to treat because of difficulties in efficiently delivering the vector to all cells, and it is likely that even small tumours will show a high percentage of relapse at later times because not all of the cells are transduced with the vector. Treatment with the tumour suppressor gene *p53* has been disappointing. Immunotherapy with an IL-2-IL-4 or IL-12-expressing vector has resulted in the cure of some small established tumours, but it is unclear if it will be equally efficacious for larger tumours. Thus, although initial results with gene therapy are encouraging, further studies to improve the efficacy of gene transfer and to eradicate larger tumours will be needed.

Safety

Concerns as to safety of gene therapy relate to: (1) generation of replication-competent virus with altered phenotype and/or host range; (2) activation of an oncogene or inactivation of the tumour suppressor gene due to insertional mutagenesis; and (3) potential immunogenicity resulting from expression of foreign proteins. The first concern relates exclusively to viral vectors and can be avoided by meticulous evaluation of packaging cell lives for the presence of wild-type virus. The second concern relates primarily to a retroviral vector, since most non-viral vectors and adenoviral vectors are not integrated into the host genome. While there is always the theoretical possibility that insertion of genetic material into the genome by viral vectors may occur at a site which would have a deleterious effect, this very rarely occurs.

Future Prospects

Gene therapy is in its infancy. While cancer is not necessarily an inherited disease, it is clearly a disease of genes and thus susceptible to therapy utilizing genetic tools. Vector development will result in vectors with the ability to efficiently target genes to tumours with a resultant increase in efficiency and reduction in toxicity. Tumour regression has been observed in Phase I trials by several investigators for immunotherapy/cytokine, drug sensitivity and tumour suppressor/antisense protocols. Since the application of gene therapy agents so far has been limited to patients with advanced, incurable cancer, interpreting response rates has been difficult. If data currently being generated in animal models of human hepatocellular and colorectal cancer can be reproduced in human disease, there is hope that gene therapy will someday be a standard component in the treatment of these lethal diseases.[70]

References

1. Roth JA, Cristiano RJ. Gene therapy for cancer: What have we done and where we going? [Review] *J Natl Cancer Inst* 1997; **89**:21–39.
2. Blaese RM. Gene therapy for cancer. *Sci Am* 1997; **276**:111–115.
3. Colombo M. Hepatocellular carcinoma. *J Hepatol* 1992; **15**:225–236.
4. Scheele J, Stangl R, Attendorf HA. Hepatic metastases from colorectal carcinoma: Impact of surgical resection on the natural history. *Br J Surg* 1990; **77**:1241.
5. Smith AE. Viral vectors in gene therapy. *Annu Rev Microbiol* 1995; **49**:807–838.
6. Bao J-J, Zhang W-W, Kuo MT. Adenoviral delivery of recombinant DNA into transgenic mice bearing hepatocellular carcinomas. *Human Gene Ther* 1996; **7**:355–365.
7. Arbuthnot PB, Bralet MP, Le Jossic C, Dedieu JF, Perricaudet M, Brechot C, Ferry N. *In vitro* and *in vivo* hepatoma cell-specific expression of a gene transferred with an adenoviral vector. Human Gene Ther 1996; **7**:1503–1514.

8. Blaese M, Blankenstein T, Brenner M, Cohen-Haguenauer O, Gansbacher B, Russell S, Sorrentino B, Velu T. Vectors in cancer therapy: How will they deliver? *Cancer Gene Ther* 1995; **2**:291–297.

9. Jones N, Shank T. Isolation of adenovirus type III host strain deletion mutants defective in transformation of rat embryo. *Cell* 1979; **17**:683–689.

10. Ilan Y, Droguett G, Chowdhury NR, Li Y, Sengupta K, Thummala NR, Davidson A, Chowdhury JR, Horwitz MS. Insertion of the adenoviral E3 region into a recombinant viral vector prevents antiviral humoral and cellular immune responses and permits long-term gene expression. *Proc Natl Acad Sci USA* 1997; **94**:2587–2592.

11. Kay MA, Holterman A-X, Meuse L, Gown A, Ochs HD, Linsley PS, Wilson CB. Long-term hepatic adenovirus-mediated gene expression in mice following CTLA41g administration. *Nature Genetics* 1995; **11**:191.

12. Taylor I, Bennett R, Sherriff S. The blood supply of colorectal liver metastases. *Br J Cancer* 1979; **39**:749–756.

13. Schaffner F, Popper H. Capillarization of hepatic sinusoids in man. *Gastroenterology* 1963; **44**:239–242.

14. Wills KN, Huang WM, Harris MP, Machemer T, Maneval DC, Gregory RJ. Gene therapy for hepatocellular carcinoma: chemosensitivity conferred by adenovirus-mediated transfer of the HSV-1 thymidine kinase gene. *Cancer Gene Ther* 1995; **2**:191–197.

15. Kanai F, Lan K-H, Shiratori Y *et al*. In vivo gene therapy for α-fetoprotein-producing hepatocellular carcinoma by adenovirus-mediated transfer of cytosine deaminase gene. *Cancer Res* 1997; **57**:461–465.

16. Kay MA, Li Q, Liu TJ, Leland F, Toman C, Finegold M, Woo SL. Hepatic gene therapy: persistent expression of human alpha 1-antitrypsin in mice after direct gene delivery in vivo. *Human Gene Ther* 1992; **3**:641–647.

17. Hafenrichter DG, Wu X, Rettinger SD, Kennedy SC, Flye MW, Ponder KP. Quantitative evaluation of liver-specific promoters from retroviral vectors after *in vivo* transduction of hepatocytes. *Blood* 1994; **10**:3394–3404.

18. Okuyama T, Huber RM, Bowling WM, Pearline R, Kennedy SC, Flye MW, Ponder KP. Liver-directed gene therapy: A retroviral vector with a complete LTR and the ApoE enhancer-α₁-antitrypsin promoter dramatically increases expression of human α₁-antitrypsin in vivo. *Human Gene Ther* 1996; **7**:637–645.

19. Wilson JM, Chowdhury NR, Grossman M, Wajsman R, Epstein A, Mulligan RC, Chowdhury JR. Temporary amelioration of hyperlipidemia in low density lipoprotein-deficient rabbits transplanted with genetically modified hepatocytes. *Proc Natl Acad Sci USA* 1990; **87**:8437.

20. Grossman M, Radar DJ, Muller DWN, *et al*. A pilot study of ex vivo gene therapy for homozygous familial hypercholesterolemia. *Nature Medicine* 1995; **1**:1148–1154.

21. Miller DG, Adam MA, Miller AD. Gene transfer by retroviral vectors occurs only in cells that are actively replicating at the time of infection. *Mol Cell Biol* 1990; **10**:4239–4242.

22. Rettinger SD, Kennedy SC, Wu X, Saylors RL, Hafenrichter DG, Flye MW, Ponder KP. Liver directed gene therapy: Quantitative evaluation of promoter elements using *in vivo* retroviral transduction. *Proc Natl Acad Sci USA* 1994; **91**:1460–1464.

23. Bowling WM, Kennedy S, Cai SR, Duncan JR, Gao C, Flye MW, Ponder KP. Portal branch occlusion safely facilitates *in vivo* retroviral vector transduction of rat liver. *Human Gene Ther* 1996; **7**:2113–2121.

24. Bosch A, McCray PB Jr., Chang SM, Ulich TR, Simonet WS, Jolly DJ, Davidson BL. Proliferation induced by keratinocyte growth factor enhances *in vivo* retroviral-mediated gene transfer to mouse hepatocytes. *J Clin Invest* 1996; **98**:2683–2687.

25. Hurford RK, Dranoff G, Mulligan RC, Tepper RI. Gene therapy of metastatic cancer by *in vivo* retroviral gene targeting. *Nature Genetics* 1995; **10**:430.

26. Nabel GL, Chang AE, Nabel EG *et al*. Immunotherapy for cancer by direct gene transfer into tumors. *Human Gene Ther* 1994; **5**:57–77.

27. Kaneko S, Hallenbeck P, Kotani T, Nakabayashi H, McGarrity G, Tamaoki T, Anderson WF, Chiang YL. Adenovirus-mediated gene therapy of hepatocellular carcinoma using cancer-specific gene expression. *Cancer Res* 1995; **55**:5283–5287.

28. Richards CA, Austin EA, Huber BE. Transcriptional regulatory sequences of carcinoembryonic antigen: Identification and use with cytosine deaminase for tumor-specific gene therapy. *Human Gene Ther* 1995; **6**:881–893.

29. Weichselbaum RR, Hallahan DE, Beckett MA, Mauceri HJ, Lee H, Sukhatme BP, Kufe AW. Gene therapy targeted by radiation preferentially radiosensitizes tumor cells. *Cancer Res* 1994; **54**:4266–4269.

30. Koeberl DW, Alexander IE, Halbert CL, Russell DW, Miller AD. Persistent expression of human clotting factor IX from mouse liver after intravenous injection of adeno-associated virus vectors. *Proc Natl Acad Sci USA* 1997; **94**:1426–1431.

31. Huber BE, Richards CA, Krenitsky TA. Retroviral-mediated gene therapy for the treatment of hepatocellular carcinoma: An innovative approach for cancer therapy. *Proc Natl Acad Sci USA* 1991; **88**:8039–8043.

32. Freeman SM, Abboud CN, Whartenby KA, Packman CH, Koeplin DS, Moolten FL, Abraham GN. The 'Bystander Effect': Tumor regression when a fraction of the tumor mass is genetically modified. *Cancer Res* 1993; **53**:5274–5283.

33. Borrelli E, Heyman R, Hsi M, Evans RM. Targeting of an inducible toxic phenotype in animal cells. *Proc Natl Acad Sci USA* 1988; **85**:7572–7576.

34. Caruso M, Panis Y, Gagandeep S, Houssin D, Salzmann J-L, Klatzmann D. Regression of established macroscopic liver metastases after *in situ* transduction of a suicide gene. *Proc Natl Acad Sci USA* 1993; **90**:7024–7028.

35. Bischoff JR, Kirn DH, Williams A, Heise C, Horn S, Muna M, Ng L, Nye JA, Sampson-Johannes A, Fattaey A, McCormick F. An adenovirus mutant that replicates selectively in *p53*-deficient human tumor cells. *Science* 1996; **274**:373–376.

36. Heise C, Sampson-Johannes A, Williams A, McCormick F, Von Hoff DD, Kirn DH. ONYX-015, an E1B gene-attenuated adenovirus, causes tumor-specific cytolysis and antitumoral efficacy that can be augmented by standard chemotherapeutic agents. *Nature Medicine* 1997; **3**:639–645.

37. Anderson MW, Reynolds SH, You M, Maronpot RM. Role of proto-oncogene activation in carcinogenesis. *Environ Health Perspect* 1992; **98**:13–24.

38. Lin Y, Brunt EM, Bowling WM, Hafenrichter DG, Kennedy SC, Flye MW, Ponder KP. *Ras*-transduced dimethylnitrosamine-treated hepatocytes develop into cancers of mixed phenotype *in vivo*. *Cancer Res* 1995; **55**:5242–5250.

39. Mukhopadhyay T, Tainsky M, Cavender AC, Roth JA. Specific inhibition of K-ras expression and tumorigenicity of lung cancer cells by antisense RNA. *Cancer Res* 1991;**51**:1744–1748.

40. Zhang Y, Mukhopadhyay T, Donehower LA, Georges RN, Roth JA. Retroviral vector-mediated transduction of K-ras antisense RNA into human lung cancer cells inhibits expression of the malignant phenotype. *Hum Gene Ther* 1993; **4**:451–460.

41. Georges RN, Mukhopadhyay T, Zhang Y, Yen N, Roth JA. Prevention of orthotopic human lung cancer growth by intratracheal instillation of a retroviral antisense K-ras construct. *Cancer Res* 1993; **53**:1743–1746.

42. Danerin KM, Volpert OV, Tainsky MA *et al*. Control of angiogenesis in fibroblasts by *p53* regulation of of thrombospondin-1. *Science* 1994;**265**:1582–1584.

43. Bookstein R, Demers W, Gregory R, Maneval D, Park J, Wills K. *p53* gene therapy *in vivo* of hepatocellular and liver metastatic colorectal cancer. *Sem Oncol* 1996; 23:66–77.

44. Greenblatt MS, Bennett WP, Hollstein M *et al.* Mutations in the *p53* tumor suppressor gene. Clues to cancer etiology and molecular pathogenesis. *Cancer Res* 1994; 54:4855–4878.

45. Kikuchi-Yanoshita R, Konishi M, Ito S *et al.* Genetic changes of both *p53* alleles associated with the conversion from colorectal adenoma to early carcinoma in familial adenomatous polyposis and nonfamilial adenomatous polyposis patients. *Cancer Res* 1992; 52:3965–3971.

46. Yang Z-Y, Perkins ND, Ohno T, Nabel EG, Nabel GJ. The p21 cyclin-dependent kinase inhibitor suppresses tumorigenicity *in vivo*. *Nature Medicine* 1995; 1:1052–1056.

47. Rosenberg SA, Anderson WF, Blaese M *et al.* The development of gene therapy for the treatment of cancer. *Ann Surg* 1993; 218:455.

48. Tepper RI, Pattengale PK, Leder P. Murine interleukin-4 displays potent anti-tumor activity *in vivo*. *Cell* 1989; 57:503–512.

49. Dranoff G, Jaffe E, Lazenby A, Golumbek T, Labitsky HI, Brose K, Jackson B, Hamada H, Pardol D, Mulligan RC. Vaccination with irradiated tumor cells engineered to secrete murine granulocyte macrophage colony stimulating factor stimulates potent specific and long-lasting anti-tumor immunity. *Proc Natl Acad Sci USA* 1993; 90:3539–3543.

50. Forni G, Fujiwara H, Martina F, Hamaoka T, Jemma C, Caretto P, Giovarelli M. Helper strategy and tumor immunology: expansion of helper lymphocytes and utilization of helper lymphokines for experimental and clinical immunotherapy. *Cancer Metastasis Rev* 1988; 7:289–309.

51. Vieweg J, Gilboa E. Considerations for the use of cytokine-secreting tumor cell preparations for cancer treatment. *Cancer Invest* 1995; 13:193–201.

52. Schwartz RH. Costimulation of T lymphocytes: the role of CD28, CTLA4 and B7/BB1 in interleukin-2 production and immunotherapy. *Cell* 1992; 71:1065–1068.

53. June CH, Bluestone JA, Nadler LM, Thompson CB. The B7 and CD28 receptor families. *Immunol Today* 1994; 15:321–331.

54. Lukacs KV, Lowrie DB, Stokes RW, Colston MJ. Tumor cells transfected with bacterial heat shock gene lose tumor genicity and induce protection against tumors. *J Exp Med* 1993; 178:343–348.

55. Rock KL, Fleischacker C, Gambell S. Peptide priming of cytolytic T cell immunity *in vivo* using β_2-microglobulin as an adjuvant. *J Immunol* 1993; 150:1244–1252.

56. Cole DJ, Weil DP, Shilyansky J, Custer M, Kauskami Y, Rosenberg SA. Characterization of the functional specificity of a cloned T cell receptor heterodimer recognizing the MART-1 melanoma antigen. *Cancer Res* 1995; 55:748–752.

57. Huang YW, Baluna R, Vitetta ES. Adhesion molecules as targets for cancer therapy. *Histology Histopathol* 1997; 12:467–477.

58. Lee KS, Rha SY, Kim SJ, Kim JH, Roh JK, Kim BS, Chung HC. Sequential activation and production of matrix metalloproteinase-2 during breast cancer progression. *Clin Exp Metastasis* 1996; 14:512–519.

59. Wang Y, Becker D. Antisense targeting of basic fibroblast growth factor and fibroblast growth factor receptor-1 in human melanomas blocks intratumoral angiogenesis and tumor growth. *Nature Medicine* 1997; 3:887.

60. O'Reilly MS, Boehm T, Shing Y, Fukai N, Vasios G, Lane WS, Flynn E, Birkhead JR, Olsen BR, Folkman J. Endostatin: an endogenous inhibitor of angiogenesis and tumor growth. *Cell* 1997; 88:(2)277–285.

61. O'Reilly MS, Holmgren L, Shing Y, Chen C, Rosenthal RA, Moses M, Lane WS, Cao Y, Sage EH, Folkman J. Angiostatin: a novel angiogenesis inhibitor that mediates the suppression of metastases by a Lewis lung carcinoma [see comments]. *Cell* 1994; 79(2):315–328.

62. Xu GW, Sun ZT, Forrester K, Wang XW, Coursen J, Harris CC. Tissue-specific growth suppression and chemosensitivity promotion in human hepatocellular carcinoma cells by retroviral-mediated transfer of the wild-type *p53* gene. *Hepatology* 1996; 24:1264–1268.

63. Kuriyama S, Nakatani T, Masui K, Sakamoto T, Tominaga K, Yoshikawa M, Fukui H, Ikenaka K, Tsujii T. Bystander effect caused by suicide gene expression indicates the feasibility of gene therapy for hepatocellular carcinoma. *Hepatology* 1995; 22:1838–1846.

64. Huber BE, Austin EA, Richards CA, Davis ST, Good SS. Metabolism of 5-fluorocytosine to 5-fluorouracil in human colorectal tumor cells transduced with the cytosine deaminase gene: Significant antitumor effects when only a small percentage of tumor cells express cytosine deaminase. *Proc Natl Acad Sci USA* 1994; 91:8302–8306.

65. Macri P, Gordon JW. Delayed morbidity and mortality of albumin/SV40 T-antigen transgenic mice after insertion of an α-fetoprotein/herpes virus thymidine kinase transgene and treatment with ganciclovir. *Human Gene Ther* 1994; 5:175–182.

66. Gene therapy is advancing toward use as cancer treatment. *Oncology News Int* 1997; 6:2,27.

67. Huber BE, Austin EA, Good SS, Knick VC, Tibbels S, Richards CA. *In vivo* antitumor activity of 5- fluorocytosine on human colorectal carcinoma cells genetically modified to express cytosine deaminase. *Cancer Res* 1993; 53:4619–4626.

68. Huang H, Chen SH, Kosai K, Finegold MJ, Woo SLC. Gene therapy for hepatocellular carcinoma: long-term remission of primary and metastatic tumors in mice by interleukin-2 gene therapy *in vivo*. *Gene Ther* 1996; 3:980–987.

69. Caruso M, Pham-Nguyen K, Kwong YL, Xu B, Kosai KI, Finegold M, Woo SL, Chen SH. Adenovirus-mediated interleukin-12 gene therapy for metastatic colon carcinoma. *Proc Natl Acad Sci USA* 1996; 93:11302–11306.

70. Rosenberg SA, Blaese RM, Brenner MK *et al.* Human gene marker/therapy clinical protocols. *Human Gene Ther* 1996; 7:2287–2313.

The Role of Nuclear Medicine in the Treatment of Liver Metastases

Marco Chinol and Giovanni Paganelli

14

Introduction

Although there is the prospect of long-term survival following hepatic resectional surgery,[1,2] the majority of patients presenting with metastatic disease require to be considered for other treatment options, given that the mean survival without treatment is <6 months and the median survival time is 1.5 months.[3-5] The results of both systemic and regional chemotherapy have been disappointing[6] and, although external radiation therapy has seen a resurgence of interest, there are concerns regarding its effect, both on the gastrointestinal tract and on the liver.[7,8] Of the novel approaches currently being employed in the management of hepatic metastases, it is clear that nuclear medicine is likely to lead to substantial developments in the management of metastatic disease.

Therapeutic Approaches in Nuclear Medicine

In the early 1980s, hepatic arterial administration of beta-emitting radionuclides bound to various particles was proposed as a therapeutic modality, based on the principle that hepatic tumours derive their blood supply by this route.[9,10] With the advent of hybridoma technology for the production of monoclonal antibodies (MAbs) of predefined specificity,[11] investigators have evaluated the radiolabeled MAbs over the past two decades.[12] Radioiodine labelled monoclonal antibodies raised against carcinoembryonic antigen (CEA) have been shown to target tumours, including hepatic metastase, in >80% of colorectal cancer patients indicating that despite antigen and cell heterogenicity within a tumour, deposition of radioactivity occurs. Unfortunately, only a tiny fraction of the injected radioactivity, and in most cases barely sufficient for tumour radio-detection, localizes in the lesion and generally is unsufficient to cause the death of tumour cells.[13] These limitations have shifted the emphasis toward other strategies such as pretargeting for delivering a therapeutic dose to tumour without damaging normal tissues.[14-16] One of such strategy, is based on the avidin–biotin system.[17-19] The combined use of avidin/biotin and MAb has been shown not only to enhance the effect of MAb at the binding site but also allow separate delivery of the MAb and the radioactive label.[20]

The observation that various tumours contain high numbers of somatostatin receptors has spurred the recent development of a new analogue of somatostatin, octreotide, which can be easily radio-labelled with a variety of radionuclides. It has shown high hepatobiliary excretion accompanied by augmented accumulation in liver metastases.[21-23]

Locoregional Therapy with Beta-emitting Radionuclides

Intra-Arterial Administration

Historically, an intra-arterial approach was the first nuclear medicine technique to be pursued for the treatment of hepatic malignancies.[24,25] The radionuclide employed was yttrium-90 (^{90}Y) which possesses the ideal characteristics for this therapeutic application. It has a half-life of 64 hours and a pure high-energy beta emission with a maximum energy of the beta particles of 2.2 MeV (mean energy of 0.93 MeV) which allow a maximum solf-tissue penetration of 1.1 cm (average 0.25 cm). The initial challenge was to bind the radionuclide firmly to an inert particulate material with a size that, once infused into the arterial supply of the liver, would lodge in the end capillaries of hepatic parenchyma. One of the first clinical trials reported the use of ^{90}Y-labelled resin microspheres in 15 patients with hepatic malignancies.[26] The arterial supply to the liver was catheterized and a dose of ^{90}Y, calculated to deliver 50 Gy to the whole organ, was bound to particles with a size of $15 \pm 5 \mu m$. Of the 12 patients who were successfully treated, 8 died of disseminated disease within six months. Four patients remained alive with a performance status of 70–80% on the Karnofsky scale with follow-up periods of 6, 6, 9 and 12 months post-treatment.

Some consideration on the potential benefits of this therapy emerged from the study. Vascularity of the hepatic tumours played a significant role in obtaining beneficial results with the greater concentration of radioactivity within the lesions being achieved in the tumours with greater vascularity. In this study, all the survivors had metastases that were well vascularized while serial angiograms revealed relatively avascular metastases amongst the group of patients who died.

The initial enthusiasm for this technique, however, was dampened by the inability of the tumours to retain completely the ^{90}Y in the liver until its decay. Part of the administered activity was found to leach from ceramic, resin or plastic materials and the ^{90}Y released from the particles, being a bone-seeker element, caused myelosuppression leading to poor clinical outcomes.[27]

More recently, a new particulate agent in which the ^{90}Y was incorporated in glass microspheres was tested in the clinical setting. A trial involving 23 patients with hepatic metastases was conducted to assess the hepatic parenchymal changes following intra-arterial administration of 50–150 Gy of ^{90}Y-bound agent.[28] A correlation between the parenchymal changes, determined by computed tomography (CT), and radiation dose was observed. All 3 patients who received the highest dose of 150 Gy showed marked severe parenchymal changes indicating that this treatment may be a viable option in the therapy of unresectable hepatic malignancies. In addition, the current preparation of ^{90}Y bound to glass microspheres seemed to have overcome the disadvantages of free yttrium, as there have been no reports of bone-marrow toxicity or pulmonary fibrosis from centers using this new agent.[27]

Intratumoral Administration

In an attempt to deliver higher radiation doses to hepatic lesions, direct intratumoral administration of radiolabelled agent has been recently explored. Thirty-three patients with liver tumours and were not candidates for surgery due to the lesion location, size or unfavourable clinical conditions, were injected with 74–92.5 MBq of ^{90}Y bound to glass microspheres directly into the tumours under real-time ultrasound guidance.[29] For tumours >3 cm in diameter, two or three injections were given and, in most cases the procedure was repeated at intervals of 3–4 weeks in order to deliver doses to the entire tumour. Only 6 patients died during the follow-up period of 12–32 months and most were already at the end stage of their disease at the commencement of the therapy. The 27 surviving patients showed a dramatic improvement in their clinical condition and hepatic ultrasonography showed that 91% of the 32 foci treated showed evidence of tumour shrinkage. The radioactive material remained in its injected location as a 'point source' until radioactivity decay as shown by serial Bremsstrahlung scintigraphy thus delivering a killing dose of 28–75 Gy to the periphery of the lesions where surviving tumour cells are more frequently found. The most appealing feature of this therapeutic modality has been that the tumour received almost all the radiation, whereas the adjacent normal liver tissues and other organs received very little, thus ensuring both safety and therapeutic efficacy, as demonstrated by the favourable outcome of this trial.

In conclusion, the locoregional approach allows delivery of radiation doses to tumours that are up to four times higher than those delivered to the normal liver tissues[30] but has the drawback of requiring a surgical procedure to place the radioactive material in to the lesions.[31]

Systemic Therapy with Radiolabeled Monoclonal Antibodies

General Considerations on Radioimmunotherapy

The concept of linking a specific antitumour antibody to a cytotoxic agent has an appealing simplicity, since the toxicity to normal tissue is limited. In this form of tumour therapy, monoclonal antibodies have been conjugated with chemotherapeutic agents, biological toxins or radionuclides.[32]

Radioimmunotherapy (RIT) produces its antitumour effect primarily as a result of the radioactivity associated with the radiolabelled antibody, which emits continuous exponentially decreasing low-dose-rate irradiation. In some situations, the antibody itself may contribute to tumour cell killing. Important determinants of RIT are the antibody (specificity, affinity, avidity, dose and immunoreactivity), the radionuclide (emission properties and chemical stability of the radioimmunoconjugate), the targeted antigen (location, density, heterogeneity of expression, stability and modulation), and the characteristics of the targeted tumour including intrinsic radiosensitivity, proliferative rate, volume and tumour bed.[33]

The range of radioisotopes which can be chosen for the production of radiolabelled antibody is ever increasing. Although the main mode of killing tumour cells is generally by damaging DNA, each radioisotope has a characteristic type and rate of decay that must be considered for its applicability for radioimmunotherapy. Furthermore the chemistry involved in conjugating antibody to the radioisotope is quite varied. Several radioisotopes, in particular ^{131}I and ^{125}I, can be directly conjugated to the antibody. Others involve the binding of a chelator to the antibody with subsequent conjugation to the radioisotope. Radiometals like ^{90}Y, ^{111}In and ^{186}Re are coupled by this technique. The most important aspect of all the binding techniques is to avoid altering the antigen binding region of the antibody to ensure optimal tumour concentration.

One of the main therapeutic advantages of radiolabeled MAbs is their potential to overcome the problem of tumour heterogeneity. Since the radionuclides can penetrate up to several millimetres of tissues, the emissions can kill tumour cells which are antigen-negative and have no radiola-

belled antibody localised on their surface (the cross-fire effect).

Systemic RIT

Patients with liver metastases arising from colorectal carcinomas present with greatly elevated serum levels of carcinoembryonic antigen (CEA). The therapeutic use of radiolabeled anti-CEA MAbs has been investigated in several experimental xenograft studies.[34] At a clinical level, the majority of the studies with anti-CEA MAbs have been directed toward the radioimmunolocalization of a variety of CEA-expressing tumours. The first anti-CEA MAb was developed in 1981 and showed about 50% localization in a series of 31 patients with colorectal carcinomas.[35] Other 26 anti-CEA MAbs were investigated by the same group and one of them, named 'antibody 35', was labelled with ^{123}I and tested in 12 patients with known liver metastases. In 10 out of 12 patients, the lesions accumulated the radioactive label and two of them, with normal liver CT scans, ultrasound and with evidence of antibody uptake, had the scintigraphic findings confirmed at surgery.[36] Anti-CEA MAbs have only been used in a pilot trial which included 7 patients who each received 3.7–7.4 GBq of ^{131}I-labelled MAb through the hepatic artery. Despite excellent images showing an intense uptake, there was no tumour response.[37] Therefore a trial involving 20 patients was carried out with the purpose of measuring the real uptake per gram of metastases which became available at surgery 3–8 days after the i.v. injection of ^{131}I-labelled anti-CEA MAb.[38] The amount of ^{131}I activity 0.55–1.48 GBq and antibody 15–60 mg were chosen in order to simulate a RIT trial. The uptake per gram of metastases ranged from 0.33 to 6.6×10^{-3}% of the injected dose. Encouraging results were observed in terms of tumour to normal liver ratios of radiolabelled MAb indicating that it is possible to administer large amounts of ^{131}I-MAb without hepatic toxicity. On the other hand, bone marrow would be the only site of acute radiotoxicity and a dose of 11.1 GBq was calculated as the maximum injectable without great risk of aplasia. Therefore, a dose tolerable to the bone marrow, would probably not be sufficient to effect macroscopic non-resectable metastases, but it may have a potential effect upon microscopic metastases.

Another antigen which is expressed in approximately 85% of colonic adenocarcinomas and in their

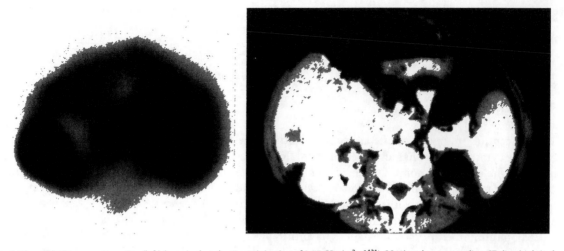

Figure 14.1. SPECT transverse section (left) (acquired on day 7 postinjection of 2.77 GBq/m^2 of ^{131}I-CC49) and corresponding CT slice (right) of a patient with metastatic colorectal cancer. A focal metastatic lesion in the inferior portion of the right lobe of the liver is evident in both the SPECT and CT images. This 3-cm lesion was not clearly identified in the planar images performed on the same day. (Reprinted from *Cancer Investigation* 1994; 12(6): 555, by courtesy of Marcel Dekker, Inc.)

liver metastases is the tumour-associated glycoprotein TAG-72.[39] The anti-TAG-72 MAb, called 'B72.3', is one of the most widely studied antibodies.[40] Radiolocalization of ^{131}I-B72.3 in patients with metastatic colorectal carcinomas has been demonstrated. A new generation of anti-TAG MAb with higher affinity and superior reactivity with tumour cells, has recently been tested in 18 patients with measurable metastatic colorectal carcinoma.[41] The MAb CC49 (20 mg) was labelled with ^{131}I in amounts varying from 0.55 GBq/m^2 to 2.77 GBq/m^2 and administered intravenously. Whole-body images and SPECT (single photon emission computed tomography) of the abdomen were obtained on day 3 and 7 postinjection (Figure 14.1) and compared with pretreatment CT scans. Moreover a subset of patients with primary-tumour histology with high expression of TAG-72 antigen was identified. The authors concluded that in patients with significant TAG-72 tumour expression, there was an excellent targeting (94%) of the lesions with therapeutic doses of ^{131}I-CC49 with respect to lesions detected with CT scanning.

One of the limitations of immunotherapy using murine antibodies is the tendency to develop an immune response. In an effort to overcome this, chimaeric mouse/human antibodies have been generated by recombinant DNA technology in order to decrease the amount of xenoprotein while maintaining antitumour specificity. In a Phase I study, ^{131}I-labelled chimaeric B72.3 was slowly infused to a group of 12 patients with liver metastases from colon cancer.[42] The dose administered ranged from 0.66 GBq/m^2 to 1.33 GBq/m^2. The only toxicity noted in this trial was bone-marrow suppression which was observed at a dose of 1.0 GBq/m^2. The expectation of being able to perform repeated infusions of this humanized MAb was not met, since 58% of the patients developed an immune response to the chimaeric B72.3. A second infusion, performed in several patients, resulted in a dramatic shortening of the plasma half-life and prevention of radioimmunolocalization in metastases previously clearly detected. Thus, the chimaeric B72.3 tested in this trial, showed limited utility as a means of delivering multiple therapeutic doses of ^{131}I, but the use of other chimaeric human isotypes, chimaeric antibody fragments or novel genetically engineered molecules may produce a breakthrough in this therapeutic modality.

Local (Intrahepatic) RIT

A therapeutic trial involving the intrahepatically administration of radiolabelled anti-CEA antibodies has been initiated for the treatment of hepatic metastases secondary to carcinoma of the colon. The protocol involves the concurrent administration (via the hepatic artery) of an anti-CEA MAb, labelled with ^{131}I, with biodegradable starch microspheres to achieve temporary stasis of hepatic blood flow.[43]

This followed the successful treatment of a 69-year-old man in whom hepatic metastases were noted at the time of hemicolectomy for adenocarcinoma of the colon. Initially, the lesions were localized using a tracer dose of ^{131}I-MAb. Then, following hepatic artery catheterization, a dose of 3.3 GBq of ^{131}I bound to 20 mg of MAb was slowly infused over 1 h. After this first treatment, the patient had a good clinical response and a CT scan of the liver, performed one month later, showed up to 30% reduction in size of some metastases. Unfortunately, about 6 weeks after antibody-guided therapy, his condition deteriorated. He was treated again with 4.0 GBq of ^{131}I in 20 mg of MAb administered as a 5-min bolus concurrently with 15 ml (60 mg/ml) of starch microspheres. Follow-up isotope scans showed high uptake of radioactive label in the lesions. There was marked improvement in his clinical condition and serum CEA levels fell to within the normal range in the first month after therapy. A repeat CT scan showed a decrease in size of the liver metastases and the surgeon who performed the original operation, observed during laparotomy that the liver metastases, particularly in the left lobe, had diminished considerably in size. Overall, this new and specific method for the treatment of hepatic metastases showed the potential to enhance the targeting of ^{131}I-labelled-anti-CEA MAb with minimal toxicity.

New Strategies: The Pretargeting Approach

Various groups have investigated the concept of tumour pretargeting based on the separate administration of MAbs and radiolabelled isotopes.[14,15,44] The injection can be delayed to a time when most of the primary MAb has been cleared from blood and normal tissues, and therefore, this strategy can achieve higher tumour to non-tumour ratios.

In pretargeting systems, MAbs first require their tagging to enable recognition by a second molecule. Four different types of tagged targeting vehicles for the use in pretargeting strategies have been described in the literature:

- biotin-conjugated or biotinylated antibodies;
- streptavidin-conjugated or streptavidinylated antibodies;
- bifunctional MAbs (Bs-MAbs); and
- monoclonal antibody–oligonucleotide conjugates

The biotinylation of MAbs is easily accomplished, and four or five biotin molecules can be incorporated per antibody molecule without loss of immunoreactivity and the use of a long spacer arm between the protein-binding site and biotin reduces steric hindrance of the subsequent avidin–biotin reaction.[45]

The conjugation of streptavidin to MAb results in a molecular weight 40% greater than that of native MAb and therefore shows slower pharmacokinetics than MAb alone.[46]

Bispecific antibodies with two different antigen-specific binding sites, one for the tumour-associated antigen and one for the radioactive effector compound, have been proposed.[14] Unpredictable pharmacokinetic properties due to the many chemical manipulations required in the production of coupled Fab' fragments, can partially be overcome by using Bs-MAbs produced by hybrid hybridomas.[47]

The attachment of oligonucleotides to MAbs, typically binds three to five oligonucleotides per antibody molecule, and although it fully preserves their specificity, it reduces the immunoreactivity by approximately 50% due to steric hindrance or charge interference. Being DNA-based conjugates, these targeting structures also need careful preservation since they lose stability more rapidly than other MAb conjugates.[48]

Once the tagged MAbs have targeted the preselected tumour antigens, a second conjugate that will recognize with high selectivity the tag on the first MAb, is administered. Theoretically, this is best done at a time when the highest concentration of tagged MAbs are found on and in the tumour. The remaining tagged MAbs, which do not selectively bind to tumour antigens, must be cleared from the normal tissues and blood and be excreted. The second molecule needs to be cleared rapidly from the normal tissues and blood after achieving its highest concentration on tumour-bound antibodies.

Second conjugates are most often radiolabelled avidin, streptavidin or biotin molecules directed at the biotinylated or avidinylated MAbs. This pretargeting technique, thus takes advantage of the avidin–biotin system, which has long and widely been used for *in vitro* applications like immunocytochemistry, enzyme-linked immunosorbent assay (ELISA) and molecular biology. Due to the flexibility of this system, several protocols have been devised for its application in clinical trials.[49] Two major methods are presently used in the clinical practice.

Two-step Strategy

This approach has been initially proposed based on the *in vitro* conjugation of streptavidin to the antibody which is administered first, followed by the injection of radiolabeled biotin (2–3 days later). A preliminary report on 10 patients with lung cancer showed decreased activity levels in all normal organs and in blood and clear images were obtained as little as 2-h postinjection of ^{111}In-labelled biotin.[18] An alternative approach has also been used to target intraperitoneal tumours. When biotinylated MAbs are injected intraperitoneally, there is a rapid accumulation of antibodies in peritoneal tumour deposits while most of the immunoglobulins which

remain unbound leave the peritoneal cavity via the lymphatic system and eventually enter the blood pool. This first step involving biotinylated MAbs is then followed 1–2 days later by the administration of radiolabelled streptavidin (Figure 14.2), thus exploiting, at best, the specific binding of the biotinylated antibody onto the tumour.[50]

Three-step Strategy

The locoregional approach described above is feasible when tumour is confined to the peritoneal cavity or in other locoregional applications. In the presence of widespread disease, a systemic injection of the tracer is nonetheless required. A three-step approach has been designed for these cases, where conjugates need to be cleared not only from a well-defined body cavity, but from the entire blood pool (Figure 14.3).

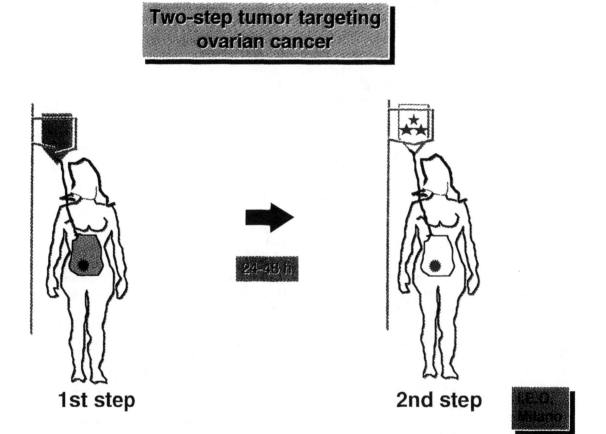

Figure 14.2. Two-step strategy. Biotinylated antibodies are injected intraperitoneally and allowed to localize into the target (first step). Then 1–2 days later, radioactive streptavidin is injected intraperitoneally to target the tumour.

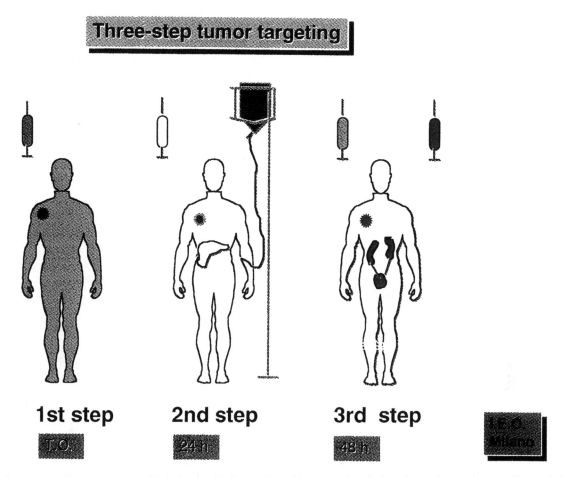

Figure 14.3.   Three-step strategy. Biotinylated antibodies are injected intravenously and allowed to localize into the target (first step). One day later, avidin/streptavidin are injected intravenously (second step). After 24 hours, when unbound streptavidin and circulating avidin–antibody complexes have been cleared from circulation, radiolabelled biotin is administered intravenously (third step).

Biotinylated MAbs are first injected (step 1) followed by injection of avidin/streptavidin one day later (step 2). The second injection is intended to remove excess circulating biotinylated antibodies in the form of cold complexes via avidin (fast clearance) and secondly to target tumour cells with streptavidin (slower clearance). Thereafter, radiolabelled biotin which will selectively bind to streptavidin and thus to the tumour, is injected (step 3).

The three-step approach is designed to remove the excess of circulating biotinylated MAbs as cold complexes, which are taken up and metabolized by the liver. This is the major factor in background reduction and is obtained prior to label injection. Moreover, the rapid blood clearance of the radiolabelled biotin allows imaging to be performed only 90–120 min after injection and with only very low background activity. In addition, another great advantage of this strategy is that of signal

amplification, which may occur if avidin binds more than one, and up to four molecules of radioactive biotin per molecule of avidin.

The Clinical Applications of the Avidin–Biotin System to the Therapy of Liver Metastases and Locoregional Recurrences from Colorectal Carcinomas

A total of 11 patients with advanced metastatic colorectal carcinomas and increased circulating CEA levels were studied at the European Institute of Oncology in Milan with a new three-step protocol. The patients received 30–40 mg of biotinylated anti-CEA monoclonal antibody (FO23C5, Sorin Biomedica, Saluggia, Italy) by intravenous injection, followed 24 hours later with 20–30 mg of avidin as a rapid bolus chase, and 50 mg of streptavidin in

100 ml of saline solution as a slow infusion. A second chase of 10–25 mg of biotinylated human serum albumin was administered 18–24 hours after the first chase and 10 min prior to the injection of 2.0 mg of ^{90}Y labeled biotin. The labeling of biotin with 1850–3700 MBq of ^{90}Y (labelling yield >95%) was achieved through the macrocyclic chelating agent 1,4,7,10-tetraazacyclododecane-N,N′,N″,N‴-tetraacetic acid (DOTA) attached to biotin via a non-cleavable linker (NeoRx Corporation, Seattle, USA) by dissolving the compound in ammonium acetate 1.0 M (pH = 7.0) and incubating at room temperature for 1 hour and at 80°C for 15 min. The final preparation was spiked with 0.5 mg of biotin-DOTA labeled with 74–111 MBq of indium-111 in order to follow the *in vivo* biodistribution. An aliquot of the injection mixture was withdrawn as standard for calculating the activity in the injected dose. Blood and urine samples were obtained at various time points up to 48 hours after injection. The percentage of the injected dose in these fluids was determined with the use of a gamma-counter.

The variation of the biodistribution in patients was obtained by the analysis of SPECT images, as well as by static and whole-body scintigraphic images, acquired at 1, 15, 24 and 40 hours after administration, using a gamma-camera equipped with a medium energy general-purpose collimator. The uptake of radioactivity in various organs was determined by the drawing of regions of interest in static, whole-body and SPECT images.

The absorbed dose in critical organs was determined by considering the activity integrated over time, the studied mass evaluated by CT or MRI, and the 'S' values of the MIRD (medical internal radiation dosimetry) formalism properly modified. The mean dose in the bone marrow was calculated from the 'S' values of the MIRD formalism, taking into account the different contributions of the ^{90}Y in the blood present in the whole body, in the trabecular and cortical bone, as well as the free ^{90}Y eventually localized in the bone. The mean doses in kidneys and liver were 450 ± 210 and 150 ± 130 cGy, respectively, while the dose delivered to the tumour was of 860 ± 450 cGy. All patients revealed the same activity profile in blood and this resulted in a mean absorbed dose of 80 ± 50 cGy in bone marrow.

The therapy was well tolerated by all patients and no acute toxicity was observed. None of the patients developed HAMA (human antimouse antibody) and only one showed an anti-avidin immune response. All patients, however, developed an immune response to streptavidin. Hematological toxicity was not observed, up to six weeks after treatment.

The blood clearance of ^{90}Y-DOTA–biotin was similar to that observed in the pilot study in which only avidin was used, with the slow component of elimination showing a $t_{1/2}$ of 1.4 ± 0.4 hours. Approximately 70% of the injected dose of labelled biotin was cleared from the body by the kidneys.

Of 9 patients evaluated with a follow-up of 2–12 months, 2 had minor responses, 4 cases were classified as stable disease and 3 as progressive disease. In particular, 1 patient who presented with multiple lung and liver metastases, revealed decreasing CEA levels, from an initial 60 ng/ml to 2.6 ng/ml four weeks following treatment. A second patient, who presented with diffuse liver metastases showed a regression of some lesions of >50% in size, while a third patient showed total regression of one of his liver metastases (Figure 14.4).

In summary, the preliminary data obtained from the use of this pretargeting technique have shown that high doses of ^{90}Y can be administered safely in humans with low bone-marrow toxicity and that some cytotoxic effects to tumours and particularly their metastases can be achieved. Moreover, the use of streptavidin instead of avidin seems to increase the dose delivered to the tumour. However, the immunogenicity of streptavidin is a problem which requires further consideration.

New Radiopharmaceuticals Based on Receptor Binding

A wide variety of human tumours contain high concentration of somatostatin receptors, which enable *in vivo* localization of the primary tumour and its metastases by scintigraphy with radiolabelled somatostatin analogues.[22] However, the extremely short biological half-life of somatostatin has prevented its clinical application. Therefore peptide analogues have been developed that possess the same pharmacological properties as somatostatin, but which clear much more slowly from the circulation. One of them, octreotide, has been the first commercially available analogue, and is far more effective than somatostatin in the suppression of growth hormone secretion.[21] Octreotide has been labelled with ^{123}I and ^{111}In and used to

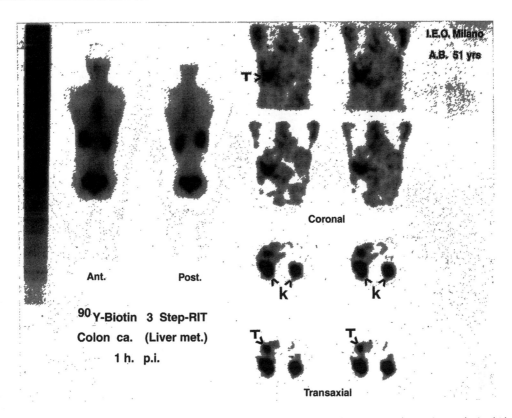

Figure 14.4. On the left, anterior and posterior whole-body planar images of a patient with metastatic colon carcinoma obtained 1 hour after the injection of ^{90}Y-DOTA–biotin (spiked with ^{111}In). The majority of the activity is excreted through the kidneys, masking the uptake of the liver metastasis localized in the right lobe. On the right, the tomographic images clearly show the uptake in the liver metastasis (T = tumour; K = kidney).

image somatostatin receptor-positive tumours in humans.[51] Besides neuroendocrine tumours, somatostatin receptors have also been identified in tumours of the central nervous system, breast, lung and lymphoid tissue and gastrointestinal tract.

A recent comparative scintigraphic study using three different radiolabelled anologues was conducted in 21 patients with histologically verified intestinal carcinoid tumours. Ten of them had known liver metastases that were imaged in seven patients.[52] A commercially available analogue (pentetreotide) can be tagged with ^{111}In through the chelating agent DTPA which is coupled with the phenylalanine in position 1 of the octreotide analogue. Since DTPA is known to bind other therapeutic useful radiometals such as ^{90}Y, it would be possible to treat with ^{90}Y-DTPA pentetreotide patients showing an accumulation in the tumour of the ^{111}In-labelled compound.

Recent studies have shown that the *in vivo* stability of the yttrium complexes can be largely improved by using macrocyclic chelating agents

such as the 12-membered ring compound DOTA.[53] These observations have prompted the synthesis of several derivatives of DOTA for linkage to pentetreotide in order to achieve a better and stable binding with ^{90}Y[54].

In our Division of Nuclear Medicine we have successfully imaged one patient with primitive pancreatic tumour which had metastatized to the liver with a three-step pretargeting approach using an antichromogranin A (CgA) MAb directed against a 49-kDa glycoprotein produced by endocrine cells.[55] The same patient was also studied with the commercial product pentetreotide labelled with ^{111}In. The liver metastases were clearly visualized in both studies (Figure 14.5). The expression of somatostatin receptors and the secretion of chromogranins by liver metastases makes of great interest to perform such comparative studies on the same patients since the two methods seem to be complementary.[56]

We expect to treat patients with positive staining by the anti-CgA MAb with therapeutic doses of ^{90}Y

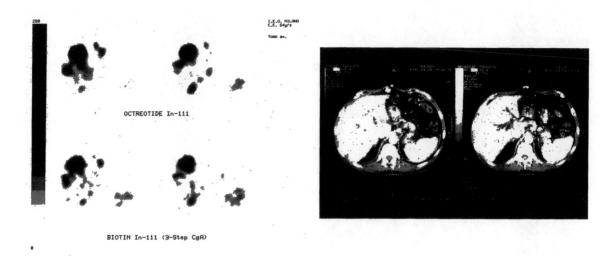

Figure 14.5. On the right, a CT scan of the abdomen showing multiple liver metastases from a carcinoid tumour originating in the pancreas. On the left, a comparison between [111]-In-pentetreotide and three-step immunoscintigraphy using the anti-CgA MAb. Both tracers show excellent uptake in the liver lesions.

and subsequently with the new DOTA-pentetreotide derivatives labelled with [90]Y.

References

1. Adson MA. Hepatic metastases in perspective. *AJR* 1983; **140**:695–700.
2. Saenz NC, Cady B, McDermott WV Jr *et al.* Experience with colorectal carcinoma metastatic to the liver. *Surg Clin North Am* 1989; **69**:361–370.
3. Jaffe BM, Donegan WL, Watson F *et al.* Factors influencing the survival in patients with untreated hepatic metastases. *Surg Gynec Obstet* 1968; **127**:1–11.
4. Bengmark S, Hafstrom L. The natural history of primary and secondary malignant tumors of the liver. The prognosis for patients with hepatic metastases from colonic and rectal carcinoma by laparotomy. *Cancer* 1969; **23**:198–202.
5. Ramming KP, Sparks FC, Eilber FR. Management of hepatic metastases. *Semin Oncol* 1977; **4**:71–80.
6. Huberman MS. Comparison of systemic chemotherapy with hepatic arterial infusion in metastatic colorectal carcinoma. *Semin Oncol* 1983; **10**:238–247.
7. Wharton JT, Delclos L, Gallager S *et al.* Radiation hepatitis induced by abdominal irradiation with the cobalt-60 moving strip technique. *AJR* 1973; **117**:73–80.
8. Turek-Maischeider M, Kazem I. Palliative irradiation for liver metastases. *JAMA* 1975; **232**:625–628.
9. Blanchard RJW. Treatment of liver tumours with yttrium-90 microspheres. *Can J Surg* 1983; **26**:442–443.
10. Harbert JC, Ziessman HA. Therapy with intraarterial microspheres. In: *Nuclear Medicine Annual* Freeman LM, Weissman HS (eds) 1987: 295–319. New York, Raven Press.
11. Kohler G, Milstein C. Continuous culture of fused cells secreting antibody of predifined specificity. *Nature* 1975; **256**:465–467.
12. Zalutsky MR. *Antibodies in Radiodiagnosis and Therapy*, 1989; Boca Raton, Florida, CRC Press.
13. Epenetos AA, Snook D, Durbin H *et al.* Limitations of radiolabeled monoclonal antibodies for localization of human neoplasms. *Cancer Res* 1986; **46**:3183–3191.
14. Goodwin DA, Meares CF, McCall M *et al.* Pre-targeted immunoscintigraphy of murine tumors with indium-111-labeled bifunctional haptens. *J Nucl Med* 1988; **29**:226–234.
15. LeDoussal JM, Martin M, Gautherot E *et al. In vitro* and *In vivo* targeting of radiolabeled monovalent and divalent haptens with dual specificity monoclonal antibody conjugates: enhanced divalent hapten affinity for cell-bound antibody conjugate. *J Nucl Med* 1989; **30**:1358–1366.
16. Goodwin DA. Tumor pretargeting: almost the bottom line. *J Nucl Med* 1995; **36**:876–879.
17. Hnatowich DJ, Virzi F, Rusckowski M. Investigations of avidin and biotin for imaging applications. *J Nucl Med* 1987; **28**:1294–1302.
18. Kalofonos HP, Rusckowski M, Siebecker DA *et al.* Imaging of tumor in patients with indium-111-labeled biotin and streptavidin-conjugated antibodies: preliminary communication. *J Nucl Med* 1990; **31**:1791–1796.
19. Paganelli G, Malcovati M, Fazio F. 1990; Monoclonal antibody pre-targeting techniques for tumour localization: the avidin-biotin system. *Nucl Med Commun* 1991; **12**:211–234.
20. Fazio F, Paganelli G. Antibody-guided scintigraphy: targeting of the 'magic bullet'. *Eur J Nucl Med* 1993; **20**:1138–1140.
21. Bauer W, Briner U, Doepfner W *et al.* SMS 201–995: a very potent and selective octapeptide analogue of somatostatin with prolonged action. *Life Sci* 1982; **31**:1133–1140.
22. Krenning EP, Kwekkeboom DJ, Bakker WH *et al.* Somatostatin receptor scintigraphy with [^{111}In-DTPA-D-Phe[1]]- and [^{123}I-Tyr[3]]-octreotide: the Rotterdam experience with more than 1000 patients. *Eur J Nucl Med* 1993; **20**:716–731.
23. Anderson CJ, Pajeau TS, Edwards WB *et al. In vitro* and *in vivo* evaluation of copper-64-octreotide conjugates. *J Nucl Med* 1995; **36**:2315–2325.
24. Grady ED, Sale W, Nicolson WP Jr. Intra-arterial radioisotopes to treat cancer. *Am Surg* 1960; **26**:678–683.
25. Nolan TR, Grady ED, Crumbley AJ *et al.* Intravascular particulate radioisotope therapy: clinical observations of 76 patients with advanced carcinoma treated with 90-yttrium particles. *Am Surg* 1969; **35**:181–192.

26. Mantravadi RV, Spigos DG, Tan WS et al. Intraarterial yttrium 90 in the treatment of hepatic malignancy. Radiology 1982; 142:783–786.

27. Herba MJ, Illescas FF, Thirlwell MP et al. Hepatic malignancies: improved treatment with intraarterial Y-90. Radiology 1988; 169:311–314.

28. Marn CS, Andrews JC, Francis IR et al. Hepatic parenchymal changes after intraarterial Y-90 therapy: CT findings. Radiology 1993; 187:125–128.

29. Tian JH, Xu BX, Zhang JM et al. Ultrasound-guided internal radiotherapy using yttrium-90-glass microspheres for liver malignancies. J Nucl Med 1996; 37:958–963.

30. Grady ED. Internal radiation therapy of hepatic cancer. Dis Colon Rectum 1979; 22:371–375.

31. Botet JF, New treatment approaches to liver tumors. J Nucl Med 1996; 37:963–964.

32. Wilder RB, DeNardo GL, DeNardo SJ. Radioimmunotherapy: recent results and future directions. J Clin Oncol 1996; 14:1383–1400.

33. Goldenberg DM. Cancer Therapy with Radiolabeled Antibodies, 1995; Boca Raton, Florida, CRC Press.

34. Goldenberg DM, Preston DF, Primus FJ et al. Photoscan localisation of GW-39 tumours in hamsters using radiolabelled anticarcinoembryonic antigen immunoglobulin. Cancer Res 1974; 34:1–9.

35. Berche C, Mach JP, Lumbroso J et al. Tomoscintigraphy for detecting gastrointestinal and medullary thyroid cancers: first clinical results using radiolabelled monoclonal antibodies against carcinoembryonic antigen. Br Med J 1982; 285:1447–1451.

36. Delaloye B, Bischof-Delaloye A, Buchegger F et al. Detection of colorectal carcinoma by emission computerised tomography after injection of ^{123}I labelled Fab and F (ab')$_2$ fragments from monoclonal anti-carcinoembryonic antigen antibodies. J Clin Invest 1986; 77:301–311.

37. Mach JP, Buchegger F, Bischof-Delaloye A et al. Progress in diagnostic immunoscintigraphy and first approach to radioimmunotherapy of colon carcinoma. In: Radiolabeled Monoclonal Antibodies for Imaging and Therapy, Srivastava SC (ed.), 1988: 65–78. New York, Plenum.

38. Ychou M, Ricard M, Lumbroso J et al. Potential contribution of ^{131}I-labelled monoclonal anti-CEA antibodies in the treatment of liver metastases from colorectal carcinomas: pretherapeutic study with dose recovery in resected tissues. Eur J Cancer 1993; 29A:1105–1111.

39. Thor A, Ohuchi N, Szpak CA et al. The distribution of oncofetal antigen TAG-72 defined by monoclonal antibody B72.3. Cancer Res 1986; 46:3118–3124.

40. Colcher D, Esteban JM, Carrasquillo JA et al. Complementation of intracavitary and intravenous administration of a monoclonal antibody (B72.3) in patients with carcinoma. Cancer Res 1987; 47:4218–4224.

41. Kostakoglu L, Divgi CR, Hilton S et al. Preselection of patients with high TAG-72 antigen expression leads to targeting of 94% of known metastatic tumor sites with monoclonal antibody ^{131}I-CC49. Cancer Invest 1994; 12:551–558.

42. Meredith RF, Khazaeli MB, Plott WE et al. Phase I trial of iodine-131-chimeric B72.3 (human IgG4) in metastatic colorectal cancer. J Nucl Med 1992; 33:23–29.

43. Epenetos AA, Courtenay-Luck N, Dhokia B et al. Antibody-guided irradiation of hepatic metastases using intrahepatically administered radiolabelled anti-CEA antibodies with simultaneous and reversible hepatic blood flow stasis using biodegradable strarch microspheres. Nucl Med Commun 1987; 8:1047–1058.

44. Paganelli G, Riva P, Deleide G et al. In vivo labelling of biotinylated monoclonal antibodies by radioactive avidin: a strategy to increase tumor radiolocalization. Int J Cancer (Suppl) 1988; 2:121–125.

45. Paganelli G, Magnani P, Zito F et al. Three-step monoclonal antibody tumor targeting in carcinoembryonic antigen-positive patients. Cancer Res 1991; 51:5960–5966.

46. Sung C, van Osdol WW. Pharmacokinetic comparison of direct antibody targeting with pretargeting protocols based on streptavidin–biotin binding. J Nucl Med 1995; 36:867–876.

47. Suresh MR, Cuello AC, Milstein C. Bispecific monoclonal antibodies from hybrid hybridomas. Methods Enzymol 1986; 121:210–215.

48. Bos ES, Kuijpers WHA, Meesters-Winters M et al. In vitro evaluation of DNA–DNA hybridization as a two-step approach in radioimmunotherapy of cancer. Cancer Res 1994; 54:3479–3486.

49. Paganelli G, Magnani P, Siccardi AG et al. Clinical application of the avidin–biotin system for tumor targetting. In: Cancer Therapy with Radiolabeled Antibodies. Goldenberg DM (ed.), 1995; 239–254. Boca Raton, Florida, CRC Press.

50. Paganelli G, Belloni C, Magnani P et al. Two-step tumour targetting in ovarian cancer patients using biotinylated monoclonal antibodies and radioactive streptavidin. Eur J Nucl Med 1992; 19:322–329.

51. Bakker WH, Krenning EP, Breeman WA et al. In vivo use of radioiodinated somatostatin analogue: dynamics, metabolism and binding to somatostatin receptor-positive tumors in man. J Nucl Med 1991; 32:1184–1189.

52. Virgolini I, Angelberger P, Li S et al. In vitro and in vivo studies of three radiolabelled somatostatin analogues: ^{123}I-octreotide (OCT), ^{123}I-Tyr-3-OCT and ^{111}In-DTPA-D-Phe-1-OCT. Eur J Nucl Med 1996; 23:1388–1399.

53. Deshpande SV, DeNardo SJ, Kukis DL et al. Yttrium-90-labeled monoclonal antibody for therapy: labeling by a new macrocyclic bifunctional chelating agent. J Nucl Med 1990; 31:473–479.

54. Otte A, Jermann E, Behe M et al. DOTATOC: a powerful new tool for receptor-mediated radionuclide therapy. Eur J Nucl Med 1997; 24: 792–795.

55. Deftos LJ. Chromogranin A: its role in endocrine function and as an endocrine and neuroendocrine tumor marker. Endocr Rev 1991; 12:181–187.

56. Siccardi AG, Paganelli G, Pontiroli AE et al.. In vivo imaging of chromogranin A-positive endocrine tumours by three-step monoclonal antibody targeting. Eur J Nucl Med 1996; 23:1455–1459.

Palliative Care

Vittorio Ventafridda, Alberto Sbanotto and Ruth Burnhill

15

Introduction

Palliative care aims to improve the quality of life of patients, drawing attention to the global aspects of patients distress. Patients with cancer, especially those involved in active therapy and those with advanced disease, may experience severe symptom distress. This may influence physical and social function, curtail patient–caregiver interaction, and lead to emotional responses of anger, frustration or depression.[1] The poor prognosis of patients with liver metastasis strongly supports the need for a thorough evaluation of quality of life in medical and surgical trials addressing metastatic liver disease.[2] Indeed, quality of life has been proposed as one of the end-points in need of consideration for any specific cancer therapy.[3,4] The liver is a common site of metastasis from a wide range of cancers, especially those affecting the gastrointestinal tract, and its involvement accounts for >50% of deaths from colorectal cancer.[5,6] The clinical course of patients with liver metastasis is dependent on tumour behaviour and responsivness to therapy, but on the average, death occurs within six months from the diagnosis of inoperable disease. Up to the present time, no survey addresses the specific symptoms that may affect these patients. The reason for this is that symptoms deriving from the primary tumour, those from liver metastasis and those from additional metastatic sites may compound on the overall complaints of the patient.[7-9] For this reason, we will concentrate primarily on cancer patients with advanced gastrointestinal malignancies and liver metastasis.

Evaluation

Most patients with advanced malignancy experience a wide range of physical and psychological symptoms (Table 15.1). Multiple studies have investigated the impact of symptoms on the quality of life and distress of patients with advanced cancer and usually, a high prevalence of symptoms is related to a poorer quality of life. Portenoy and colleagues found that the vast majority of patients presented with multiple concurrent symptoms (mean 11.5, range 0–25) and that those with a higher number of symptoms had a greater psychological distress and a worse quality of life.[10] In another survey, Holmes *et al.* found a high

Table 15.1 Prevalence of main symptoms in patients affected by cancer (modified from Portenoy *et al.*)[17]

Symptoms	Percentage
Lack of energy	75%
Worrying	70%
Feeling sad	65%
Pain	65%
Sleepiness	60%
Nervous feeling	60%
Insomnia	50%
Xerostomia	55%
Anorexia	45%
Nausea	45%
Sweating	40%
Taste alterations	35%
Constipation	35%
Cough	30%
Weight loss	30%
Oedema	30%
Dyspnoea	25%
Vomiting	20%

Table 15.2 Important aspects in the assessment of patients

Cancer History
Past medical history (including drug allergies, abuse and
addiction)
Current symptoms
Psychosocial and financial aspects (with special attention to the
patient's knowledge of the disease process and its extent)
Global distress
Quality of life
Current medications
Physical examination
Available diagnostic data
Additional investigations needed or planned
Opinions from patients family, relatives and friends

correlation between the intensity of symptoms and the deterioration of daily life activities.[11]

Although different methods of data collection make comparison of results very difficult, most symptoms reveal a prevalence rate of >50%.[1,8,12-17] Psychosocial issues are generally evaluated poorly because of the subjective nature of symptoms and the many possible interactions among them. However, their importance for an accurate assessment of overall distress and quality of life cannot be underestimated.[17-20] In the evaluation of the patient, it is important to perform a comprehensive assessment that includes data from the past medical history, the psychosocial history, the current symptom complex, and the current medication schedule.[21] A complete medical examination and the evaluation of relevant laboratory and imaging data are also essential (Table 15.2). Several tools for the evaluation of symptoms have been described, validated and tailored for the assessment and follow up of distinct patient populations.[10,22-28] Some of these are overaly comprehensive and lengthy and require special training before their implementation. Others are simple and much easier to reproduce. Whenever possible, results should be discussed within a multidisciplinary team, so that the origin of distress, including physical, psychological, spiritual and social issues, can be identified.[29] When indicated, more specific investigations may be required to obtain a comprehensive understanding of the pathophysiology of the symptom complex. The importance of this is demonstrated by Gonzales *et al.* who evaluated the impact of a comprehensive approach to cancer pain and found that a previously undiagnosed aetiology for pain was present in 64% of patients, of which 20% were treatable with primary therapy.[30]

Ascites

Most often ascites represents a poor prognostic sign in cancer patients,[31] carrying a median survival of approximately 8-10 weeks from diagnosis.[32] Therefore, it is extremely important to achieve an adequate control of this complication with minimal hospitalizations and distress. Patients with malignant ascites usually have extensive intra-abdominal disease in the form of hepatic metastasis and/or peritoneal seedings. They may complain of abdominal swelling, respiratory discomfort, oesophageal reflux, pain, difficulty with de-ambulation and manifest symptoms of the squashed stomach syndrome.

Extensive hepatic metastasis may lead to a distortion of the normal hepatic structure and lead to a rise in portal venous pressure. In addition, the combination of poor nutrition and reduced albumin synthesis due to liver damage may result in a decreased colloid osmotic pressure. Studies conducted with intraperitoneal radiolabelled colloid have shown that in patients with widespread peritoneal disease and liver metastasis, additional fluid is lost into the peritoneal cavity due to a combination of lymphatic obstruction and of increased peritoneal fluid production.[33,34] Furthermore, factors produced by the tumour that are capable of altering the microvascular permeability have been proposed.[32]

The results from the management of ascites are often disappointing, and no gold standard treatment has been established. Current therapies vary widely from simple oral regiments to the insertion of peritoneovenous shunts. In nearly all instances, however, the treatment of ascites should begin with paracentesis, which provides both diagnostic and therapeutic value since, in many instances, the fluid does not reaccumulate. Protein content, as well as bacterial and cytological evaluations can be performed at that time. The ratio of serum to ascitic fluid content of lactate dehydrogenase, protein and carcinoembrionic antigen or other tumour markers, may be helpful when the diagnosis of malignant ascites is still uncertain.[32,35,36] Other non-neoplastic causes of ascites, such as congestive heart failure, cirrhosis, nephrosis, and less frequently, complications of radiotherapy and chemotherapy, should always be excluded. Therapeutically, paracentesis to control tense ascites, especially in those patients whose fluid re-accumulates at a relatively slow rate, is an effective procedure. Nevertheless, this approach is greatly debatable when the general condition of the patient is poor, since further protein depletion and increased debilitation of the patient will occur. Under these circumstances, paracentesis is indicated only if a substantial symptomatic advantage, i.e. relief from secondary dyspnoea, abdominal discomfort and pain, is gained from the procedure.

Medical management with diuretics is often instituted for ascites, even though it is difficult to predict which patients will respond. Good responses are seen in only 40–50% of patients.[37,38] Oral spironolactone (100–400 mg/day) and furosemide (40 mg/day) are the most commonly used drugs.[37,39,40] Water and salt restriction, used in the treatment of ascites due to cirrhosis, causes unnecessary distress and is not indicated, especially in the dying patient with malignant ascites. The introduction of radiolabelled colloids into the peritoneal cavity is used only rarely. Although response rates using this method vary between 30% and 50%, most studies are incomplete and do not include an evaluation on quality of life. Moreover, the onset of therapeutical effect is slow and usually 2–3 months are required before a maximum effect is seen.[41] Intracavitary injection of irritating agents, like bleomycin and *Corynebacterium parvum*, to induce obliteration of the space between visceral and parietal peritoneum have been proposed and 40–60% partial to complete responses have been obtained.[42,43] The intraperitoneal instillation of chemotherapeutic agents may be effective in ascites caused by gastrointestinal and ovarian carcinomatosis, and can be administered concomitantly with systemic antineoplastic agents. Commonly used agents in this method include cisplatin, 5-fluorouracil (5-FU), bleomycin and doxorubicin, and partial or complete responses range from 45 to 60% of cases.[44–47] Administration is usually through a temporarily placed catheter, which may itself be complicated by malfunction and sepsis, and which requires for its insertion a strict selection and follow-up of patients.[48,49]

In patients with rapidly recurring ascites and with a life expectancy of more than a few months, the implant of a peritoneovenous shunt should be considered. Shunts were first introduced for the management of refractory ascites in patients with either cirrhosis or malignancy.[50] The technique involves the placement of a shunt with a one-way valve that allows the collection of ascites from the abdominal cavity and drains it into the intravascular space. Usually, the superior vena cava or the right atrium are selected for intravascular placement of the catheter tip. Currently, two main types of shunts are used: the LeVeen and the Denver shunts. Both are equally effective in decreasing the amount of ascites and relieving secondary symptoms.[51,52] Some relative contraindications and special considerations to their use require mentioning. First, a serum bilirubin level >3 mg/dl in the presence of hepatic metastasis increases the risk of disseminated intravascular coagulation in the immediate postoperative period after shunt insertion.[53] Second, patients suffering from congestive heart failure may not be able to tolerate the increased preload resulting from the shunting of ascites into the intravascular space.[54] Third, in the case of infection of the ascitic fluid, a shunt should not be inserted. Fourth, shunt malfunction increases when the ascitic fluid contains a high concentration of protein or cells (e.g. blood cells) that may either clot or block the catheter. The most frequent complication is indeed shunt occlusion, which may arise in 10–40% of cases, and is usually secondary to catheter malposition, kinking or clot formation.[54–56] The long-term rate of ascites control through the use of shunts is approximately 70%.[51] This rate compares favourably with the use of intracavitary radiocolloids or chemotherapy.

Nevertheless, because peritoneovenous shunt insertion requires hospitalization and operative intervention, and because its use is associated with considerable morbidity, therapy should be reserved for few selected patients. Certainly, patients with a life expectancy of <1–2 months should not be considered candidates for shunt placement.

Cachexia–anorexia

Cancer cachexia is a syndrome characterized by anorexia, progressive wasting and weight loss.[57,58] It is more frequently seen in patients affected by lung, pancreatic and gastric cancer.[58] Current evidence suggests that it is more common in patients with solid tumours (breast cancer being the main exception) as compared to those with haematological malignancies.[59] The exact incidence of the cancer cachexia syndrome varies widely, being dependent on the precise definition of its individual symptoms and signs, primary cancer type and stage of disease. Different surveys have shown that 50–65% of patients affected with stomach, oesophagus, pancreas, colon and rectal cancer have significant weight loss and evidence of malnutrition at the time of operation.[60-62] The ECOG study led by DeWys failed to show a close relationship between extent of cancer and weight loss.[63] In patients undergoing antineoplastic treatments, chemotherapy plays an important role in weight loss through a variety of different mechanisms.[64] Weight loss can be present in about 50% of patients undergoing chemotherapy.[63] Radiotherapy also may cause weight loss, depending on the site treated and dose of radiation used.[65] Major gastrointestinal surgery usually causes weight loss and a fall in serum albumin, although part of the weight loss may due to neoplasm and organ removal, as well as fluid losses.[60,62,65] Patients admitted to palliative care services or to hospices present an higher incidence of weight loss that ranges from 55 to 80%.[13]

Anorexia affects from 30 to 80% of patients with cancer and is influenced by concomitant symptoms of xerostomia, dysphagia, taste alterations, dyspepsia, nausea, constipation and many others.[8,12-18,59,66] Psychological aspects and particularly depression can have a significant role in anorectic patients.[20,67]

A number of different mechanisms have been associated to the cachexia-anorexia syndrome and include the influence of factors like tumour necrosis factor (TNF) and other cytokines (the interleukins IL-1 and IL-6, and the interferon IFNγ), hormones, leukaemia-inhibitory factor, the abnormal production of eicosanoids, the activation of monocytes and macrophages, and the impairment of lymphocyte function through inadequate IL-2 production.[68-72] Despite extensive research into many of these mechanisms, it has proven difficult to attribute a definitive causative role of cancer cachexia and weight loss to any of the suggested mechanisms. Recently, Todorov and colleagues isolated in mice a circulatory catabolic factor. The substance identified is a proteoglycan (MW = 24 000) which produces cachexia *in vivo* by directly inducing muscle catabolism.[73] This substance has also been identified in the urine of cachectic patients with various types of neoplasms and weight losses of >1.5 kg per month. It has not been found in normal controls and in patients whose weight loss was secondary to trauma or <1.3 kg per month. Such promising findings may soon result in a better understanding of the underlying causes of cachexia and anorexia in cancer patients.

Limiting the wasting process and improving the quality of life are the main goals in the management

Table 15.3   Nutritional assessment of patients with cachexia

Clinical assessment and caloric intake
Anthropometric tests
  body weight
  skinfold thickness
  mid-arm circumference
Dynamometry
Laboratory tests
  plasma proteins
  urinary metabolite excretion
Infrared interactance test
Bioimpendance test
Research methods
  CT/MRI/ultrasound scanning
  neutron activation analysis
  whole-body potassium estimate
  total body water estimate

of patients with the cachexia–anorexia syndrome. The assessment of cachectic patients should be simple, considering primarily the clinical aspects, common anthropometric tests like body weight, the skinfold thickness test, dynamometry and a few laboratory tests (see Table 15.3). A weight loss of >10% is usually considered a mark of severe nutritional depletion. Ascites, oedema and tumour mass can all influence such assessment and food intake counts may need to be considered.[26] More complex methods of assessment are usually reserved for research.[74-78] Appetite assessment can be conducted through visual analogue scales or questionnaires[79,80] and is important in the overall assessment of quality of life in patients with advanced cancer.

Dietary counselling, as well as parental and enteral nutritional supplements have an important role in the management of anorexic and cachectic patients. The aim of the nutritional counselling is to improve the quality of life by giving the patient a greater enjoyment from eating. A comprehensive review of these issues has been undertaken by Bruera and Higginson.[81]

The pharmacological treatment of cachexia and anorexia is limited to a few medication groups. Corticosteroids, especially prednisolone, methylprednisolone and dexamethasone have been studied extensively. In one study of 116 patients affected by advanced gastrointestinal malignancies and treated with dexamethasone, a significant increase in appetite and stamina was noted. In this placebo-controlled trial, the additional effect of two different daily dosages of dexamethasone emerged after about two weeks of treatment but subsided after a total of four weeks. Side-effects were minimal except one case of gastrointestinal haemorrhage.[82] In a double-blind cross-over trial using prednisolone, Willox and colleagues reported a significant improvement in appetite and overall well-being in patients receiving chemotherapy.[83] In another, Bruera et al. showed that methylprednisolone twice a day significantly reduced pain and analgesic consumption. In addition, performance status, appetite and food intake improved significantly. The effect on appetite, however, was no longer present three weeks after the beginning of the trial.[79] Two other multicentre studies have evaluated the use of intravenous methylprednisolone, with similar results. In the first study, preterminal cancer patients obtained a significant increase in quality of life indexes with daily intravenous doses of 125 mg of methylprednisolone for a total of eight weeks.[84] In the second study, female patients with terminal cancer receiving the same daily dosage of methylprednisolone, reported an improved quality of life for the duration of the study.[85]

Although the exact mechanism of action of corticosteroids in patients with advanced and terminal disease is not known, these medications are currently used for a wide range of symptoms arising in these patients.[86-88] The side-effects of corticosteroids cannot be neglected, especially after prolonged use, and in cancer patients, weakness, delirium, proximal myopathy, osteoporosis and immunodepression have all been reported.

Synthetic progesterone derivatives including medroxyprogesterone acetate (MPA) and more recently, megestrol acetate have been shown to improve appetite and possibly non-fluid weight gain in advanced cancer patients, particularly those affected by breast cancer.[89-91] In several recently conducted controlled studies, megestrol acetate has been shown to have a significant effect on appetite.[92-95] Two of these studies have additionally reported a favourable effect on weight gain in a subgroup of patients.[93,95] A recent, multicenter randomized, double-blinded trial that studied the effect of 500 mg of oral MPA given twice daily to patients affected by advanced non-hormone-sensitive cancers, including gastrointestinal tumours failed to show a significant increase in quality of life evaluated through the European Organization for Research and Treatment Quality of Life Questionnaire (EORTC-QLQ-C30), but confirmed the beneficial effect on appetite and weight.[96]

The mechanisms of action of MPA and megestrol acetate are not yet known, but are possibly similar to other steroid agents. Weight gain appears to be principally due to increase in body fat stores and only in part due to hydration of the fat-free mass.[97] Most studies have reported only limited side effects secondary to MPA or megestrol acetate use.

Additional agents used in the treatment of cachexia and anorexia include hydrazine sulphate,[98,99] cyproheptadine,[100] cannabinoids[101] and pentoxifylline.[102] None of these agents have so far been shown to be effective in improving the cachexia–anorexia syndrome. More recently, eicosapentaenoic acid (EPA) has been proposed for treatment, owing to its ability to inhibit tumour-produced lipid-mobilizing factor and to reduce protein degradation.[103] Clinical controlled studies are now underway to determine its effectiveness in advanced cancer patients.

In summary, the management of the cachexia-anorexia syndrome should start by attempting to increase the oral intake through frequent, small, palatable, high-protein meals, and by attempting to reduce concurrent symptoms that may potentially interfere with the patients appetite. For this, the support of a dietitian is highly desirable. Secondarily, a pharmacological approach based on megestrol acetate, starting with a dose of 160 mg/day and titrating it up according to the patients response, can be initiated. When life expectancy is short and/or other problems suggest the use of steroids (e.g. pain or neurologic complications), dexamethasone can be recommended as an additional agent.

Nausea and Vomiting

Nausea and vomiting affect from 20 to 70% of patients with advanced or terminal cancer, especially those with breast and stomach cancer.[1,15,66,104] Prevalence of nausea and vomiting during the last six weeks of illness is reported to be around 40%.[66] Dunlop evaluated the gastrointestinal symptoms in a group of 50 patients with advanced cancer, and nausea was ranked as the eighth most frequent and distressing symptom.[59] Additionally, nausea was referred more frequently by female patients.

In the chronic nausea syndrome, symptoms persist for more than 2–4 weeks in the absence of defined aetiologies, like radiotherapy, chemother-

Table 15.4 Main emetic pathways and centres

Cortex	Taste, smell, raised intracranial pressure, and anxiety stimulate this area
Chemoreceptor trigger zone (CTZ)	Opioids, chemotherapy, metabolites, and direct irradiation stimulate this area. Dopamine and 5-HT$_3$ are the main neurotransmitters involved.
Cranial nerve VIII	Motion stimulates labyrinth receptors and impulses reach the CTZ, via the vestibular nuclei and cerebellum.
Gastrointestinal tract	Chemotherapy, radiotherapy, bowel obstruction, visceral metastasis and drugs can all cause central nervous system stimulation via vagal and sympathetic impulses. Dopamine and 5-HT$_3$ are the main neurotransmitters involved.
Vomiting centre	This is the central coordinating area, which integrates all stimuli deriving from the above mentioned areas. Acetylcholine and histamine are the main neurotransmitters involved at this level.

apy or postsurgical syndromes. This chronic state, as opposed to acute symptoms secondary to known causes, will be the main focus of this section. For a detailed pathophysiology of nausea and vomiting, the reader is referred to the text by Allan.[105] Additionally, Table 15.4 summarizes the main emetic centres and pathways. It may become apparent, that due to the involvement of several pathways and neurotransmitters, different antiemetics acting through different mechanisms and on different sites, may be necessary for adequate symptom relief. While nausea and vomiting related to chemotherapy and radiotherapy are generally related to a simple model of nausea, patients with advanced cancer often present a more complex clinical picture, where several factors may be involved.

A possible mechanism of chronic nausea is autonomic failure, originally described in patients affected by diabetes, chronic renal disease and neurological disorders.[106,107] Some of the common clinical characteristics of diabetic autonomic neuropathy, such as nausea, anorexia, early satiety, and cardiovascular dysfunction are also present in advanced cancer patients, especially those with a poorer performance status.[108] A possible multifactorial aetiology may be involved for autonomic failure in advanced cancer. Malnutrition itself may play a relevant role.[107] Moreover, autonomic failure, as suggested in several reports from lung cancer patients, could be the expression of a paraneoplastic syndrome.[109–111] Other causes of autonomic neuropathy are radiation damage, chemotherapeutic agents (e.g. vinca alkaloids), direct tumour involvement and HIV infection.[112,113]

Although opioid-related nausea is most commonly of short duration and responsive to most antiemetics, chronic nausea is also frequently reported. Specially those patients receiving high doses of opioids may develop severe nausea, accompanied by abdominal distension and severe constipation. Nausea in these cases may correlate to changes in position, such as seen in vestibular disturbances. Metabolite accumulation may explain the chronic nausea that develops in patients receiving long-term opioids, especially in the presence of renal insufficiency.[114]

In the evaluation of nausea and vomiting, concomitant symptoms of pain, dyspnoea and psychological disturbances should be integrated. The assessment should be dynamic and simple using visual analogue scales like the Edmonton Symptom Assessment Scale.[22] Once the intensity, frequency and associated symptoms of nausea have been recorded, commonly found causes should be sought. These include:

- Opioid therapy
- Constipation
- Bowel obstruction
- Iatrogenic causes (e.g. chemotherapy or radiotherapy)
- Metabolic imbalance
- Gastritis or peptic ulcer
- Autonomic failure
- Raised intracranial pressure
- Drugs other than opioids or antineoplastic agents (e.g. digitalis)

The management of chronic nausea is directed towards the underlying cause. Metabolic alterations including hypercalcemia, drug-related side-effects (e.g. opioids) and simple constipation are common causes of chronic nausea. Once the underlying factors are corrected, the pharmacological treatment of chronic nausea relies upon a 'step by step' approach. The initial treatment is with prokinetic agents that include metoclopramide, domperidone and cisapride. Multiple trials have studied the efficacy of prokinetic agents in gastroparesis.[115,116] In addition to the peripheral anti-emetic properties, metoclopramide has a central anti-emetic action. Since domperidone does not cross the blood–brain barrier, its action is exclusively peripheral and therefore, its central extrapyramidal side-effects, are minimal. The action of cisapride is through the reduction of gastroduodenal reflux and through an increase of intestinal peristalsis. Because all pro-kinetic agents stimulate gastrointestinal peristalsis, they are contraindicated in the presence of gastro-intestinal obstruction, where an increase in pain and vomiting may be seen.

Neuroleptics, such as phenothiazides and buty-rophenones, comprise an additional group of clini-cally used antiemetic agents. The strong effect of sedation limits their use. Haloperidol is the agent most often used, especially for chronic nausea related to opioids, where its main central mechan-ism of action results particularly useful.

Occasionally, adjuvant agents such as cortico-steroids, anticonvulsants, antidepressants, neurolep-tics and others are required. Corticosteroids are among the most widely used adjuvant agents. In addition to their non-specific anti-emetic effect, they may exert a direct anti-inflammatory effect that may be useful in those conditions characterized by oedema (e.g. in brain metastases or during radio-therapy or chemotherapy). Octreotide, a synthetic analogue of somatostatin, may be effective in gastrointestinal obstructive and subobstructive conditions, where it reduces the amount of gastrointestinal secretions and increases fluid re-absorption.[117]

Pereira and Bruera have proposed the following therapeutic ladder for the management of chronic nausea:[118] First, oral or subcutaneous metoclo-pramide (10 mg), administered every 4 hours is used. Second, oral or parenteral dexamethasone is added for its synergistic effects.[119] If the second step results ineffective after 2–3 days of treatment, higher doses (60–120 mg/day) of metoclopramide plus dexamethasone are administered.[120] When metoclopramide is contraindicated or if the previ-ous steps have failed to control the nausea, addi-tional agents, such as haloperidol or cisapride are used. The new 5-hydroxytryptamine 5-HT$_3$ antagonists, ondansetron and ganisetron, may be indicated when the usual anti-emetics have failed. Clinical experience with these agents is limited and high costs have strongly limited their use.[121]

Pain

Pain is a common symptom in patients with metastatic cancer. Its incidence in >75% of all patients is dependent on tumour type and stage of disease. Between 40 and 50% of all cancer patients with pain report it as moderate to severe, while another 25% describe it as very severe.[122,123]

The prevalence of pain in patients with liver metastases is not known. In primary liver cancer, >70% of patients present pain of various inten-sity.[124] Considering liver and biliary cancers together, prevalence of pain ranges from 65 to 100%, with a mean of 79%.[123] Pain in cancer patients may be directly or indirectly due to the following causes:

- disease progression and related pathology;
- invasive diagnostic and therapeutic procedures;
- side-effects of chemotherapy or radiotherapy;
- associated infections;
- skeletal and muscular pain related to immobility.

The nerve supply of the liver is via branches of the vagus and splanchnic nerves that originate mainly from the coeliac ganglia. Afferent sympathetic fibres transmit the pain signals to the central nervous system. The pathophysiological mechan-ism of liver pain is explained by the growth of metastatic lesions causing distension of the liver and stretching of the liver capsule. The rate of hepatic enlargement may play an important role in the production and intensity of perceived pain, as gradual enlargement of metastases often does not produce any pain. In addition, liver nociceptors may possibly be stimulated by changes in hepatic venous pressure.[125]

Pain originating from the liver is typically referred as dull, aching and poorly localized. It is usually referred to the midline and/or right hypocondrial regions and can radiate to the right shoulder or to one of the lower thoracic or upper lumbar segments. Often, it may be described as a mild-to-moderate pressure or full-ness sensation of insidious onset. Pain symptoms may be compounded by concurrent tumour involvement of other tissues or organs, often from the biliary system or the peritoneum. Only about 15–20% of patients with metastatic lesions are asymptomatic.

For adequate pain management, a correct pain assessment is of utmost importance[126] and the evaluation should include all of the following aspects:

- A detailed medical history that includes previous use of analgesics and other drugs.
- An accurate account of pain characteristics and intensity.
- A physical examination that includes a focused neurologic examination.
- A psychosocial assessment.
- Appropriate diagnostic tests.
- A diagnosis of the prevalent pain syndrome.

The evaluation of pain must be made from the patients own report. Other sources of assessment that include relatives or health professionals are only partially reliable. The two main classes of evaluation tools are intensity scales, such as visual analogue, numerical and verbal scales,[127] and pain questionnaires, such as the Brief Pain Inventory,[128] the Memorial Pain Assessment Card[129] and others.[130]

Because pain in cancer patients is a dynamic problem, it is important to re-assess the patient at regular intervals in order to evaluate the effectiveness of current treatments, and record the appearance of new pains.

Currently, medical treatment is the mainstay of cancer pain management.[131] The World Health Organization has proposed a simple, validated and effective method for the control of cancer pain.[132] This method has been shown to be effective in about 90% of patients with cancer,[133] and in about 75% of patients during the terminal phase of illness.[134] The method is based on a sequential, step-wise approach (see Figure 15.1) whereby medications are administered according to the following simple principles:

- By mouth.
- By the clock.
- By the ladder.
- For the individual.
- With attention to detail.

Patients with mild-to-moderate pain are given non-steroidal anti-inflammatory drugs (NSAIDs). Patients with moderate-to-severe pain, or those failing to obtain satisfactory relief from the first step, receive an opioid for mild pain (e.g. codeine) that is generally combined with a NSAID. If pain fails to be controlled with this second step, then stronger opioids are indicated (e.g. morphine) that are again combined with a NSAID. Adjuvant medications may be added at any step in order to treat side-effects (e.g. constipation) or concurrent symptoms (e.g. anorexia). The most common analgesics used are reported in Table 15.5, while a detailed review of the WHO analgesic ladder method and other pharmacological treatments are provided by Ventafridda and colleagues.[131]

The use of subcutaneous continuous infusion via a portable syringe-driver has been used extensively in recent years. It is a simple and efficacious way of drug administration, characterized by a high bioavailability, by a reduction of side-effects from the absence of a 'bolus effect', and by a stable, 24-hour analgesic coverage.[135,136] Similar results can be obtained with continous intravenous infusion of drugs, but there are practical problems that relate to venous access and limitation of patient mobility.[137] Furthermore, subcutaneous infusion of opioids is usually considered to be equally effective in analgesic potency as intravenous infusion.[138] The indications for a continuous opioid infusion are several and include dysphagia, gastrointestinal tract obstruction, opioid-related side-effects due to bolus administration (e.g. nausea and drowsiness), and chronic nausea.[135-137] With the application of the WHO analgesic ladder, results show an 80–90% good or satisfactory pain control.[132,139,140]

Nerve blocks and neurosurgical techniques may supplement or reduce the use of systemic drugs in order to obtain satisfactory analgesia. Among surgical techniques used for cancer pain management, the coeliac plexus block is probably the most common for pain originating in the abdomen.[131] It is indicated for pain that is due to cancer infiltration of upper abdominal viscera, including pancreas, liver, gallbladder and proximal small bowel.[141] Moreover, it should be used in those patients who have failed to obtain satisfactory analgesia with medications or those who have suffered intolerable side-effects. Various surgical techniques, which give similar results, are available.[142-145] Ischia and colleagues compared three different techniques for performing coeliac blocks in a randomized trial and found no significant differences in analgesic results.[146] Two further studies compared the efficacy of pharmacological treatment versus coeliac plexus block and showed similar results with both treatments tested.[147,148] One of these studies, however, showed a lower consumption of opioids in the coeliac plexus block group.[147] This technique can be

Table 15.5   Common analgesics for cancer pain

Drug	Schedules of administration	Notes
NSAID		
Aspirin	500–1000 mg p.o. q6 h	Gastrointestinal disturbances are common. Contraindicated in bleeding dyscrasias.
Paracetamol	500–1000 mg p.o. q4–6 h	Weak anti-inflammatory action. No adverse effects on gastric mucosa and platelets
Ibuprofen	200–1000 mg p.o. q6 h	Less gastrolesive than other NSAIDs. Contraindicated in bleeding dyscrasias.
Naproxen	200–250 mg p.o. b.i.d.	Gastrointestinal disturbances are less common than with aspirin. Contraindicated in bleeding dyscrasias
Opioids for moderate pain		
Codeine	60 mg p.o. q4–6 h	Constipation is common. It has both analgesic and antitussive action. Drowsiness.
Oxycodone	5 mg p.o. q4–6 h (starting dose)	Drowsiness. Constipation. Nausea and vomiting. No antitussive activity.
Tramadol	50–100 mg p.o. q6–8 h. Parenteral (i.v./i.m./s.c.) also available.	Drowsiness. Constipation. Nausea and vomiting. It has a codeine-equivalent antitussive action.
Opioids for severe pain		
Morphine	5–10 mg p.o. q4 h (starting dose in opioid-naive patients). No maximum limiting dose. Also administrable by i.v./i.m./s.c./rectal/nebulized route	It is the most important analgesic for cancer pain. Drowsiness (especially at the beginning of therapy). Constipation. Nausea and vomiting. It has antitussive action.
Methadone	3–5 mg p.o. q8–12 h (in opioid-naive patients). Also available the i.m./i.v. administration	Drowsiness. Constipation. Nausea and vomiting. Because of its dual phase kinetics, it can accumulate, especially in elderly patients. Contraindicated in confused patients. It can be an alternative to in patients with morphine unresponsiveness.
Hydromorphone	1 mg p.o. q4 h (in opioid-naive patients). It can be administered by i.v./i.m./s.c./rectal routes	As for other opioids: drowsiness, constipation, nausea and vomiting. It can be an alternative in patients with morphine unresponsiveness.

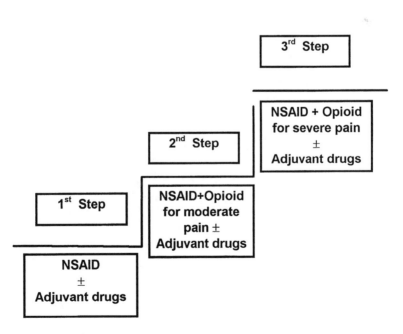

Figure 15.1.   The World Health Organization analgesic ladder (see text for explanation)

extremely efficacious in relieving true visceral pain, while somatic pain (e.g. pain due to retroperitoneal spreading) is much less sensitive. Most authors report good immediate analgesia in more than 80–90% of patients, but pain relief is usually short-lasting (average 2–4 weeks). After the effective pain relief period, most patients need some adjuvant form of pharmacological treatment, usually opioids.[146] Orthostatic hypotension is the most common side-effect of this technique and appears in approximately 50–70% of patients.[146] Less frequent side-effects include transient diarrhoea and pain at the site of injection. The most serious side-effect is that associated with accidental injection of the neurolytic solution into the subarachnoidal lumbar space or into the spinal roots.[142,149-151] Intraoperative chemical splanchnicectomy has been proposed for patients suffering pain diagnosed prior to the surgical intervention. The success rate ranges from 60 to 80% according to different authors.[152-154] A preventive analgesic effect in patients with no established pre-operative pain may equally be possible.[154] Surgical splanchnicectomy, performed through the transhiatal approach, has been reported to provide pain relief in <80% of patients.[155] Postoperative morbidity is approximately 20% and pleural-related complications comprise about 10%.[155] The less invasive thoracoscopic technique for splanchnicectomy has also been proposed and is under evaluation.[4,156] Nonetheless, all invasive techniques should be considered only as part of a continuing care programme and reserved for the few selected patients that can truly benefit from them.

A relatively common and severe pain syndrome which affects patients with gastrointestinal and ovarian cancer, often with concomitant liver metastases, is that of gastrointestinal obstruction.[157] It occurs in ≤28% of patients with colorectal cancer and in as many as 42% of patients with ovarian cancer.[158] Symptoms include continuous and/or colicky abdominal pain (respectively in about 90% and 75% of patients), nausea, vomiting, and constipation. Nasogastric suction and intravenous fluids can be useful in preparing patients for surgery, but are generally contraindicated in terminal patients. Nasogastric suction is uncomfortable and creates a physical barrier between the patient and the family. In the presence of a high-level obstruction, when pharmacological measures have failed to control the symptoms, a nasogastric tube may become unavoidable. A percutaneous venting gastrostomy is indicated in these patients if a longer survival is expected.[159,160] In patients with a poor general condition and unable to undergo surgery (e.g. with liver failure, ascites, palpable abdominal masses), non-operative pharmacological meassures, based on the concurrent use of analgesics, anti-emetics and anti-secretive drugs, should be attempted.[117,157] Results with a combined pharmacological approach are often successful and are respectful of the quality of life in these patients.[161,162]

Summary

In conclusion, the approach towards patients with advanced cancer and specifically those with liver metastases, should be global and multidisciplinary. For palliation, the control of symptoms is not sufficient in itself, as it is only part (though an important part) of the overall management and care of patients and their families. Since the aim of palliative care is the best quality of life possible for the individual patient, not only physical, but also psychosocial support should be provided and should involve the care of several professional disciplines. In the end, the success of palliative care is measured exclusively by the patient.

References

1. Coyle N, Adelhardt J, Foley KM, Portenoy RK. Character of terminal illness in the advanced cancer patient: pain and other symptoms during the last four weeks of life. *J Pain Symptom Manage* 1990; **5**(2):83–93.
2. Moinpour CM. Measuring quality of life: an emerging science. *Semin Oncol* 1994; **21**(5 Suppl 10):48–60.
3. Johnson JR, Temple R. Food and Drug Administration requirements for approval of new anticancer drugs. *Cancer Treat Rep* 1985; **69**(10):1155–1159.
4. Kosmidis P. Quality of life as a new end point. *Chest* 1996; **109**(5 Suppl):110S–2S.
5. Pickren JW. Tsukada Y, Lane WW, Liver metastases: analysis of autopsy data. In: *Liver Metastases*. Weiss L, Gilbert HA (eds), Boston, GK Hall. 1982:2–18.
6. Sugarbaker PH, Kemeny N. Treatment of metastatic cancer to the liver. In: *Cancer. Principles and Practice of Oncology*, 3rd edn De Vita VT, Hellman S, Rosenberg SA, (eds), 1989: 2275–2298. Philadelphia, JB Lippincott.
7. Given CW, Given BA, Stommel M. The impact of age, treatment, and symptoms on the physical and mental health of cancer patients. A longitudinal perspective. *Cancer* 1994; **74**(7 Suppl):2128–2138.

8. Reuben DB, Mor V, Hiris J. Clinical symptoms and length of survival in patients with terminal cancer. *Arch Intern Med* 1988; **148**(7):1586–1591.

9. Mor V, Masterson Allen S, Houts P, Siegel K. The changing needs of patients with cancer at home. A longitudinal view. *Cancer* 1992; **69**(3):829–838.

10. Portenoy RK, Thaler HT, Kornblith AB *et al*. The Memorial Symptom Assessment Scale: an instrument for the evaluation of symptom prevalence, characteristics and distress. *Eur J Cancer* 1994; **30A**(9):1326–1336.

11. Holmes S, Dickerson J. The quality of life: design and evaluation of a self-assessment instrument for use with cancer patients. *Int J Nurs Stud* 1987; **24**(1):15–24.

12. Brescia FJ, Adler D, Gray G, Ryan MA, Cimino J, Mamtani R. Hospitalized advanced cancer patients: a profile. *J Pain Symptom Manage* 1990; **5**(4):221–227.

13. Curtis EB, Krech R, Walsh TD. Common symptoms in patients with advanced cancer. *J Palliat Care* 1991; **7**(2):25–29.

14. Ventafridda V, De Conno F, Ripamonti C, Gamba A, Tamburini M. Quality-of-life assessment during a palliative care programme. *Ann Oncol* 1990; **1**(6):415–420.

15. Fainsinger R, Miller MJ, Bruera E, Hanson J, MacEachern T. Symptom control during the last week of life on a palliative care unit. *J Palliat Care* 1991; **7**(1):5–11.

16. Grosvenor M, Bulcavage L, Chlebowski RT. Symptoms potentially influencing weight loss in a cancer population. Correlations with primary site, nutritional status, and chemotherapy administration. *Cancer* 1989; **63**(2):330–334.

17. Portenoy RK, Thaler HT, Kornblith AB *et al*. Symptom prevalence, characteristics and distress in a cancer population. *Qual Life Res* 1994; **3**(3):183–189.

18. McCarthy M. Hospice patients: a pilot study in 12 services. *Palliative Med* 1990; **4**:93–104.

19. Plumb MM, Holland J. Comparative studies of psychological function in patients with advanced cancer. Self-reported depressive symptoms. *Psychosom Med* 1977; **39**(4):264–276.

20. Plumb MM, Holland J. Comparative studies of psychological function in patients with advanced cancer. II. Interviewer-rated current and past psychological symptoms. *Psychosom Med* 1981; **43**(3):243–54.

21. Ingham J, Portenoy R. Cachexia in context: the interactions among anorexia, pain and other symptoms. In: *Cachexia-Anorexia in Cancer Patients*. Bruera E, Higginson I (eds), 1996; 158–171. Oxford, Oxford University Press.

22. Bruera E, Kuehn N, Miller MJ, Selmser P, Macmillan K. The Edmonton Symptom Assessment System (ESAS): a simple method for the assessment of palliative care patients. *J Palliat Care* 1991; **7**(2):6–9.

23. Melzack R. The McGill pain questionnaire: major properties and scoring methods. *Pain* 1975; **1**:277–299.

24. Price DD, McGrath P, Rafti A *et al*. The validation of a visual analog scale or ratio scale for pain. *Pain* 1983; **17**:45–46.

25. Mahler D, Weinberg D, Wells C *et al*. The measurement of dyspnoea. *Chest* 1984; **85**:751–758.

26. Bruera E, Cowan I, Chadwick S *et al*. Caloric intake assessment in advanced cancer patients: a comparison of three methods. *Cancer Treat Rep* 1986; **70**(8):981–983.

27. Intensive treatment scheduling of nabilone plus dexamethasone vs. metoclopramide plus dexamethasone in cisplatinum-induced emesis. *Proc Am Soc Clin Oncol* 1986; 253.

28. Folstein MF, Folstein SE, McHugh PR. 'Mini-mental state'. A practical method for grading the cognitive state of patients for the clinician. *J Psychiatr Res* 1975; **12**(3):189–198.

29. Butters E, Higginson I, George R, Smits A, McCarthy M. Assessing the symptoms, anxiety and practical needs of HIV/AIDS patients receiving palliative care. *Qual Life Res* 1992; **1**(1):47–51.

30. Gonzales GR, Elliott KJ, Portenoy RK, Foley KM. The impact of a comprehensive evaluation in the management of cancer pain. *Pain* 1991; **47**(2):141–144.

31. Appelqvist P, Silvo J, Salmela L, Kostiainen S. On the treatment and prognosis of malignant ascites: is the survival time determined when the abdominal paracentesis is needed? *J Surg Oncol* 1982; **20**(4):238–242.

32. Garrison RN, Kaelin LD, Heusser LS, Galloway RH. Malignant ascites: clinical and experimental observations. *Ann Surg* 1986; **203**:644–651.

33. Lacy JH, Wieman TJ, Shively EH. Management of malignant ascites. *Surg Gynecol Obstet* 1984; **159**(4):397–412.

34. Coates G, Bush RS, Aspin N. A study of ascites using lymphoscintigraphy with ^{99m}Tc-sulfur colloid. *Radiology* 1973; **107**(3):577–583.

35. Green LS, Levine R, Gross MJ, Gordon S. Distinguishing between malignant and cirrhotic ascites by computerised stepwise discriminant functional analysis of its biochemistry. *Am J Gastroenterol* 1978; **70**:448–454.

36. Loewenstein MS, Rittgers RA, Feinerman AE *et al*. Carcinoembryonic antigen assay of ascites and detection of malignancy. *Ann Intern Med* 1978; **88**(5):635–638.

37. Sharma S, Walsh D. Management of symptomatic malignant ascites with diuretics: two case reports and a review of the literature. *J Pain Symptom Manage* 1995; **10**(3):237–242.

38. Razis DV, Athanasiou A, Dadiotis L. Diuretics in malignant effusions and edemas of generalized cancer. *J Med* 1976; **7**(6):449–461.

39. Amiel SA, Blackburn AM, Rubens RD. Intravenous infusion of frusemide as treatment for ascites in malignant disease. *Br Med J Clin Res Ed* 1984; **288**(6423):1041.

40. Greenway B, Johnson PJ, Williams R. Control of malignant ascites with spironolactone. *Br J Surg* 1982; **69**(8):441–442.

41. Jackson GL, Blosser NM. Intracavitary chromic phosphate ^{32}P) colloidal suspension therapy. *Cancer* 1981; **48**(12):2596–2589.

42. Paladine W, Cunningham TJ, Sponzo R, Donavan M, Olson K, Horton J. Intracavitary bleomycin in the management of malignant effusions. *Cancer* 1976; **38**(5):1903–1908.

43. Ostrowski MJ, Priestman TJ, Houston RF, Martin WM. A randomized trial of intracavitary bleomycin and *Corynebacterium parvum* in the control of malignant pleural effusions. *Radiother Oncol* 1989; **14**(1):19–26.

44. Hagiwara A, Takahashi T, Sawai K *et al*. Clinical trials with intraperitoneal cisplatin microspheres for malignant ascites - a pilot study. *Anticancer Drug Res* 1993; **8**(6):463–470.

45. Lind SE, Cashavelly B, Fuller AF. Resolution of malignant ascites after intraperitoneal chemotherapy in women with carcinoma of the ovary. *Surg Gynecol Obstet* 1988; **166**(6):519–522.

46. Lucas WE, Markman M, Howell SB. Intraperitoneal chemotherapy for advanced ovarian cancer. *Am J Obstet Gynecol* 1985; **152**(4):474–478.

47. Bitran JD. Intraperitoneal bleomycin. Pharmacokinetics and results of a phase II trial. *Cancer* 1985; **56**(10):2420–2423.

48. Kaplan RA, Markman M, Lucas WE, Pfeifle C, Howell SB. Infectious peritonitis in patients receiving intraperitoneal chemotherapy. *Am J Med* 1985; **78**(1):49–53.

49. Piccart MJ, Speyer JL, Markman M, ten Bokkel Huinink WW, Alberts D, Jenkins J, Muggia F. Intraperitoneal chemotherapy: technical experience at five institutions. *Semin Oncol* 1985; **12**(3 Suppl 4):90–96.

50. Leveen HH, Christoudias G, Ip M, Luft R, Falk G, Grosberg S. Peritoneovenous shunting for ascites. *Ann Surg* 1974; **180**(4):580–591.

51. Gough IR, Balderson GA. Malignant ascites. A comparison of peritoneovenous shunting and nonoperative management. *Cancer* 1993; **71**(7):2377–2382.

52. Cheung DK, Raaf JH. Selection of patients with malignant ascites for a peritoneovenous shunt. *Cancer* 1982; **50**(6):1204–1209.

53. Tempero MA, Davis RB, Reed E, Edney J. Thrombocytopenia and laboratory evidence of disseminated intravascular coagulation after shunts for ascites in malignant disease. *Cancer* 1985; **55**(11):2718–2721.

54. Lund RH, Moritz MW. Complications of Denver peritoneovenous shunting. *Arch Surg* 1982; **117**(7):924–928.

55. Lokich J, Reinhold R, Silverman M, Tullis J. Complications of peritoneovenous shunts for malignant ascites. *Cancer Treat Rep* 1980; **64**(2–3):305–309.

56. Campioni N, Pasquali Lasagni R et al. Peritoneovenous shunt and neoplastic ascites: a 5-year experience report. *J Surg Oncol* 1986; **33**(1):31–35.

57. Fearon KC, Carter DC. Cancer cachexia. *Ann Surg* 1988; **208**(1):1–5.

58. Kern KA, Norton JA. Cancer cachexia. *J Parenter Enteral Nutr* 1988; **12/bl>**(3):286–298.

59. Dunlop GM. A study of the the relative frequency and importance of gastrointestinal symptoms and weakness in patients with far advanced cancer. *Palliative Med* 1989; **63**(2):37–43.

60. Thompson BR, Julian TB, Stremple JF. Perioperative total parenteral nutrition in patients with gastrointestinal cancer. *J Surg Res* 1981; **30**(5):497–500.

61. Muller JM, Brenner U, Dienst C, Pichlmaier H. Preoperative parenteral feeding in patients with gastrointestinal carcinoma. *Lancet* 1982; **i**(8263):68–71.

62. Holter AR, Fischer JE. The effects of perioperative hyperalimentation on complications in patients with carcinoma and weight loss. *J Surg Res* 1977; **23**(1):31–43.

63. DeWys WD, Begg C, Lavin PT et al. Prognostic effect of weight loss prior to chemotherapy in cancer patients. Eastern Cooperative Oncology Group. *Am J Med* 1980; **69**(4):491–497.

64. Mitchell EP, Schein PS. Gastrointestinal toxicity of chemotherapeutic agents. *Semin Oncol* 1982; **9**(1):52–64.

65. Sloan GM, Maher M, Brennan MF. Nutritional effects of surgery, radiation therapy, and adjuvant chemotherapy for soft tissue sarcomas. *Am J Clin Nutr* 1981; **34**(6):1094–1102.

66. Reuben DB, Mor V. Nausea and vomiting in terminal cancer patients. *Arch Intern Med* 1986; **146**(10):2021–2023.

67. Wagemans MF, Bakker EN, Zuurmond WW, Spoelder EM, Van Loenen AC, De Lange JJ. Intrathecal administration of high-dose morphine solutions decreases the pH of cerebrospinal fluid. *Pain* 1995; **61**(1):55–59.

68. Beutler B, Cerami A. Cachectin and tumour necrosis factor as two sides of the same biological coin. *Nature* 1986; **320**(6063):584–588.

69. Strassmann G, Fong M, Kenney JS, Jacob CO. Evidence for the involvement of interleukin-6 in experimental cancer cachexia. *J Clin Invest* 1992; **89**(5):1681–1684.

70. Matthys P, Dijkmans R, Proost P et al. Severe cachexia in mice inoculated with interfero-gamma-producing tumor cells. *Int J Cancer* 1991; **49**(1):77–82.

71. Mori M, Yamaguchi K, Honda S et al. Cancer cachexia syndrome developed in nude mice bearing melanoma cells producing leukemia-inhibitory factor. *Cancer Res* 1991; **51**(24):6656–6659.

72. Heber D, Tchekmedyian NS. Pathophysiology of cancer: hormonal and metabolic abnormalities. *Oncology* 1992; **49**(Suppl 2):28–31.

73. Todorov P, Cariuk P, McDevitt T, Coles B, Fearon K, Tisdale M. Characterization of a cancer cachectic factor. *Nature* 1996; **379**(6567):739–742.

74. Lukaski HC. Methods for the assessment of human body composition: traditional and new. *Am J Clin Nutr* 1987; **46**(4):537–556.

75. Presta E, Wang J, Harrison GG, Bjorntorp P, Harker WH, Van Itallie TB. Measurement of total body electrical conductivity: a new method for estimation of body composition. *Am J Clin Nutr* 1983; **37**(5):735–739.

76. Sjostrom L, Kvist H. Regional body fat measurements with CT-scan and evaluation of anthropometric predictions. *Acta Med Scand* (Suppl) 1988; **723**:169–177.

77. Cohn SH, Vaswani AN, Yasumura S, Yuen K, Ellis KJ. Assessment of cellular mass and lean body mass by noninvasive nuclear techniques. *J Lab Clin Med* 1985; **105**(3):305–311.

78. Mazess RB, Barden HS, Bisek JP, Hanson J. Dual-energy X-ray absorptiometry for total-body and regional bone-mineral and soft-tissue composition. *Am J Clin Nutr* 1990; **51**(6):1106–1112.

79. Bruera E, Roca E, Cedaro L, Carraro S, Chacon R. Action of oral methylprednisolone in terminal cancer patients: a prospective randomized double-blind study. *Cancer Treat Rep* 1985; **69**(7–8):751–754.

80. Loprinzi CL, Michalak JC, Schaid DJ et al. Phase III evaluation of four doses of megestrol acetate as therapy for patients with cancer anorexia and/or cachexia. *J Clin Oncol* 1993; **11**(4):762–776.

81. Bruera E, Higginson I (eds) *Cachexia–Anorexia in Cancer Patients*, 1996 Oxford, Oxford University Press.

82. Moertel CG, Schutt AJ, Reitemeier RJ, Hahn RG. Corticosteroid therapy of preterminal gastrointestinal cancer. *Cancer* 1974; **33**(6):1607–1609.

83. Willox JC, Corr J, Shaw J, Richardson M, Calman KC, Drennan M. Prednisolone as an appetite stimulant in patients with cancer. *Br Med J Clin Res Ed* 1984; **288**(6410):27.

84. Della Cuna GR, Pellegrini A, Piazzi M. Effect of methylprednisolone sodium succinate on quality of life in preterminal cancer patients: a placebo-controlled, multicenter study. The Methylprednisolone Preterminal Cancer Study Group. *Eur J Cancer Clin Oncol* 1989; **25**(12):1817–1821.

85. Popiela T, Lucchi R, Giongo F. Methylprednisolone as palliative therapy for female terminal cancer patients. The Methylprednisolone Female Preterminal Cancer Study Group. *Eur J Cancer Clin Oncol* 1989; **25**(12):1823–1829.

86. Ettinger AB, Portenoy RK. The use of corticosteroids in the treatment of symptoms associated with cancer. *J Pain Symptom Manage* 1988; **3**(2):99–103.

87. Farr WC. The use of corticosteroids for symptom management in terminally ill patients. *Am J Hosp Care* 1990; **7**(1):41–46.

88. Needham PR, Daley AG, Lennard RF. Steroids in advanced cancer: survey of current practice [see comments]. *BMJ* 1992; **305**(6860):999.

89. Tchekmedyian NS, Tait N, Moody M, Aisner J. High-dose megestrol acetate. A possible treatment for cachexia. *JAMA* 1987; **257**(9):1195–1198.

90. Cavalli F, Goldhirsch A, Jungi F et al. Randomized trial of low- versus high-dose medroxyprogesterone acetate in the treatment of postmenopausal patients with advanced breast cancer. In: *Role of Medroxyprogesterone Acetate in Endocrine-Related tumors*. Pellegrini A, Robustelli della Cuna G (eds) 1984: 79–89. New York, Raven Press.

91. Downer S, Joel S, Allbright A. et al. A double blind placebo controlled trial of medroxyprogesterone acetate (MPA) in cancer cachexia. *Br J Cancer* 1993; **67**(5):1102–1105.

92. Bruera E, Macmillan K, Kuehn N, Hanson J, MacDonald RN. A controlled trial of megestrol acetate on appetite, caloric intake, nutritional status, and other symptoms in patients with advanced cancer. *Cancer* 1990; **66**(6):1279–1282.

93. Loprinzi CL, Ellison NM, Schaid DJ *et al.* Controlled trial of megestrol acetate for the treatment of cancer anorexia and cachexia. *J Natl Cancer Inst* 1990; **82**(13):1127–1132.

94. Tchekmedyian NS, Hickman M, Siau J, Greco FA, Keller J, Browder H, Aisner J. Megestrol acetate in cancer anorexia and weight loss. *Cancer* 1992; **69**(5):1268–1274.

95. Feliu J, Gonzalez Baron M, Berrocal A, *et al.* Usefulness of megestrol acetate in cancer cachexia and anorexia. A placebo-controlled study. *Am J Clin Oncol* 1992; **15**(15):436–440.

96. Simons JP, Aaronson NK, Vansteenkiste JF, *et al.* Effects of medroxyprogesterone acetate on appetite, weight, and quality of life in advanced-stage non-hormone-sensitive cancer: a placebo-controlled multicenter study. *J Clin Oncol* 1996; **14**(4):1077–1084.

97. Loprinzi CL, Schaid DJ, Dose AM, Burnham NL, Jensen MD. Body-composition changes in patients who gain weight while receiving megestrol acetate. *J Clin Oncol* 1993; **11**(1):152–154.

98. Loprinzi CL, Goldberg RM, Su JQ *et al.* Placebo-controlled trial of hydrazine sulfate in patients with newly diagnosed non-small-cell lung cancer. *J Clin Oncol* 1994; **12**(6):1126–1129.

99. Loprinzi CL, Kuross SA, O'Fallon JR, *et al.* Randomized placebo-controlled evaluation of hydrazine sulfate in patients with advanced colorectal cancer. *J Clin Oncol* 1994; **12**(6):1121–1125.

100. Kardinal CG, Loprinzi CL, Schaid DJ, *et al.* A controlled trial of cyproheptadine in cancer patients with anorexia and/or cachexia. *Cancer* 1990; **65**(12):2657–2662.

101. Nelson K, Walsh D, Deeter P, Sheehan F. A phase II study of delta-9-tetrahydrocannabinol for appetite stimulation in cancer-associated anorexia. *J Palliat Care* 1994; **10**(1):14–18.

102. Goldberg RM, Loprinzi CL, Mailliard JA, *et al.* Pentoxifylline for treatment of cancer anorexia and cachexia? A randomized, double-blind, placebo-controlled trial. *J Clin Oncol* 1995; **13**(11):2856–2859.

103. Beck SA, Smith KL, Tisdale MJ. Anticachectic and anti-tumor effect of eicosapentaenoic acid and its effect on protein turnover. *Cancer Res* 1991; **51**(22):6089–6093.

104. Ventafridda V, Ripamonti C, De Conno F, Tamburini M, Cassileth BR. Symptom prevalence and control during cancer patients' last days of life. *J Palliat Care* 1990; **6**(3):7–11.

105. Allan SG. Nausea and vomiting. In: *Oxford Textbook of Palliative Medicine*. Doyle D, Hanks GWC, MacDonald N (eds), 1993: 282–290. Oxford, Oxford Medical Publications.

106. Hosking DJ, Bennett T, Hampton JR. Diabetic autonomic neuropathy. *Diabetes* 1978; **27**(10):1043–1055.

107. Henrich WL. Autonomic insufficiency. *Arch Intern Med* 1982; **142**(2):339–344.

108. Bruera E, Chadwick S, Fox R, Hanson J, MacDonald N. Study of cardiovascular autonomic insufficiency in advanced cancer patients. *Cancer Treat Rep* 1986; **70**(12):1383–1387.

109. Schuffler MD, Baird HW, Fleming CR *et al.* Intestinal pseudo-obstruction as the presenting manifestation of small-cell carcinoma of the lung. A paraneoplastic neuropathy of the gastrointestinal tract. *Ann Intern Med* 1983; **98**(2):129–134.

110. Park D, Johnson R, Crean G. Orthostatic hypotension in bronchial carcinoma. *BMJ* 1972; **3**:510–511.

111. Mamdani MB, Walsh RL, Rubino FA, Brannegan RT, Hwang MH. Autonomic dysfunction and Eaton Lambert syndrome. *J Auton Nerv Syst* 1985; **12**(4):315–320.

112. Roca E, Bruera E, Politi PM, Barugel M, Cedaro L, Carraro S, Chacon RD. Vinca alkaloid-induced cardiovascular autonomic neuropathy. *Cancer Treat Rep* 1985; **69**(2):149–151.

113. Villa A, Foresti V, Confalonieri F. Autonomic neuropathy and HIV infection [Letter]. *Lancet* 1987; **ii**(8564):915.

114. Hagen NA, Foley KM, Cerbone DJ, Portenoy RK, Inturrisi CE. Chronic nausea and morphine-6-glucuronide. *J Pain Symptom Manage* 1991; **6**(3):125–128.

115. Ricci DA, Saltzman MB, Meyer C, Callachan C, McCallum RW. Effect of metoclopramide in diabetic gastroparesis. *J Clin Gastroenterol* 1985; **7**(1):25–32.

116. Shivshanker K, Bennett RW, Jr., Haynie TP. Tumor-associated gastroparesis: correction with metoclopramide. *Am J Surg* 1983; **145**(2):221–225.

117. Mercadante S. The role of octreotide in palliative care. *J Pain Symptom Manage* 1994; **9**(6):406–411.

118. Pereira J, Bruera E. Chronic nausea. In: *Cachexia–Anorexia in Cancer Patients*, Bruera E, Higginson I (eds), 1996: 23–37. Oxford, Oxford University Press.

119. Bruera ED, Roca E, Cedaro L, Chacon R, Estevez R. Improved control of chemotherapy-induced emesis by the addition of dexamethasone to metoclopramide in patients resistant to metoclopramide. *Cancer Treat Rep* 1983; **67**(4):381–383.

120. Bruera E, Brenneis C, Michaud M, MacDonald N. Continuous Sc infusion of metoclopramide for treatment of narcotic bowel syndrome [Letter]. *Cancer Treat Rep* 1987; **71**(11):1121–1122.

121. Cole RM, Robinson F, Harvey L, Trethowan K, Murdoch V. Successful control of intractable nausea and vomiting requiring combined ondansetron and haloperidol in a patient with advanced cancer. *J Pain Symptom Manage* 1994; **9**(1):48–50.

122. Daut RL, Cleeland CS. The prevalence and severity of pain in cancer. *Cancer* 1982; **50**(9):1913–1918.

123. Bonica JJ, Cancer Pain. In: *The Management of Pain*, 2nd edn. Bonica JJ (ed.). 1990: 400–460. Phailadelphia, Lea and Febiger.

124. Sung JL, Wang TH, Yu JY. Clinical study on primary carcinoma of the liver in Taiwan. *Am J Dig Dis* 1967; **12**(10):1036–1049.

125. Tiniakos DG, Lee JA, Burt AD. Innervation of the liver: morphology and function. *Liver* 1996; **16**:151–160.

126. Foley KM. Pain syndromes in patients with cancer. In: *International Symposium on Pain of Advanced Cancer*. Bonica JJ, Ventafridda V, (eds), 1979: 59–75. New York, Raven Press.

127. Jensen MP, Karoly P, Braver S. The measurement of clinical pain intensity: a comparison of six methods. *Pain* 1986; **27**(1):117–126.

128. Daut RL, Cleeland CS, Flanery RC. Development of the Wisconsin Brief Pain Questionnaire to assess pain in cancer and other diseases. *Pain* 1983; **17**(2):197–210.

129. Fishman B, Pasternak S, Wallenstein SL, Houde RW, Holland JC, Foley KM. The Memorial Pain Assessment Card. A valid instrument for the evaluation of cancer pain. *Cancer* 1987; **60**(5):1151–1158.

130. Deschamps M, Band PR, Coldman AJ. Assessment of adult cancer pain: shortcomings of current methods. *Pain* 1988; **32**(2):133–139.

131. Ventafridda V, Caraceni A, Sbanotto A. Cancer Pain Management. *Pain Rev* 1996; **3**:153–179.

132. World Health Organization. *Cancer Pain Relief*. 1. 1986. Geneva, World Health Organization.

133. Ventafridda V, Caraceni A, Gamba A Field-testing of the WHO Guidelines for Cancer Pain Relief: summary report of demonstration projects. In *Second International Congress on Cancer Pain*, Foley KM, Bonica JJ, (eds), 1990:451–464. New York, Raven Press.

134. Grond S, Zech D, Schug SA, Lynch J, Lehmann KA. Validation of World Health Organization guidelines for cancer pain relief during the last days and hours of life. *J Pain Symptom Manage* 1991; **6**(7):411–422.

135. Ventafridda V, Spoldi E, Caraceni A, Tamburini M, De Conno F. The importance of subcutaneous morphine administration for cancer pain control. *Pain Clinic* 1986; 1:47–55.

136. Bruera E, Brenneis C, Michaud M, *et al.* Use of the subcutaneous route for the administration of narcotics in patients with cancer pain. *Cancer* 1988; 62(2):407–411.

137. Portenoy RK, Moulin DE, Rogers A, Inturrisi CE, Foley KM. I.v. infusion of opioids for cancer pain: clinical review and guidelines for use. *Cancer Treat Rep* 1986; 70(5):575–581.

138. Moulin DE, Kreeft JH, Murray Parsons N, Bouquillon AI. Comparison of continuous subcutaneous and intravenous hydromorphone infusions for management of cancer pain [see comments]. *Lancet* 1991; 337(8739):465–8.

139. Walker VA, Hoskin PJ, Hanks GW, White ID. Evaluation of WHO analgesic guidelines for cancer pain in a hospital-based palliative care unit. *J Pain Symptom Manage* 1988; 3(3):145–149.

140. Zech DF, Grond S, Lynch J, Hertel D, Lehmann KA. Validation of World Health Organization Guidelines for cancer pain relief: a 10-year prospective study. *Pain* 1995; 63(1):65–76.

141. Black A, Dwyer B. Coeliac plexus block. *Anaesth Intensive Care* 1973; 1(4):315–318.

142. Thompson GE, Moore DC, Bridenbaugh LD, Artin RY. Abdominal pain and alcohol celiac plexus nerve block. *Anesth Analg* 1977; 56(1):1–5.

143. Singler RC. An improved technique for alcohol neurolysis of the celiac plexus. *Anesthesiology* 1982; 56(2):137–141.

144. Ischia S, Luzzani A, Ischia A, Faggion S. A new approach to the neurolytic block of the coeliac plexus: the transaortic technique. *Pain* 1983; 16(4):333–341.

145. Montero Matamala A, Vidal Lopez F, Aguilar Sanchez JL, Donoso Bach L. Percutaneous anterior approach to the coeliac plexus using ultrasound. *Br J Anaesth* 1989; 62(6):637–640.

146. Ischia S, Ischia A, Polati E, Finco G. Three posterior percutaneous celiac plexus block techniques. A prospective randomized study in 61 patients with pancreatic cancer pain. *Anesthesiology* 1992; 76(4):534–540.

147. Ventafridda GV, Caraceni AT, Sbanotto AM, Barletta L, De Conno F. Pain treatment in cancer of the pancreas. *Eur J Surg Oncol* 1990; 16(1):1–6.

148. Mercadante S. Celiac plexus block versus analgesics in pancreatic cancer pain. *Pain* 1993; 52(2):187–192.

149. Davies DD. Incidence of major complications of neurolytic coeliac plexus block. *J R Soc Med* 1993; 86(5):264–266.

150. Van Dongen RT, Crul BJ. Paraplegia following coeliac plexus block. *Anaesthesia* 1991; 46(10):862–863.

151. Jabbal SS, Hunton J. Reversible paraplegia following coeliac plexus block. *Anaesthesia* 1992; 47(10):857–858.

152. Gardner AM, Solomou G. Relief of the pain of unresectable carcinoma of pancreas by chemical splanchnicectomy during laparotomy. *Ann R Coll Surg Engl* 1984; 66(6):409–411.

153. Sharp KW, Stevens EJ. Improving palliation in pancreatic cancer: intraoperative celiac plexus block for pain relief. *South Med J* 1991; 84(4):469–471.

154. Lillemoe KD, Cameron JL, Kaufman HS, Yeo CJ, Pitt HA, Sauter PK. Chemical splanchnicectomy in patients with unresectable pancreatic cancer. A prospective randomized trial. *Ann Surg* 1993; 217(5):447–455.

155. Bali B, Deixonne B, Rzal K *et al.* Bilateral splanchnicectomy by transhiatal approach in pain of pancreatic origin. 37 cases. *Presse Med* 1995; 24(20):928–932.

156. Worsey J, Ferson PF, Keenan RJ, Julian TB, Landreneau RJ. Thoracoscopic pancreatic denervation for pain control in irresectable pancreatic cancer. *Br J Surg* 1993; 80(8):1051–1052.

157. Ripamonti C. Management of bowel obstruction in advanced cancer. *Curr Opin Oncol* 1994; 6(4):351–357.

158. Ripamonti C, De Conno F, Ventafridda V, Rossi B, Baines MJ. Management of bowel obstruction in advanced and terminal cancer patients. *Ann Oncol* 1993; 4(1):15–21.

159. Malone JM, Jr., Koonce T, Larson DM, Freedman RS, Carrasco CH, Saul PB. Palliation of small bowel obstruction by percutaneous gastrostomy in patients with progressive ovarian carcinoma. *Obstet Gynecol* 1986; 68(3):431–433.

160. Campagnutta E, Cannizzaro R, Gallo A, Zarrelli A, Valentini M, De Cicco M, Scarabelli C. Palliative treatment of upper intestinal obstruction by gynecological malignancy: the usefulness of percutaneous endoscopic gastrostomy. *Gynecol Oncol* 1996; 62(1):103–105.

161. Steadman K, Franks A. A woman with malignant bowel obstruction who did not want to die with tubes. *Lancet* 1996; 347(9006):944.

162. Mangili G, Franchi M, Mariani A, Zanaboni F, Rabaiotti E, Frigerio L, Bolis PF, Ferrari A. Octreotide in the management of bowel obstruction in terminal ovarian cancer. *Gynecol Oncol* 1996; 61(3):345–348.

Index

Clinical Oncology

NEW Personal Subscription Rate only £92.00!

An International Cancer Journal

Clinical Oncology is a well-established international journal covering all aspects of the clinical management of cancer patients, reflecting the current multi-disciplinary approach to therapy.

Clinical Oncology is the journal of the Faculty of Clinical Oncology of the Royal College of Radiologists and is edited by a Board of recognised experts drawn from all major disciplines involved in cancer treatment.

Published for all clinicians with an active interest in the treatment of cancer, Clinical Oncology contains:

- Original articles on every type of malignant disease, embracing all modalities used in cancer therapy:
  - ▶ Reporting the results of clinical trials
  - ▶ Describing innovations on cancer treatment
  - ▶ Analysing the results of established treatments and practices

- Papers reflecting the Royal College of Radiologists' role in training and continuing education in oncology:
  - ▶ Signed editorials, discussing current issues in oncology
  - ▶ Articles presenting current controversies in cancer therapy
  - ▶ Authoritative reviews and updates on a wide range of clinical topics

The Journal also includes correspondence which allows a forum for individual comment. Case reports detail single patients or small series to illustrate scientific points of general interest. Book reviews offer informed criticism of major oncological publications.

FREE Subscription to Clinical Oncology on the Internet

Clinical Oncology is available FREE electronically for all subscribers to the print journal. The LINK is a new online service on the Internet, publishing about 250 Springer journals. Electronic versions of the journals are linked to the print editions, combining proven quality with user-friendly accessibility and retrievability. For further details see our web site:

http//:link.springer.de

Invitation to Contribute

Manuscripts for publication and all other editorial communication should be sent to:

Dr W.G. Jones
Editor, Clinical Oncology
Royal College of Radiologists
38 Portland Street
London W1N 4JQ, UK

Subscription Order Form / Sample Copy Request

Clinical Oncology ISSN: 0936 - 6555

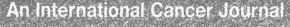

☐ Please send me a FREE sample copy
☐ Please enter my subscription to Volume 10 (6 issues) 1998
☐ Institutional rate: £210.00
☐ Personal rate: £92.00
☐ Eurocard / Access / Mastercard
☐ Visa / Barclaycard / Bankamericard
☐ American Express

Card No. _____ Valid until _____

☐ Please bill me

☐ Cheque made payable to: Springer-Verlag London Ltd.

VAT No (if registered) _____

Available from:
Springer-Verlag London Ltd.
Sweetapple House, Catteshall Road
Godalming, Surrey GU7 3DJ, United Kingdom
Tel: +44 (0)1483 418822   Fax: +44 (0)1483 415151
Email: postmaster@svl.co.uk

PLEASE PRINT CLEARLY

Name _____

Address _____

_____

_____ Postcode _____

Signature _____

Date _____

Printed by Publishers' Graphics LLC
MO20120905-077